Colour Atlas of
First Pass Functional
Imaging of the Heart

Colour Atlas of First Pass Functional Imaging of the Heart

Edited by

N. Schad
Professor of Radiology
City Hospital Passau
Technical University of Munich
West Germany

E. J. Andrews, Jr. and J. W. Fleming
Co-Directors, Nuclear Cardiology
Florida Heart Center – Medical Center Clinic
West Florida Regional Medical Center
Pensacola, Florida, USA

Springer-Science+Business Media, B.V. 1985

Published in the UK and Europe by
MTP Press Limited
Falcon House
Lancaster, England

British Library Cataloguing in Publication Data

Colour atlas of first pass functional imaging
of the heart.
1. Angiocardiography   2. Radioisotopes
in medical diagnosis
I. Schad, N.   II. Andrews, E. J.   III. Fleming, J. W.
616.1'207575   RC683.5.A5

Published in the USA by
MTP Press
A division of Kluwer Boston Inc
190 Old Derby Street
Hingham, MA 02043, USA

Library of Congress Cataloging in Publication Data

Main entry under title:

Colour atlas of first pass functional imaging of
the heart.

Bibliography: p.
Includes index.
1. Radioisotope scanning—Atlases.   2. Heart—Diseases
—Diagnosis—Atlases.   I. Schad, Nikolaus, 1924–
II. Andrews, E. J. (E. James)   III. Fleming, J. W.
(Jack W.)   [DNLM: 1. Heart—radionuclide imaging—atlases.
WG 17 C719]
RC683.5.R33C65   1984   616.1'207575   84–20183

ISBN 978-94-010-8664-6   ISBN 978-94-009-4888-4 (eBook)

DOI 10.1007/ 978-94-009-4888-4

Copyright © Springer Science+Business Media Dordrecht 1985
Originally published by 1985 MTP Press Limited
Softcover reprint of the hardcover 1st edition 1985

Contents

Foreword

For many years, clinicians have relied on cardiac catheterization to provide the most reliable information on cardiac anatomy and function. There is a definite need, however, to obtain this same information at more frequent intervals with minimal trauma to patients.

Consequently, primarily over the last decade, great strides have been made in developing non-invasive methods to accurately assess cardiac function. Many of these methods utilize radioisotopes to allow us to obtain computerized images of the cardiac structure. The methods by which we acquire and process these images are continuously evaluated and modified so as to improve their sensitivity and specificity in settings that allow us to most closely mimic the patient's everyday physical demands.

First pass radionuclide angiography is one non-invasive method that provides quantitative measures of biventricular function and regional wall motion. More recent technical advances include the development of computer programs to analyze regional haemodynamic parameters such as the functional images presented in this text, parametric imaging methods such as phase analysis, calculation of absolute ventricular volumes, and assessment of diastolic function.

This technique is particularly useful for examining parameters at peak stress, which is the time that changes of the most pertinent diagnostic relevance will be revealed. It is particularly useful in those individuals with equivocal symptoms, or those who are asymptomatic but with significant risk factors, who may exhibit abnormal findings only at peak stress, for whom this test can provide a very useful screening tool. Additionally, this procedure allows us to serially and non-traumatically examine the effects of medical and surgical therapy in those patients with identified cardiovascular disease.

Over the past decade, the applications and the utility of first pass radionuclide angiography have been well accepted. New radioisotopes that allow multiple studies at one setting and newer mobile cameras will also serve to further increase utilization of the technique. However, differences, and disagreement, in methods of background elimination, image and data processing, exercise protocol and patient positioning, sensitivity and specificity will be found among the many laboratories that perform first pass studies. The majority of differences can primarily be categorized into two camps based on those users who seek quantitative data (e.g. ejection fraction, end-diastolic and end-systolic volumes, etc.) and those who prefer the information provided by quantitative images, such as the functional images described by the authors. Many will recognize these preferences as the natural biases usually exhibited by cardiologists seeking numbers compared to radiologists trained to interpret pictures.

However, putting these differences aside, of prime importance to clinicians is whether or not we can accurately diagnose the presence of disease or, with assurance, be able to diagnose its absence based on the data obtained from first pass radionuclide angiography. From the early days when Borer et al. (1977) reported a 100% sensitivity and specificity for the test, which to date has not been reproduced by other investigators, we have all been striving to improve the predictive value of the test. Most users today would agree that the sensitivity of exercise ventriculography is in the range of 85–95% with a specificity ranging between 60–70% (Pitt et al., 1983). Rozanski et al. (1983) have reported that we may be underestimating specificity due to referral biases and feel the true specificity in their laboratory to be about 79%. Dr. Schad and his colleagues in this book report that they are able to get higher values for sensitivity and specificity utilizing functional images of radionuclide angiography data in their laboratory. Current cameras make it difficult and laborious for most laboratories to process functional images without additional computer capability as developed by Dr. Schad. The development of new, higher count rate camera systems with improved computer capability, however, could result in functional imaging taking a rapid step forward. This should make it possible for others to utilize the technique and reproduce these favorable results.

To further understanding and acceptability, the editors of this book, Drs Schad, Andrews, and Fleming, have very effectively communicated their approach to analyzing first pass radionuclide angiography. They utilize colour-coded images of regional haemodynamic information based on temporal changes in cardiac function, which they have classified as functional images. They have provided very minute details as to the technical considerations inherent in processing functional images in regard to background elimination, the isolation of left ventricular counts, and the determination of left ventricular indices. Dr. Schad eloquently describes the rationale of functional imaging as well as the interpretation and haemodynamic significance of each functional image. He also elaborates the advantages of functional imaging compared to conventional cine images geared to obtaining quantitative data.

Contributing authors allow us to examine the applications of functional images to different disease states and to evaluate the effects of different therapeutic modalities such as coronary angioplasty, intracoronary thrombolysis, and cardiac transplantation providing vital information for physicians in the continued, appropriate management of these patients.

This book provides very practical, descriptive information on functional imaging for a broad audience including cardiologists and cardiovascular surgeons, internists, nuclear medicine physicians and radiologists, technologists, and academic investigators. The information in this book adds to our understanding of the complexities of cardiac anatomy and function and provides another method by which we can hope to define pathological processes in an effort to better manage and benefit patients with cardiovascular disease. However, as with all technological advances and reported research findings, it is vitally important to have results duplicated by other investigators. The authors report laudable results. With the advent of improved technology, the door will be opened for others to more readily apply these techniques, to reproduce these results and, thus, to allow the method to gain more widespread clinical applicability.

Borer, J. S., Bacharach, S. L., Green, M. V., Kent, K. M., Epstein, S. E. and Johnston, G. S. (1977). Real-time radionuclide angiography in the non-invasive evaluation of global and regional left ventricular function at rest and during exercise in patients with coronary artery disease. N. Engl. J. Med., **296**, 839

Pitt, B., Kalff, V., Rabinovitch, M. A., Buda, A. J., Colfer, H. T., Vogel, R. A. and Thrall, J. H. (1983). Impact of radionuclide techniques on evaluation of patients with ischemic heart disease. J. Am. Coll. Cardiol., **1**, 63

Rozanski, A., Diamond, G. A., Berman, D., Forrester, J. S., Morris, D. and Swan, H. J. C. (1983). The declining specificity of exercise radionuclide ventriculography. N. Engl. J. Med., **309**, 518

Donald H. Schmidt, MD

Professor of Medicine
University of Wisconsin Medical School
Head, Cardiovascular Disease Section
Mount Sinai Medical Center
Milwaukee, Wisconsin, USA

Introduction

Radionuclide angiocardiography provides a unique clinical opportunity for studying the function of the heart non-invasively. Most methods utilize the viewing of cinematographic analogue images which require repeated playback of single scenes particularly when details are of diagnostic interest. During cine display some information may be missed and interobserver variation can be a problem. In contrast, the processed functional image has a fundamental advantage in that one single image represents information about regional changes in the right or left ventricle during systole and diastole. All regional changes during the preselected time interval are mapped in functional images, and abnormalities become immediately visible and easy to analyse.

Regional wall motion abnormalities may be associated with regional myocardial ischaemia as well as a variety of pathological conditions. The method is quite sensitive to changes in myocardial function not previously appreciated such as early changes of developing cardiomyopathy or residuals of remote myocarditis. Coronary artery disease often is more diffuse than is appreciated by coronary arteriography. Thus, the clinician must use the information from functional imaging as another parameter in clinical decision making. The necessity has therefore emerged to present an atlas of these functional images as they are seen in a variety of pathological conditions.

This atlas represents an introduction to functional imaging and a few examples of studies obtained in common pathological conditions. These relate the collective experience in the United States and Europe of nearly 20 thousand patients studied with first pass radionuclide functional imaging. After some technical notes and detailed descriptions of the normal functional images, representative images seen in some clinical conditions are presented. These discussions are written by different groups based upon their special work and fields of interest. Chapters dealing with postoperative results and follow-up are presented by the cardiac surgeons who are very interested in the outcome of their surgery. They have always been very supportive in the development of better techniques for functional imaging. Since the evaluation for ischaemic heart disease and cardiomyopathy is such a pressing clinical problem these chapters will be of special interest.

It is a privilege to edit the contributions of such a group of outstanding physicians and scientists. We would like to express our gratitude to all who have helped make this publication possible and to Mr Bloomer who encouraged us to collect the material. We hope that this basic atlas will be of general interest and that it will serve as a guide for interpretation of functional images in the evaluation of patients with cardiac disease with the goal of helping physicians make better clinical decisions.

N. Schad, E. J. Andrews, Jr. and J. W. Fleming
October 1984

Acknowledgments

Our grateful appreciation to:

The Medical Education and Research Foundation of Pensacola, Florida, for their support and encouragement.

All the physicians and other members of the Departments of Nuclear Cardiology and Electrocardiology without whose support this work would have not been possible.

Dennis Heuiser, R.T., for processing and excellent technological assistance.

Timothy P. Becks and Susan Morgan, Media Services, West Florida Regional Medical Center, for their help in photography and illustrations.

Pam Cornell, Joan Martin and the other Medical Secretaries of the Medical Center Clinic for their assistance in typing the manuscript.

Karen Guttke, for her patience and endurance in organizing materials and case studies.

All members of the nuclear cardiology and angiographic section in Passau who helped to examine, evaluate and collect the presented cases.

Contributors

Andrews, E. J., Jr.
M.D., Co-Director, Nuclear Cardiology, Florida Heart Center; Director, Nuclear Medicine, Medical Center Clinic – West Florida Regional Medical Center, Pensacola, Florida, USA; Adjunct Associate Professor of Radiology, Department of Radiology, University of Florida, Gainesville, Florida, USA

Bortolotti, U.
M.D., Senior Surgeon, Cardiac Surgery Center, University of Padua, Italy

Bougionkas, G.
M.D., Cardiac Surgeon, Department of Cardiac Surgery, University of Tessaloniki; former surgeon at the Herzchirugische Klinik der Ludwig-Maximilian University, Munich, West Germany

Bruzzone, F.
M.D., Cardiologist, Department of Cardiovascular Diseases (Prof. Caponnetto), University of Genova, Italy

Fleming, J. W.
M.D., Co-Director, Nuclear Cardiology, Florida Heart Center; Director, Cardiology, Medical Center Clinic – West Florida Regional Medical Center, Pensacola, Florida, USA; Clinical Associate Professor of Medicine, College of Medicine, University of Florida, Gainesville, Florida, USA

Galluci, V.
M.D., Professor of Surgery, Director of Cardiac Surgery Center, University of Padua, Italy

Hatz, R.
Cand. Med., Herzchirurgische Klinik der Ludwig-Maximilian University, Munich, West Germany

Hemmer, W.
M.D., Surgeon, Herzchirurgische Klinik der Ludwig-Maximilian University, Munich, West Germany

Kemkes, B. M.
M.D., Priv. Doz. Herzchirurgische Klinik der Ludwig-Maximilian University, Munich, West Germany

Kreuzer, E.
M.D., Professor of Surgery, Herzchirurgische Klinik der Ludwig-Maximilian University, Munich, West Germany

Luther, M.
M.D., Priv. Doz. Dozent of the first Clinic of Internal Medicine, City Hospital Pasing, Munich, West Germany

Mello, M. M.
R.T., Chief Technologist, Nuclear Cardiology, Florida Heart Center, West Florida Regional Medical Center, Pensacola, Florida, USA

Milano, A.
M.D., Surgeon, Cardiac Surgery Center, University of Padua, Italy

Nickel, O.
Physicist, Nuclear Medicine Department, University of Mainz; former physicist at the section of Nuclear Cardiology; City Hospital of Passau, Munich, West Germany

Peters, B. M.
Technical Assistant, Herzchirurgische Klinik der Ludwig-Maximilian University, Munich, West Germany

Phillips, D. F.
M.D., Director, Section of Coronary Angioplasty, Florida Heart Center; Cardiologist, Medical Center Clinic – West Florida Regional Medical Center, Pensacola, Florida, USA; Formerly, Director, Section of Coronary Angioplasty, Cleveland Clinic Foundation, Cleveland, Ohio, USA

Reble, B.
M.D., Surgeon, Herzchirurgische Klinik der Ludwig-Maximilian University, Munich, West Germany

Reichart, B.
M.D., Chris. Barnard Professor of Surgery, Cardiac and Thoracic Surgery, Groote Schuure Hospital, University of Kapstadt; former Herzchirurgische Klinik (Prof. W. Klinner) der Ludwig-Maximilian University, Munich, West Germany

Romeo, F.
M.D., Senior Cardiologist, Cattedra 2° Malattie Apparato Cardiovascolare (Prof. Reale), University of Rome, Italy

Schad, N.
M.D., Professor of Radiology, Nuclear Cardiology, City Hospital of Passau (Prof. Breit) Teaching Hospital of Technical University, Munich, West Germany

Weikl, A.
M.D., Senior Cardiologist, Cardiac Clinic, University of Erlangen; former Senior Cardiologist, City Hospital of Nürnberg, West Germany

1

Technical Notes

O. NICKEL

Cardiac functional imaging has been made possible through sophisticated developments in electronics, computer technique and nuclear chemistry. Because the techniques are complex, it is very important for the physician to understand the basic technical principles of the procedures.

DATA ACQUISITION AND IMAGE PROCESSING EQUIPMENT

First pass studies of the heart require high speed capabilities of the gamma-camera and computer system. A schematic overview of a system used for cardiac radionuclide imaging is shown in Figure 1.1. The central component of the system is a minicomputer (or microcomputer) with a memory capacity of at least 64 kbyte. The acquisition of one image from the gamma-camera is done within a separate buffer memory which stores each scintillation of the

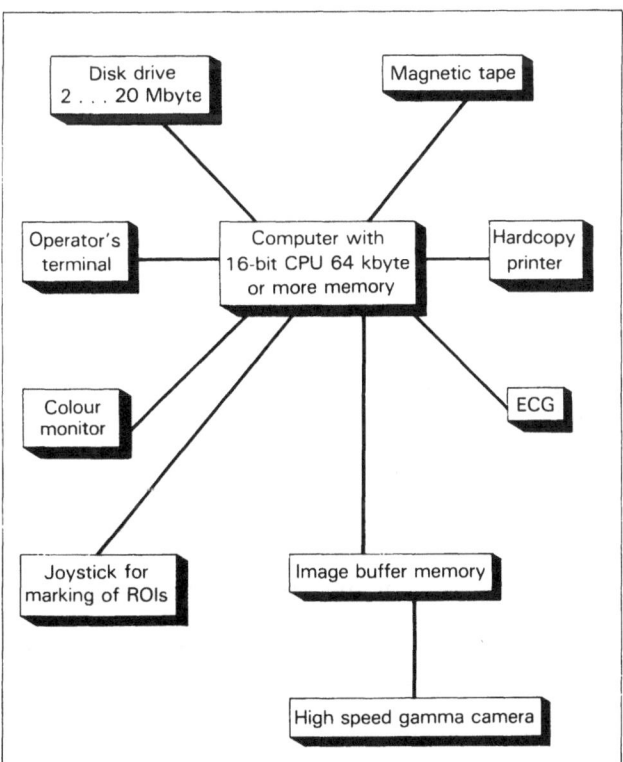

Figure 1.1 Schematic diagram of the data acquisition and processing equipment.

camera corresponding to its x and y value in a matrix. This is done in less than 1 microsecond which means that a maximum countrate of more that 1 million cps is possible. After a given accumulation of time, e.g. 20 or 40 ms, the content of this buffer is transferred to a disk which then allows the next image to be acquired.

The gamma-camera itself should have a very high countrate capability with a saturation countrate above 200 000 cps. Most conventional Anger-type cameras reach saturation below 100 000 cps and are, therefore, not suited for first pass cardiac imaging. The multicrystal camera* has been the camera best suited for this purpose, reaching saturation at approximately 300 000–450 000 cps. During acquisition, it is possible to record the electrocardiogram simultaneously. This allows correlation of data acquisition with the occurrence of the R-wave. This becomes important during data processing.

The disk drive should have enough capacity to store the raw data of two first-pass studies. A capacity of 2 Mbyte is the lowest acceptable level, if a matrix of 14×21 picture elements (pixels) is to be used (such as is done by the multicrystal camera). Other systems use matrix sizes of 32×32 pixels which require the minimum capacity of 5–10 Mbyte.

For long term storage of studies a magnetic tape unit is helpful which also allows the acquisition of a large number of studies without subsequent processing. This is especially useful where a large number of patients are examined daily. The operator controls the system via a terminal with a keyboard and video monitor. The images are displayed on a colour monitor and can be documented by a hardcopy printer, video-imager, or Polaroid film. A joystick (or lightpen) is required to do manual corrections during the processing of the images.

RADIONUCLIDES

In order to obtain high countrates, it is necessary to use a radio-isotope with an activity of 20–30 mCi. The half-life ($T_{\frac{1}{2}}$) of the isotope should be short in order to keep the radiation dose to the patient as low as possible. Two isotopes commonly used for routine work are ^{99m}Tc ($T_{\frac{1}{2}} = 6$ h) and ^{195m}Au ($T_{\frac{1}{2}} = 30$ seconds).

* System 70 and 77 (Baird Co.), Bedford, Massachussetts, USA.

The use of pertechnetate Tc 99 m has long been documented as safe with years of clinical experience. The biological $T_{\frac{1}{2}}$ is reduced even further by conjugating ^{99m}Tc with DTPA. ^{195m}Au is available through the use of a generator (Panek et al., 1982), similar to ^{99m}Tc, but due to the very short half-life the isotope must be injected directly from the generator into the patient, which is more difficult. The short $T_{\frac{1}{2}}$ of the gold isotope has several advantages.

(1) The radiation dose to the patient is very low (approximately one eighth that of ^{99m}Tc). Radiation exposure to the technical staff performing the study is likewise reduced ($\approx 50\%$).
(2) Subsequent injections can be carried out every 3 minutes without significant interference from background activity. This allows first pass studies to be performed in several projections, at several levels of exercise, or before and after the administration of medication (Dymond et al., 1982a; Mena et al., 1982).

It has been well documented that the countrate achievable with ^{195m}Au is comparable to that of ^{99m}Tc. With the multicrystal camera, a mean maximum countrate of about 300 000 cps has been achieved with ^{99m}Tc as well as with ^{195m}Au (Schad et al., 1984a). A series of images obtained from a first pass study using ^{195m}Au is shown in Figure 1.2.

IMAGE PROCESSING TECHNIQUES

There are three important considerations which must be addressed in order to obtain images of ventricular function which are of diagnostic quality: (1) statistical noise due to relatively low total counts in a 20–40 ms acquisition time must be reduced, (2) the ventricular border must be accurately defined (edge definition) and (3) background activity from the lung and other cardiac chambers must be eliminated (subtraction). In order to obtain standardized and reproducible results, an automatic computer program has been developed to handle these considerations.

Total image counts can be increased by the summation of images obtained during equal cardiac phases (Schad, 1977). These summed images form one 'representative cycle'. In creating a representative cycle of the left ventricle, the point of arrival of the bolus in the left ventricle is first determined by analysis of the time–activity curve. This curve (Figure 1.3) has two peaks, the first for the right ventricle, and the second for the left ventricle (LV). Five to ten cycles used for summation can be selected depending upon the length of the washout. Precise determination of each cardiac cycle is possible by using the electrocardiogram (e.c.g.) (R-wave) information which is stored with each image.

During transit through the heart, the bolus of activity does not remain compact but becomes more spread out. When there is maximum activity in the LV, some activity still remains in the lung. On the representative cycle image (summation), this background activity still persists.

Figure 1.4 shows the summation of seven raw-

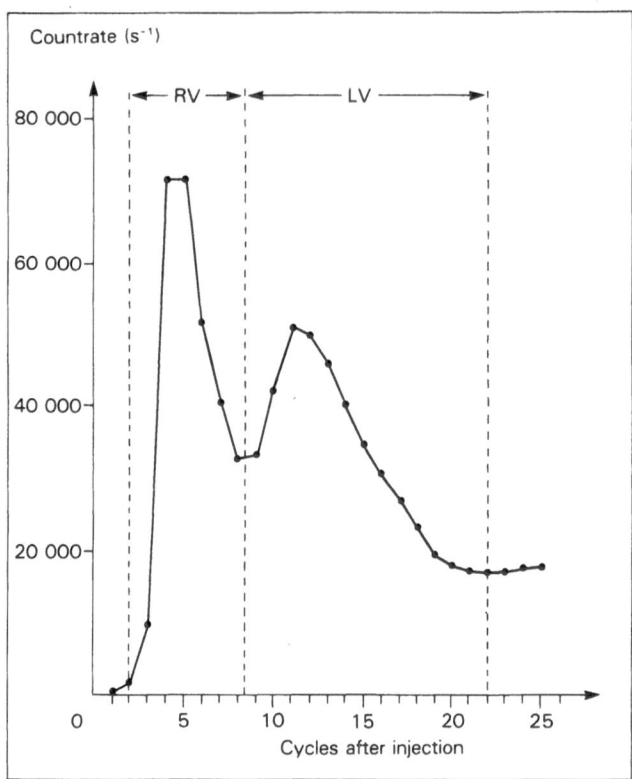

Figure 1.3 Time–activity curve measured over the right and left heart chambers.

data images of the LV obtained with each occurrence of an R-wave corresponding to the beginning of systole. This image still contains counts from the background activity. In order to measure the amount of background activity surrounding the heart, the cardiac border must first be determined. This is done by contrast enhancement through functional (parametric) images. The region limited to only the LV can be visualized by subtracting the end-systolic from the end-diastolic image (Figure 1.5). Because activity does not change significantly outside of the ventricle during systole, only the changes of activity within the ventricle are appreciated. Theoretically, this image could be used for border definition, but it is 'noisy', which could lead to error. This is especially true if the ventricle does not have a normal contraction pattern (e.g. ischaemia).

For this reason, an additional feature of the LV image is utilized, the spatial gradient image (Figure 1.6). This image represents the amount of change in activity from one image point to another in the direction of maximum change. The gradient is high at the cardiac border and aorta, and it is low outside of the heart and in the centre of the ventricle. This image provides good contrast at the border of the heart, especially if contraction is weak and the ventricle is enlarged.

By summation of the original image, the stroke volume image, and the spatial gradient image, a 'contrast-enhanced' image results which now can be used for border definition (Figure 1.7). The LV border can now be defined by a constant intensity level. The intensity–distribution histogram provides a sophisticated way to obtain an appropriate intensity level. The histogram in Figure 1.8 shows the number of pixels having intensities in the range

2

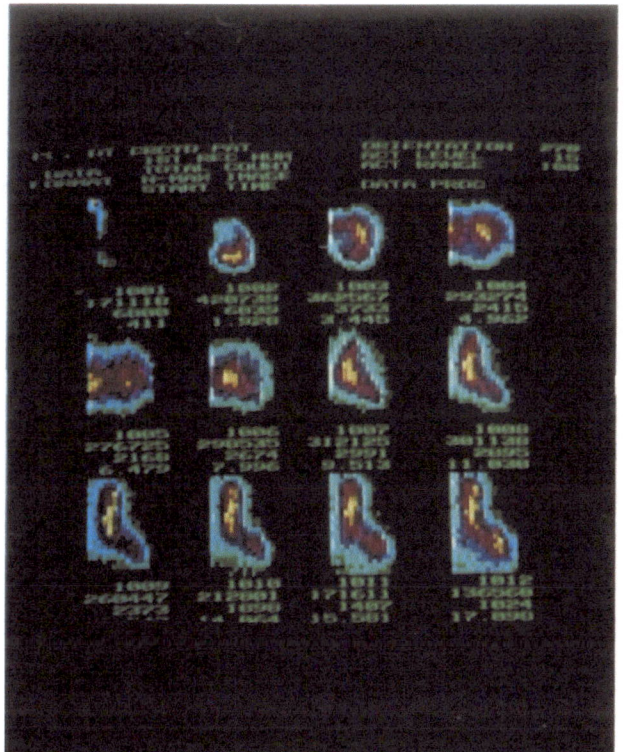

1.2

1.4

1.5

1.6

1.7

Figure 1.2 Series of images during the first transit of an ^{195m}Au bolus through the heart. Each image is accumulated within a time of 1.5 s.

Figure 1.4 Sum of seven images of the left ventricle synchronized by the R-waves (corresponding to the beginning of systole).

Figure 1.5 Difference of the first minus the last systolic image (stroke–volume image).

Figure 1.6 Image of the regional spatial intensity gradients of the first systolic image. The intensity of each pixel gives the square of the regional gradient. High gradients are around the ventricular border and along the aorta.

Figure 1.7 Sum of the original image (Figure 1.4), the stroke–volume image (Figure 1.5) and the gradient image (Figure 1.6). This gives a strong contrast enhancement of the left ventricle against the background.

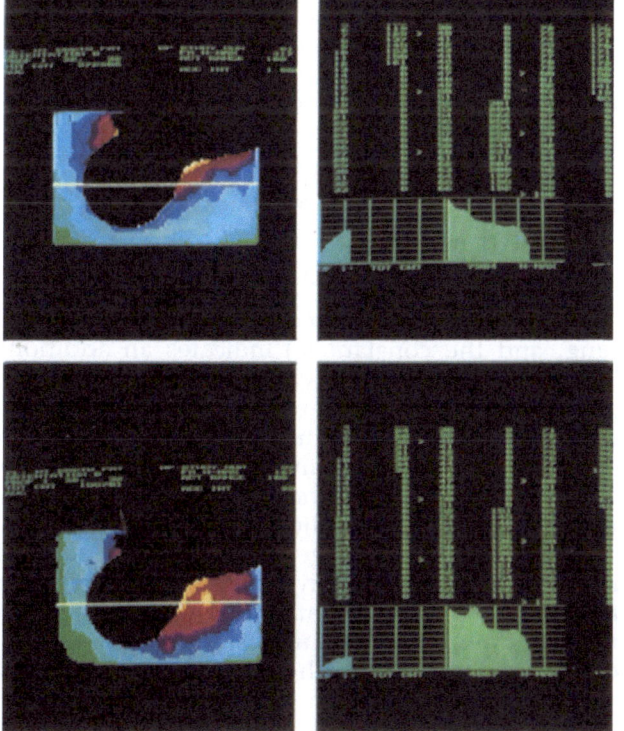

1.9

1.10

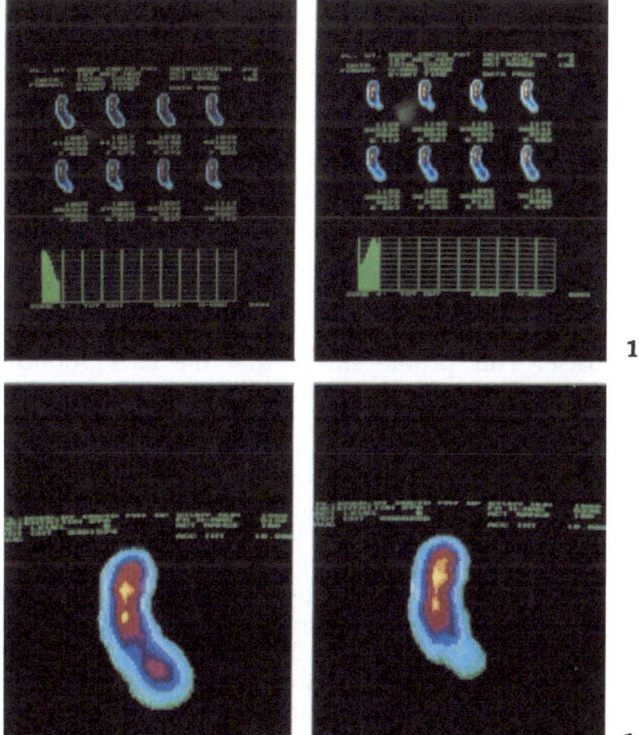

1.12

1.13

1.14

1.15

Figure 1.9 Background outside the heart cavities with profile curve.

Figure 1.10 Distribution of radiation from the lung with profile curve.

Figure 1.12 Background-corrected systolic images of left ventricle with suppression of background noise. Below: Time–activity curve of ventricular activity during systole (ventricular volume curve).

Figure 1.13 Background-corrected diastolic images of LV. Below: Time–activity curve during diastole.

Figure 1.14 End-diastolic image of left ventricle.

Figure 1.15 End-systolic image of left ventricle.

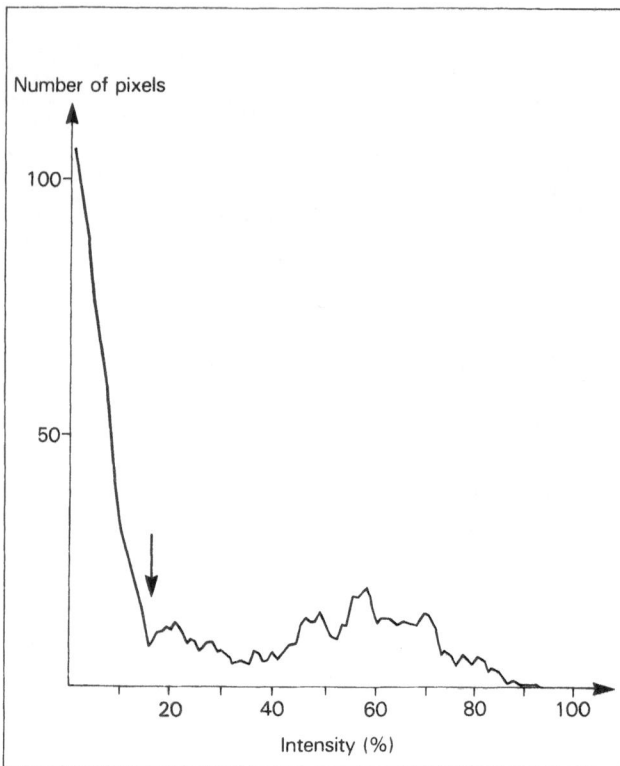

Figure 1.8 Intensity-distribution histogram of the contrast enhanced image (Figure 1.6). The cut-off level, where the distinction between background and heart cavity can be made, is indicated by an arrow.

from 0% to 100% of the maximum intensity (along the x-axis). The number of pixels are high on the low intensity side between 0% and 10%. This part characterizes the background around the heart. A minimum occurs between 10% and 20%. This latter level can be defined as the ventricular border. However, this border is not yet taken as the final border but is used to measure the background activity around the ventricle. This measurement should be carried out as close as possible to the ventricle without including intraventricular activity in the determination.

Figure 1.9 shows the distribution of background radiation around the left ventricle and aorta together with a profile slice through the centre of the ventricle. This profile shows that the background is varying around the ventricular border. An analysis of these variations leads to the conclusion that the radiation arises from the residual activity within the lung. An image of the lung (Figure 1.10), which is acquired when the pulmonary veins are washing out, and the left ventricle has not yet washed in, shows a similar profile curve, but the intensity is much higher. To calculate this 'washout' factor, the fact that background activity consists of more than just radiation from the lung must be taken into account. This can be demonstrated by comparison of the background above the anterior ventricular wall and below the inferior wall with the corresponding points on the lung image. The relative differences between the two points are not the same: the intensity on the lung image is high above the anterior wall and nearly vanishes below the inferior wall. The difference between these two points of background is not as large, which indicates an additional background contribution.

This additional component can be handled by analysis of many points distributed in equal steps around the ventricle (in a horseshoe configuration). By measuring the intensities of the lung image and the background image at these points, a pair of values (x_i, y_i) is obtained for each point which can be compared. On a two-dimensional plot of the values (x_i, y_i) for each point (Figure 1.11), there is a linear

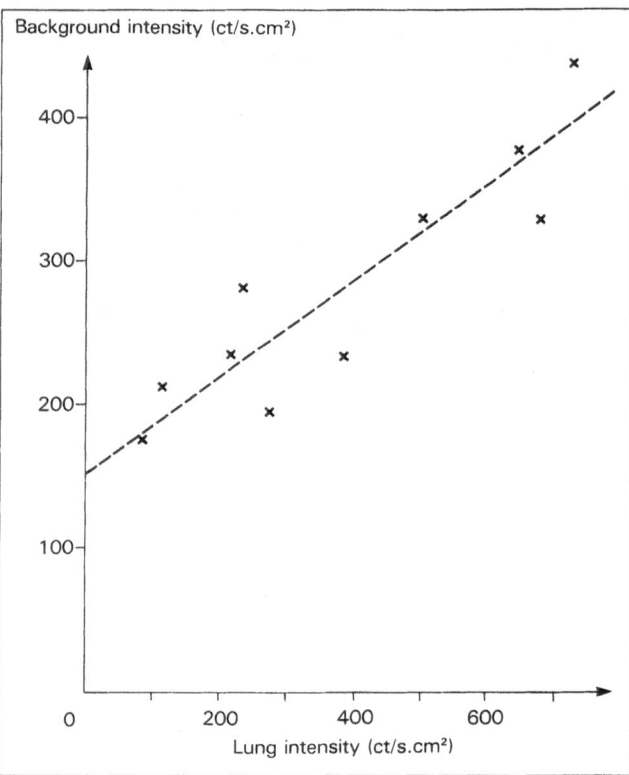

Figure 1.11 Plot of the measured data points for background and lung intensity around the left ventricle.

correlation between the x_i and y_i. In other words, y_i is a good approximation of a linear function of x resulting in the formula:

$$y = a + bx$$

The factor b is the desired 'washout' factor of the lung, and the constant (a) indicates an additional background component which is more or less homogeneously distributed around the ventricle and contributes to each pixel the same background intensity (a). The background image can now be calculated according to the above formula from the parameters a and b and the lung image.

This background image is subtracted from each image of the representative cycle. The definition of the border is now repeated using the same technique as before (with the intensity histogram), or by definition of a level which is between 15% and 20% relative to the maximum ventricular intensity. All pixels having intensities below this level must be suppressed in order to avoid excessive 'noise' around the ventricle.

The final results of these procedures are shown in Figures 1.12–1.15. The representative cycle processed in this way gives a good foundation for the evaluation of functional images as well as for the measurement of global functional parameters.

MEASUREMENT OF EJECTION FRACTION AND VOLUME

The volume of the left ventricle is directly proportional to the countrate (background-corrected) measured over the ventricle. However, for accurate results, this area must be carefully defined. This definition is done automatically at the ventricular border as described before, but some correction at the valve plane is required. Also, movement of the valves during systole should be taken into account which means that different regions of interest must be defined for end-diastole and end-systole.

The ejection fraction is given by:

$$EF = (EDV - ESV) / EDV,$$

where EDV = end-diastolic volume
= $K \times$ end-diastolic counts,
ESV = end-systolic volume
= $K \times$ end-systolic counts.

The proportionality constant K is equal for ED and ES which means that EDV and ESV in the above formula can be replaced by the corresponding countrates.

The measurement of absolute volumes is more difficult because the proportionality constant is dependent upon many factors which include: (1) concentration of radioactivity in the blood, (2) absorption of radiation by the patient (chest wall) and (3) sensitivity of the gamma-camera. Therefore, geometrical measurements were initially tried using the same formula (area/length) that has been established for volume determination by contrast-cineangiography (Rerych et al., 1978b). However, due to the limited resolution of the gamma-camera, outline definition is not exact, and this method gives only a rough estimate of volume.

Another method has been developed which uses ventricular countrate for calculation of volume (Nickel et al., 1982). If the total countrate of the left ventricle or any activity-filled chamber is divided by the maximum count-density (in the centre of the chamber), a 'normalized total countrate' (NTC) results which is independent of the concentration of radioactivity and the absorption of radiation by the patient. It has been found experimentally using balloon models that NTC is a linear function of volume:

$$NTC = a + bV$$

The factor (b) is geometrically related to the camera, and the constant (a) is related to the distance from the chamber (LV) to the camera. From these experiments, an empirical formula for the calculation of ventricular volume was derived which includes the distance from the ventricle to the camera. The results of volume measurements using this method have been compared to contrast-cineangiographic measurements in more than 100 cases, and close correlation was found. The correlation coefficient was 0.95 in a group of 70 cases in which an anterior projection was used, and 0.88 in a group of 40 cases using a right anterior oblique projection. The standard error of the estimate was 15 ml and 20 ml respectively.

The methods described above are easily performed, require little processing time, and can be done by an automatic computer program. Helpful and reliable information is obtained concerning cardiac function.

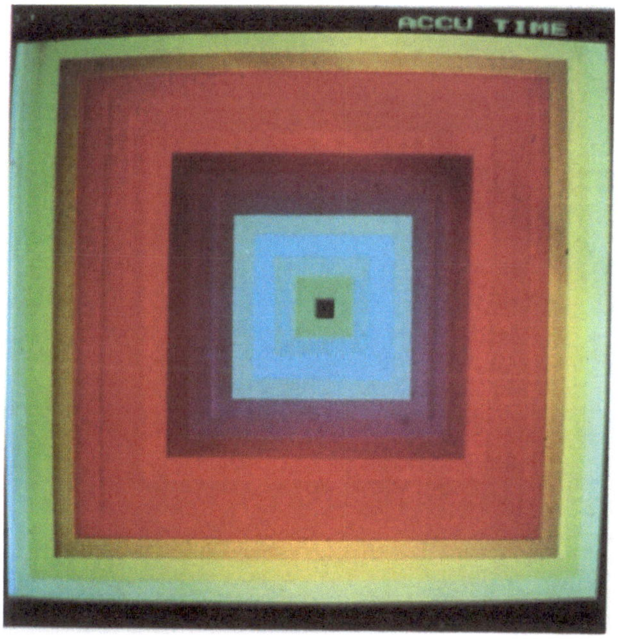

Figure 1.16 Colour spectrum related to count rate utilized for producing ventricular pictures by Baird System-77 camera.

2

Functional Imaging

N. SCHAD AND F. BRUZZONE

The representative cardiac cycle (RC) is obtained by phasic summation of a series of images of several heart cycles during the washout phase of the left (or right) ventricle (Schad, 1976, 1977). Every image of the RC covers a time interval of 20 to 50 ms according to the pre-selected accumulation interval during acquisition. To resolve shortlasting events such as end-systole with high heart rates (exercise studies) a short time interval of 20 to 25 ms per image is used. After edge detection, background measurement and subtraction each image of the RC represents the distribution of regional volumes (counts) within the left (or right) ventricle and the aorta (pulmonary artery) at a particular moment of the cardiac cycle.

The volume (counts) of each cylinder (voxel) measured by the gamma-camera through the heart is represented as a number of a pixel, and for easier interpretation subsequently colour-coded (grey shades on print-outs). Thus, each image of the RC corresponds to a distribution of numbers. Spatial and temporal changes of these numbers, i.e. volumes, of the left (or right) ventricle during a given cardiac phase reflect regional wall function. In routine analysis volume changes during systolic contraction are evaluated. Changes occurring during the first rapid filling phase of diastole are also of particular interest (Figure 2.1). Generally, regional changes during a time interval between two images of the cardiac cycle can be simply demonstrated by subtracting the two images. In fact, by subtracting the end-systolic (ES) from the end-diastolic (ED) image an image of regional distribution of stroke volumes is generated, and by further dividing this image by the end-diastolic one the regional ejection fraction image is obtained (Schad, 1976, 1977). Subtraction, however, increases regional statistical noise disproportionally because the statistical fluctuation derives from the sum of both images but relates to their difference ($[\sqrt{(ED-ES)/ED}]-ES$). Hence within regions where changes are minimal, for example where ventricular ejection is poor, statistical fluctuations are high on the subtraction image. Correspondingly, these regions are 'noisy', poorly delineated, and difficult to separate from surrounding areas, and their function is not easily evaluated. However, it is precisely these regions which are the most important in regional diagnosis. Furthermore, by concentrating on only the two endpoints of the cardiac cycle one loses all information about what occurs throughout the entire period of ventricular contraction or relaxation (Schad and Nickel, 1978).

To overcome these drawbacks, all regional changes during a total cardiac phase or part of that phase can be fitted (via least squares) to a given mathematical function so that an automatic smoothing of the data occurs. A linear and a cosine fit have been adopted. Since for assessment of regional ventricular performance regional changes during contraction (relaxation) are decisive for strategy of treatment, images are processed presenting these changes. These are called 'functional' (or parametric) images, because they reflect function during a given phase of the cardiac cycle (Schad, 1976).

Basically, the following three different functional images are generated:

(1) the regional ejection fraction image (REFI),
(2) the images of regional ejection rate, and
(3) the regional mean (transit) time image.

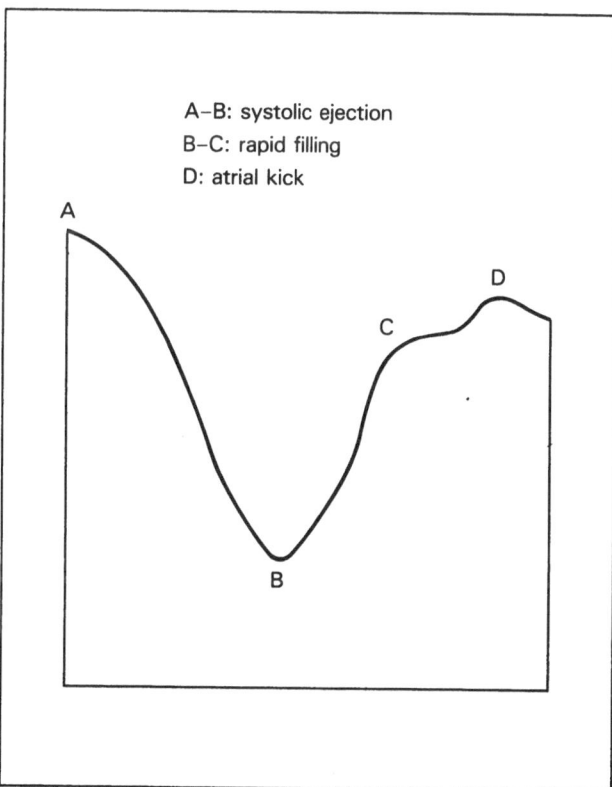

A–B: systolic ejection
B–C: rapid filling
D: atrial kick

Figure 2.1 *The activity curve of the representative cycle* of the left ventricle corresponding to its volume curve.

These functional images are processed by the use of the RC images corresponding to the entire ventricular systolic contraction, i.e. beginning with the end-diastolic and ending with the end-systolic image. The same processing, however, can be adopted for any cardiac phase, rapid diastolic filling for example. Routinely, the same three functional images are processed separately for the first and second half of systole. Thus, the first and second half systolic ejection fraction images, respectively, visualize the regional ejection fractions occurring only during the first and second half of ventricular contraction. Dysfunction limited to early systole, as frequently seen in myocardial ischaemia, can therefore be better evaluated on these 'half-half' images than on those demonstrating function during the entire systole.

Temporal masking due to varying function or degree of dysfunction during systole is avoided or reduced on the first and second half systolic functional images. These images, however, contain more random fluctuations than the corresponding image covering the entire systole. This is one more reason to generate cardiac studies with high initial count rates. When maximum count rates during first pass of the radionucleide bolus through the right heart result in less than 180 000 cps, first and second half systolic images frequently become too 'noisy' to be successfully evaluated. A further subdivision in first, second and third third systolic images, as used in contrast ventriculograms (Johnson *et al.*, 1975), would not only increase the number of images to be processed but also introduce even more random fluctuations, i.e. diagnostic uncertainties, and prolong the processing and evaluation time.

Single 'temporally smoothed' images (for example, end-diastolic and end-systolic images) can be used to process subtraction images, which contain fewer random fluctuations than the subtraction images obtained from the original RC images. The *regional ejection fraction image* thus processed presents the regional distribution of EFs for each pixel, i.e. cylinder measured through the heart. For example, on the graph (Figure 2.7) the short cylinder at the apex and the next one are completely emptied during systole, the outer contour corresponding to the end-diastolic and the inner to the end-systolic border of the left ventricle. Hence, both cylinders have a 100 per cent ejection fraction colour-coded as yellow pixels on the functional image. In contrast, the following drawn cylinders are not completely emptied during systolic contraction since residual volume (dotted line) remains in them at the end of systole. Consequently, they produce lower ejection fractions, the lowest one resulting at the base of the heart where most residual volume is located.

Thus, the normal REFI image (Figures 2.8, 2.9) shows semiannular symmetric bands of an equal range of values, which decrease from 100% EF corresponding to the shell of wall motion where all blood is displaced to low EF in the subvalvular regions where the residual volume remains at end-systole. The adopted colour-scale presents 10 steps each of 10% EF ranging from 0 to 100%. In the most used RAO view the function approximates symmetry with respect to the long axis of the ventricle, whereas in the LAO view normally some asymmetry is encountered (Figure 2.34) because the high septal area contributes less to ejection than the lateral wall, the residual volume remaining particularly in the sub-aortic region.

In regions with decreased ejection underneath wall motion disorders the high EF-bands become smaller than in normal segments, sometimes being interrupted or partly missing. Lower regional ejection fractions appear to 'advance' to the periphery of the left ventricle. Very low regional EF values point to extension of malfunction in depth. In this way functional images in one projection provide some three-dimensional information. The first/second half systolic REFI images contain many more random fluctuations (Figures 2.24, 2.25). Therefore, only defects or very low EFs can be used for diagnosis with certainty.

Regional EF images obtained after a cosine fit of ED and ES may still show relevant fluctuations leading to diagnostic uncertainties because of the subtraction process of two single images. The so-called trend images, however, which pull information from all sequential images of a certain cardiac phase and average it, present a higher image quality and less diagnostic uncertainties. Noisy areas are automatically depressed by the involved process of temporal smoothing (least squares fit), and the contrast between normal and abnormal regions is enhanced; areas with reduced or abnormal function are better delineated than on subtraction images, and the extent of malfunction becomes measureable. Therefore, trend images are diagnostically more reliable than subtraction images.

Images that show the rate of linear decrease or increase in activity or blood can be processed (Noelpp *et al.*, 1977). These images collect all information during a selected cardiac phase, for example systole (Figures 2.2, 2.3), and reflect the average rate or trend of density change during that phase for all matrix points (regional 'temporal' gradients). The computational formula for the linear decrease image is given by the sum of systolic images times $n+1$, minus the sum of weighted systolic images times 2, where n corresponds to the number of systolic images and the weight to the time interval from the first end-diastolic image on. The inverse subtraction generates the increase image. For example, on the graph (Figure 2.10) the short cylinder at the apex of the left ventricle is completely emptied during contraction with a stroke volume represented by the height of the column on the right. The rate of emptying is given by the slope of the triangle and is coded with the red colour on the functional image (Figure 2.11). The next cylinder, also completely emptied, presents the largest stroke volume and therefore the highest column on the right. Consequently, the slope of the triangle is steepest and will be coded as yellow on the functional image. The next cylinders toward the base of the heart are all only partially emptied having lower stroke volumes. Correspondingly the ejection rates are again lower.

The normal *regional ejection rate image* shows in the RAO view symmetric bands of equal ranges of value (Figures 2.11, 2.13). The shell with the maximum rate lies somewhat inside the end-diastolic contour of the ventricle where the largest volume (stroke volume) is completely displaced during systole. It can be proven that it corresponds to the inner part of the 100% shell of the REFI image (Figure 2.12) where the largest voxels are completely emptied during contraction. This region of maximum ejection rates is normally crescent-shaped. Toward the base of the heart the ejection rates decrease with the lowest values immediately below the valve plane. The regional ejection rate image practically

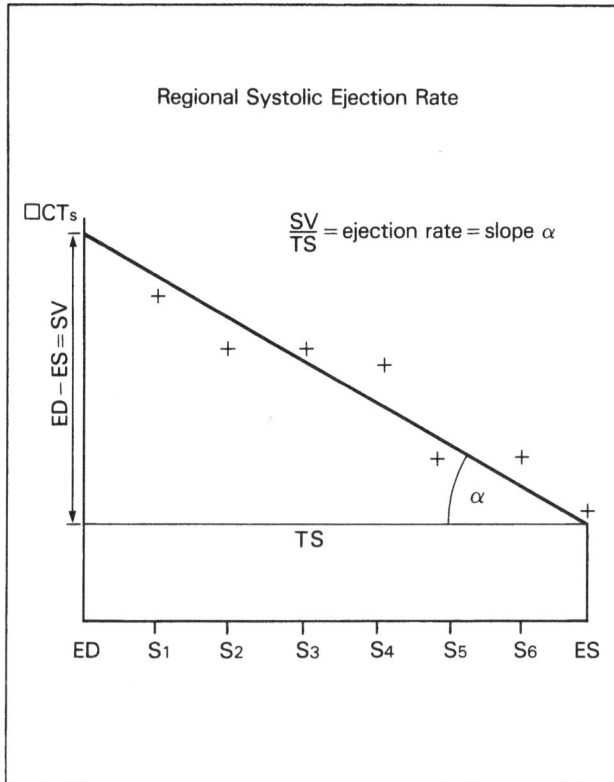

Figure 2.2 *Regional systolic ejection rate*: for every pixel the rate of decrease of activity or blood is computed by a linear least squares fit through all systolic data points. The rate represents the stroke volume (SV = ED − ES) divided by the constant time of systole (TS). Higher stroke volumes produce steeper slopes or higher rates. Where blood does not decrease during systole no decrease rates result (black areas).

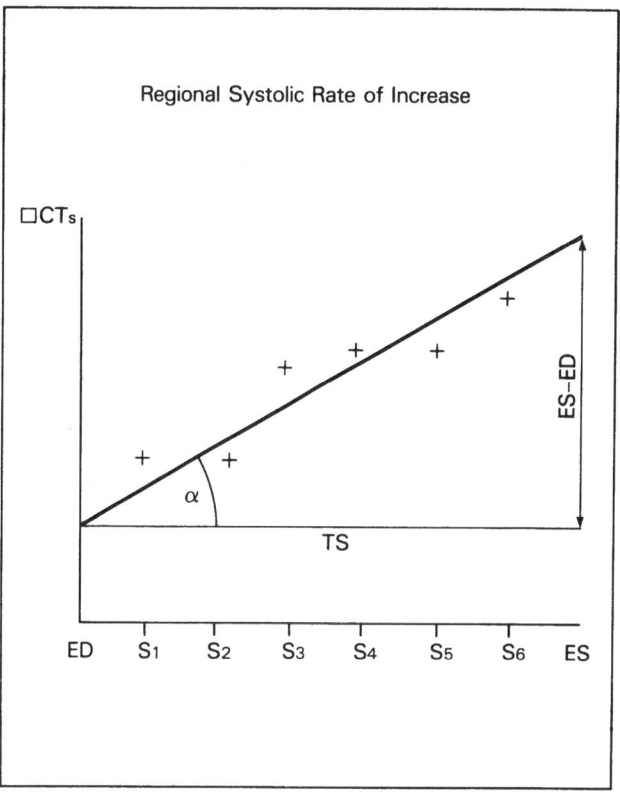

Figure 2.3 *Regional systolic rate of increase*: for each pixel the rate of increase of activity or blood is computed by a linear least squares fit through all systolic data points. The rate corresponds to the difference between end-systolic and end-diastolic counts (ES − ED) divided by the constant time of systole (TS). Regions with significant increase of blood during systole as the aorta or pulmonary outflow tract are characterized by high increase rates. Where blood does not increase during systole no increase rates result (black areas).

demonstrates the distribution of regional stroke volumes, since the stroke volume of every voxel is divided by a constant, i.e. the time of systole. Being a trend image, however, it presents much less random fluctuations than the stroke volume image derived by simple subtraction of ES from ED. As with the REFI image, in the LAO view some asymmetry of function at the septal side is normal (Figure 2.35).

Reduced regional ejection rate is characterized by interruption of high velocity band and substitution by lower values. Loss of part of the normally crescent-shaped high rate yellow band and central shifting of high rates is a very sensitive sign of dysfunction. First and second half systolic rate images are diagnostically more reliable than the corresponding REFI images because they contain less random fluctuations. During the first half of contraction maximum rates are usually located at the centre of the ventricle; during the second half, however, maximum rates are found at the periphery. (Figures 2.26, 2.27). Defects and very low rate regions can be considered as a result of pathological function.

With the processing of regional ejection rate images one usually also obtains an image that exhibits all regions where activity or blood increases during systole (Figure 2.3), i.e. the aorta and sometimes the area of entrance of pulmonary veins due to residual lung activity flowing into the left atrium (Figure 2.22). This image is very useful for detecting mitral reflux or left to right shunts.

Regional ejection rate images are based on a linear least squares fit of the systolic RC images. Systolic function at the periphery of the left ventricle normally approaches linearity whereas at the subvalvular area it assumes more the shape of a cosine function (Figure 2.6). Therefore, the linear fit of the ejection rate image may introduce some distortions into the data of the subvalvular area, whereas it is an adequate function for analysing peripheral ventricular performance. Conversely, a cosine fit could introduce some distortion of data in the peripheral regions. The great advantage of the third functional so-called *mean (transit) time image* is that no assumptions have to be made about the shape of the regional curves of systolic changes. The computational formula for the mean time image is given by the sum of weighted systolic images divided by the sum of systolic images (Schad, 1977). The mean time elapsing from end-diastole or the upslope of the curve to the centre of gravity is measured for every pixel (Figures 2.4, 2.5) and the distribution of these times is represented in one image that practically illustrates the regional persistence of blood during systole. In fact, in the normally contracting periphery (Figure 2.6) there is no end-systolic residual volume and the curve is rather linear so that a short mean time results. On the other hand, in the subvalvular region end-systolic volume is relatively high and the curve approaches a cosine function with the result of a longer mean time.

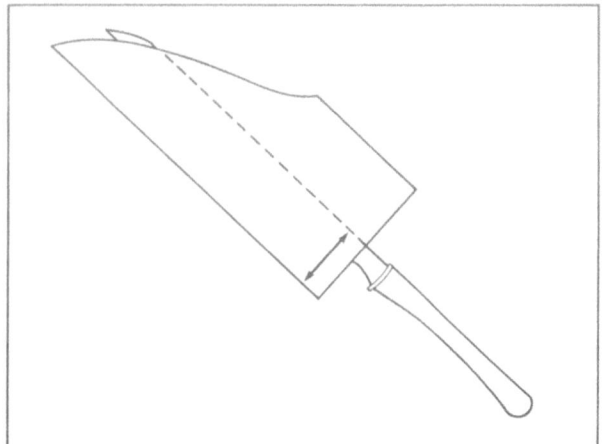

Figure 2.4 *Regional systolic mean (transit) time*: for the time–activity curve of every pixel the time when the centre of gravity of the curve occurs is computed. The centre of gravity lies where the area of the curve balances on the edge of a knife (area divided in two equal areas). The time elapsing from the start of the curve to the balancing point is the mean (transit) time. No assumptions have to be made about a particular shape or function of the curve.

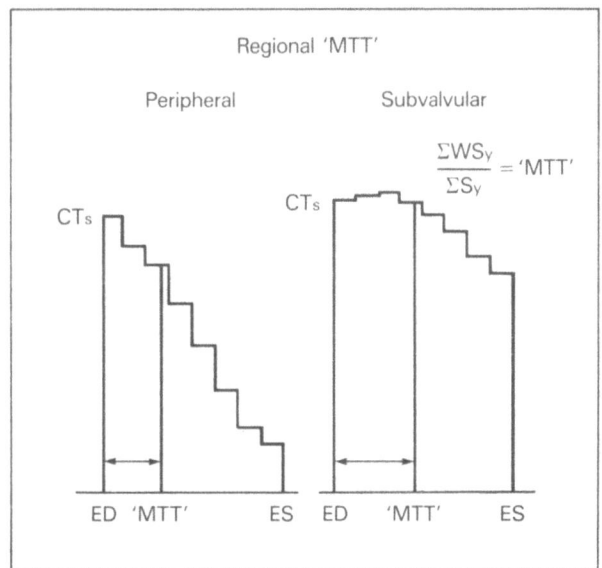

Figure 2.5 *Regional peripheral and subvalvular systolic mean times.* At the ventricular periphery (left) where activity or blood stays a short time only, short mean times result (small area under the curve). At the subvalvular regions (right) where activity or the residual volume remains for a longer time interval, longer mean times result (large area under the curve). Computational formula for mean times is given by the sum of weighted systolic images divided by the sum of images. Determination of mean times does not require any fit to a particular curve or mathematical function.

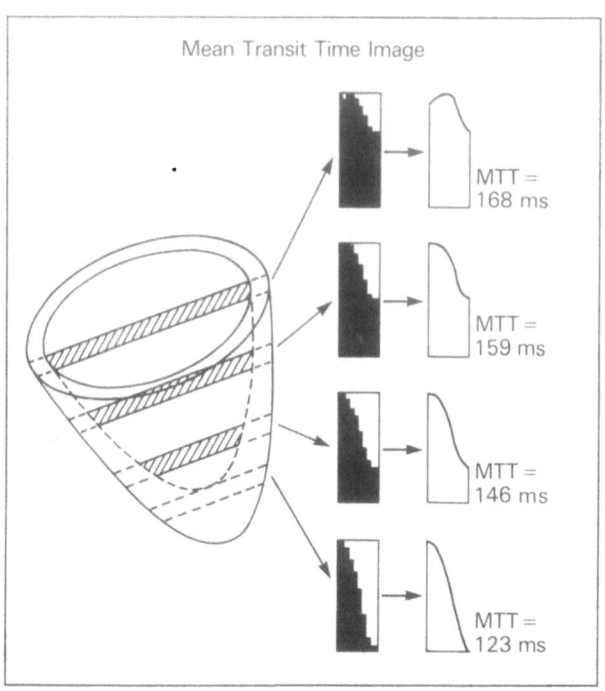

Figure 2.6 *Systolic mean (transit) times at different ventricular regions.* Outer contour of the heart corresponds to end-diastole, inner contour to end-systole. Approaching the base of the ventricle more and more blood remains in the cylinders measured through the heart at the end of contraction (dashed lines). Consequently, end-systolic count-values increase, the area under the curve enlarges and the mean times rise. in addition, there is normally a transition from a more linear curve pattern in the ventricular periphery to a cosinusoid pattern in the subvalvular region.

On the mean time image (Figures 2.14, 2.15) the longest times are seen below the valve plane where residual volume remains and the blood 'persists' longest. The shortest times result at the periphery of the ventricle from where blood is rapidly displaced toward the outflow tract during contraction. The time bands are approximately symmetrical in the RAO view; in the LAO view (Figure 2.36) the same asymmetry is observed as with the other functional images. To better discriminate differences in regional mean times a second image is generated that subdivides each level of values into eight colour-levels (Figures 2.16, 2.17, 2.21, 2.37). This second image is usually taken for evaluation.

With regional malfunction persistence of blood is prolonged or, as seen on the images, long subvalvular mean times 'advance' toward the periphery pointing to the wall dysfunction. Thus, this image can show differences in flow contributions coming from distinct wall segments during contraction. In fact, under infarcted segments very long mean times as normally encountered at the outflow tract or the aorta become visible indicating long systolic persistence of blood in these regions. Analogous images have been recently observed with nuclear magnetic resonance examinations where low flows underneath infarcts can produce intra-cavitary signals.

Drawing information from all systolic images the mean transit time image is much less subjected to random fluctuations than the subtraction image as the REFI image. Consequently, first and second half systolic mean time images are more reliable than the corresponding REFI images (Figures 2.28, 2.29). Very long times as normally only seen in the subvalvular area appearing in the periphery can be considered as the result of pathological function.

The same functional images as routinely used for left ventricular regional evaluation can be processed to examine *right ventricular regional function*. (Figures 2.18, 2.19, 2.20, 2.21, 2.23). The appearance of the

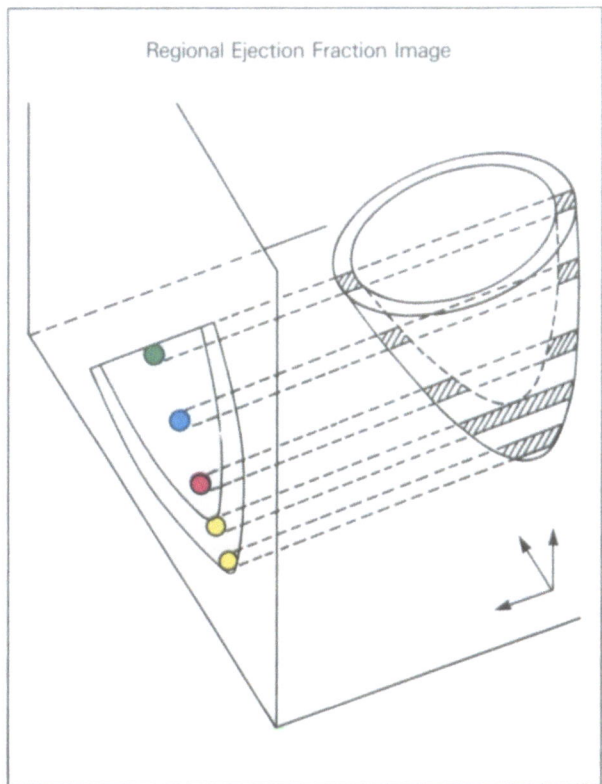

Figure 2.7 *Ejection fraction at different ventricular regions.* The outer contour of the heart corresponds to end-diastole, inner contour to end-systole. Cylinders measured through the apex of the ventricle are completely emptied and, therefore, produce the highest EFs. For details see text.

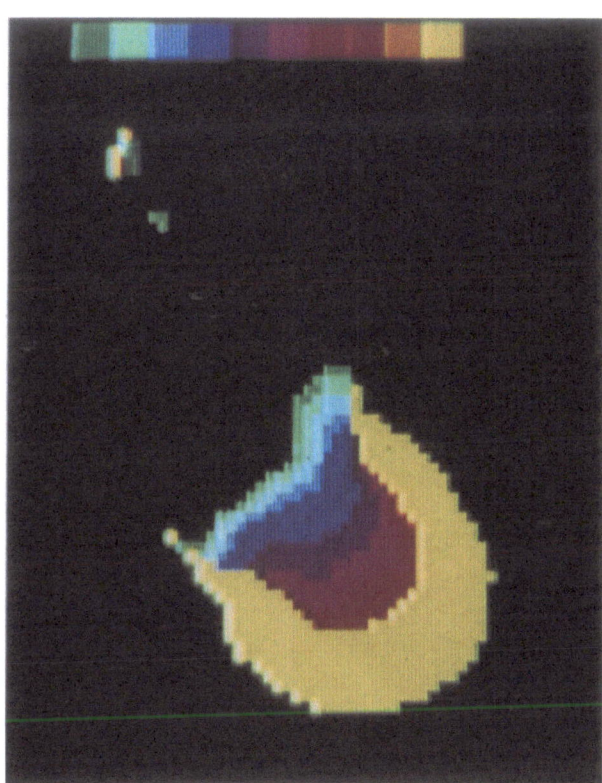

Figure 2.8 *Regional ejection fraction image at rest*, RAO view, left ventricle (colour scale 10% EF). Symmetric semi-annular EF bands, which decrease in value toward the outflow tract. Wall motion corresponds to 100% EF (yellow band).

images in the RAO view is analogous to those seen for the left ventricle. The pulmonary conus because of its very late contraction shows systolic function on the second half images only. On the image reflecting entire systole it even may show an increase of activity or blood (Figure 2.23).

All the above images illustrate regional systolic contraction of the ventricles. *Ventricular relaxation*, however, can be regionally analysed as well. The rapid filling phase of ventricular diastole is of particular interest. Images of regional rate of rapid filling (rate of increase) can be processed for the left or right ventricle (Figures 2.30, 2.31, 2.32, 2.33). Maximum rates should normally point to the apex of the ventricle when mitral valve inflow is central and ventricular compliance normal. Deviations of inflow directions are seen in ischaemia and infarcts as well as with some mitral valve prostheses. Similarly to ventricular contraction, mean time images of rapid filling can be generated. Conversely to contraction, however, the longest times result at the periphery. In the RAO view symmetrical bands should result with normal inflow and normal compliance (Figures 2.31, 2.33). Loss of symmetry would mean abnormal rapid filling.

Functional images visualize on one single image function during a selected time interval. But the count rate of the used images, border definition, background subtraction and the mathematical process involved have a substantial effect on the quality and diagnostic accuracy of the single functional images as here described. The diagnostic value of the single functional images will be discussed and illustrated in the following chapters of clinical applications.

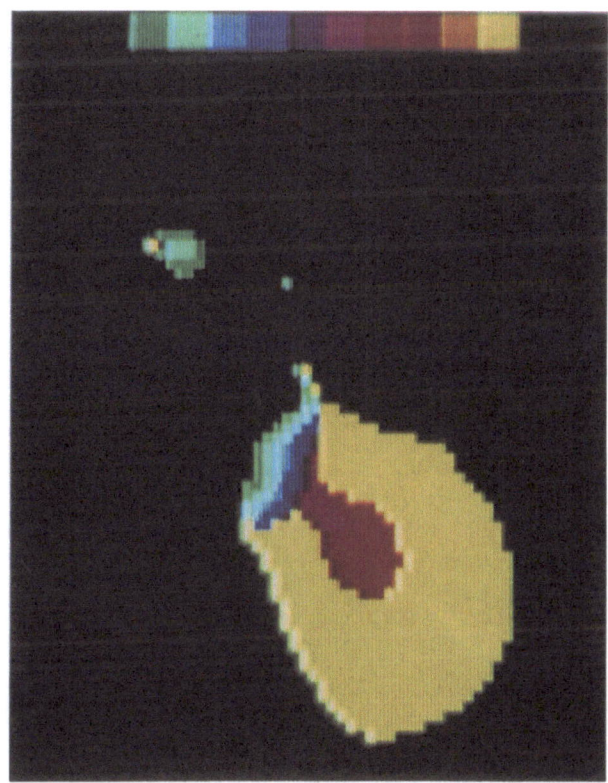

Figure 2.9 *Regional ejection fraction image at peak exercise*, RAO view, left ventricle (colour scale 10% EF). In comparison to the rest study (Figure 2.8) wall motion increases (yellow band of 100% EF) and high regional EF's advance to the outflow tract because of stronger conraction. Decrease of end-diastolic and particularly end-systolic ventricular size and volume.

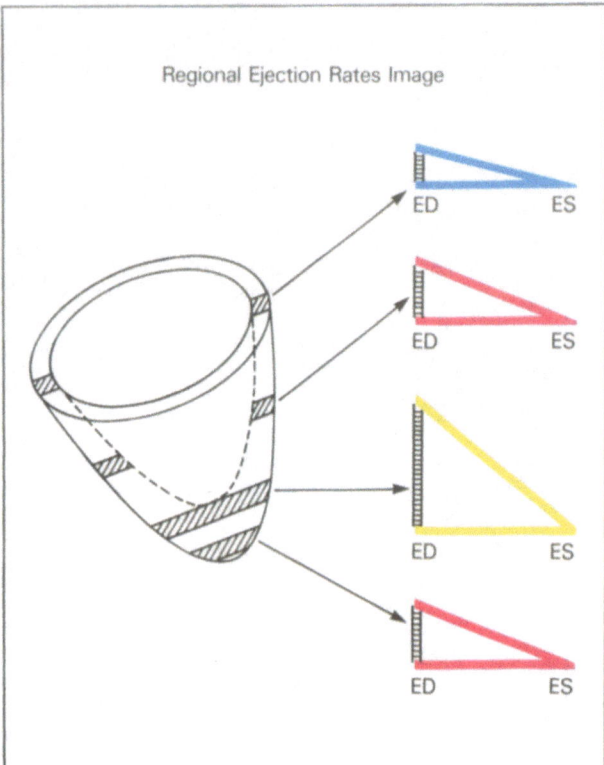

Figure 2.10 *Ejection rates at different ventricular regions,* The outer contour of the heart corresponds to end-diastole, inner contour to end-systole. Columns (right) represent stroke volumes. Highest stroke volumes and consequently steepest slopes or highest rates result near the border where the largest volumes are completely emptied during systolic contraction. For details see text.

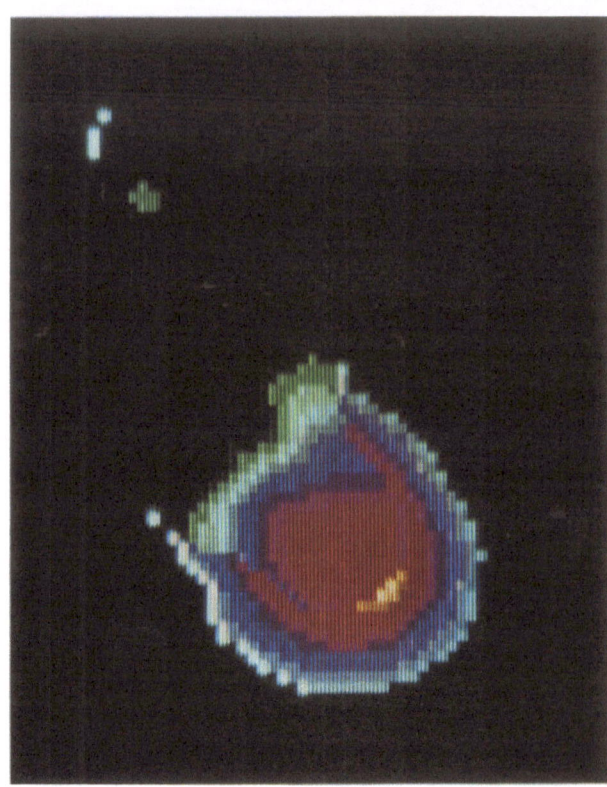

Figure 2.11 *Regional ejection rate image at rest,* RAO view, left ventricle. Functional symmetry with maximum rates where the largest volume is completely displaced (crescent-shaped yellow zone).

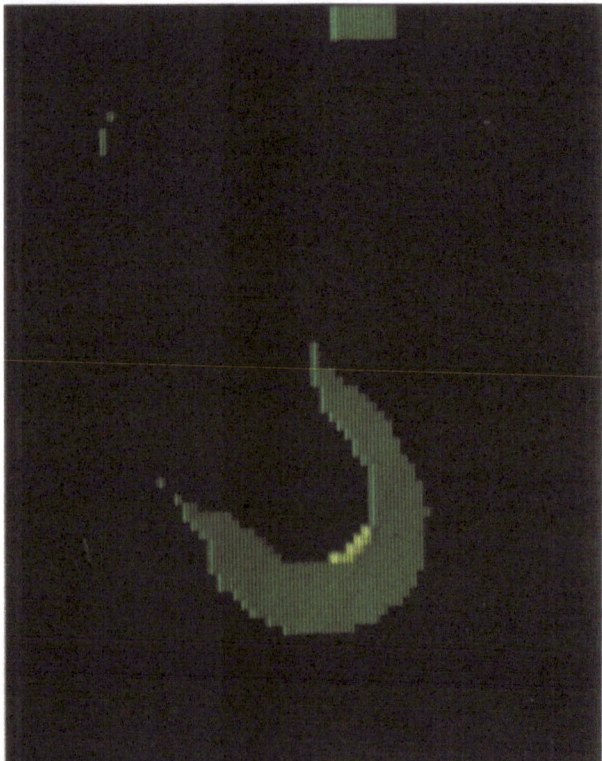

Figure 2.12 *Location of maximum ejection rates.* Compare Figure 2.8 with Figure 2.11. Maximum ejection rates result at the inner part of the 100% EF band, as can be seen by summation of the crescent-shaped zone and the 100% wall motion band (green).

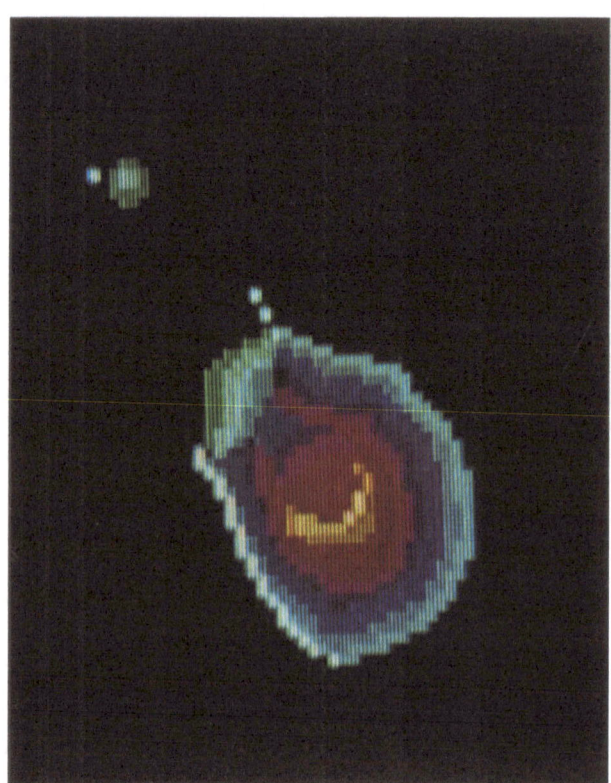

Figure 2.13 *Regional ejection rate image at peak exercise,* RAO view, left ventricle. The crescent-shaped yellow high rates shift to the outflow tract, since contraction of the left ventricle increases.

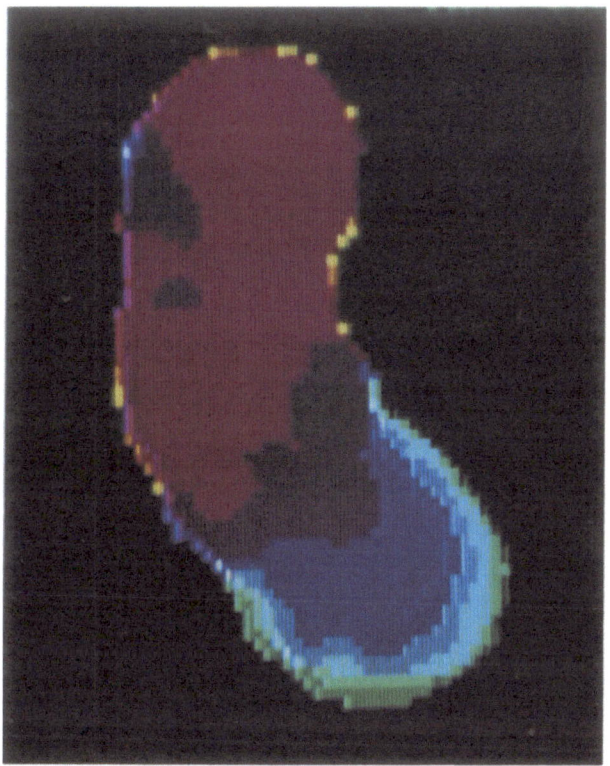

Figure 2.14 *Regional mean – (transit) – time image at rest*, RAO view, left ventricle. Low values lie at the ventricular periphery because of short persistence of activity in the region of wall motion. Increase in persistence and time values toward the outflow tract. Longest times immediately below the aortic valve and in the ascending aorta, where blood and activity remain at the end of systole.

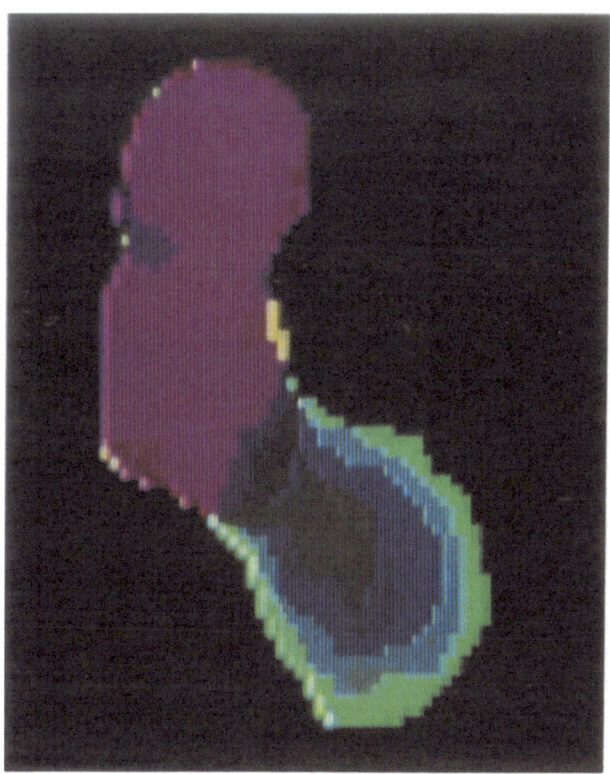

Figure 2.15 *Regional mean (transit) time image at peak exercise*, RAO view, left ventricle. With exercise the bands corresponding to shorter times advance to the outflow tract due to stronger contraction.

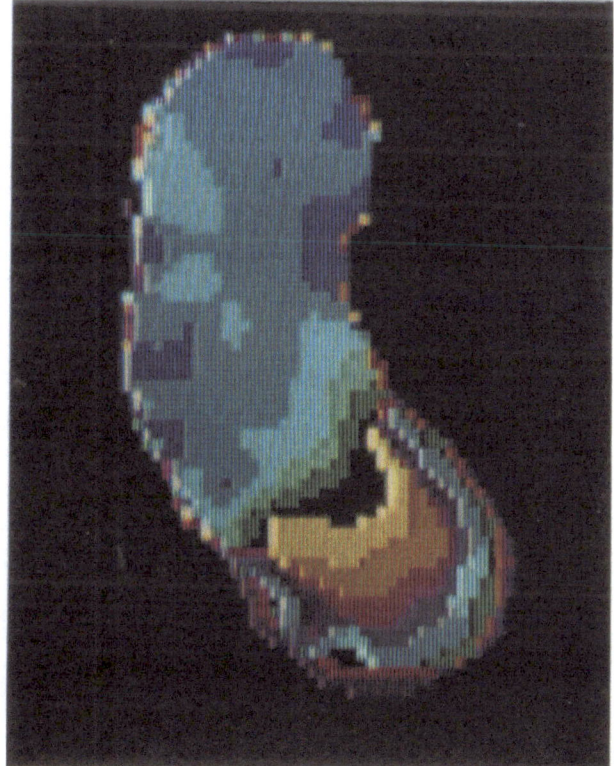

Figure 2.16 *Regional mean (transit) time image at rest*, RAO view. Same image as Figure 2.14, but with better discrimination of value-levels or colours: each colour-level is further subdivided in 8 distinct colours. For findings see under Figure 2.14.

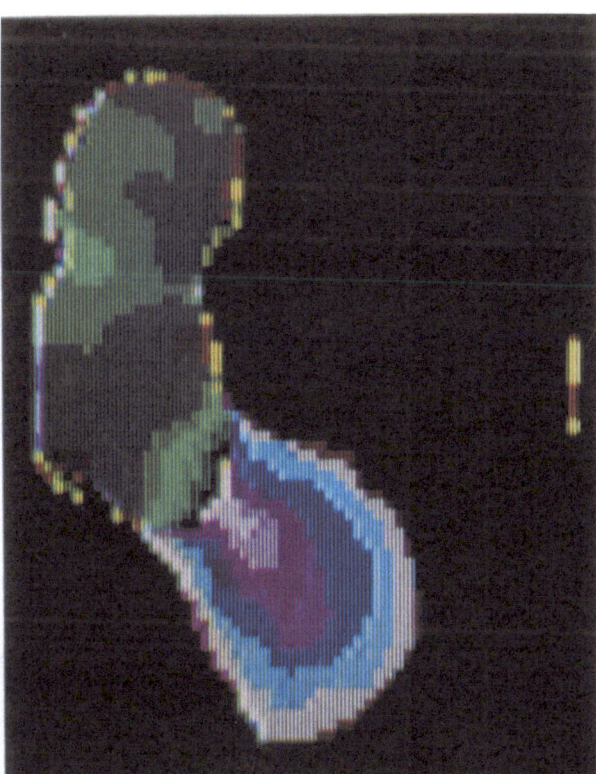

Figure 2.17 *Regional mean (transit) time image at peak exercise*, RAO view, left ventricle. Same image as Figure 2.15, but with better discrimination of value-levels or colours: each colour-level is further subdivided in 8 distinct colours. For findings see under Figure 2.15.

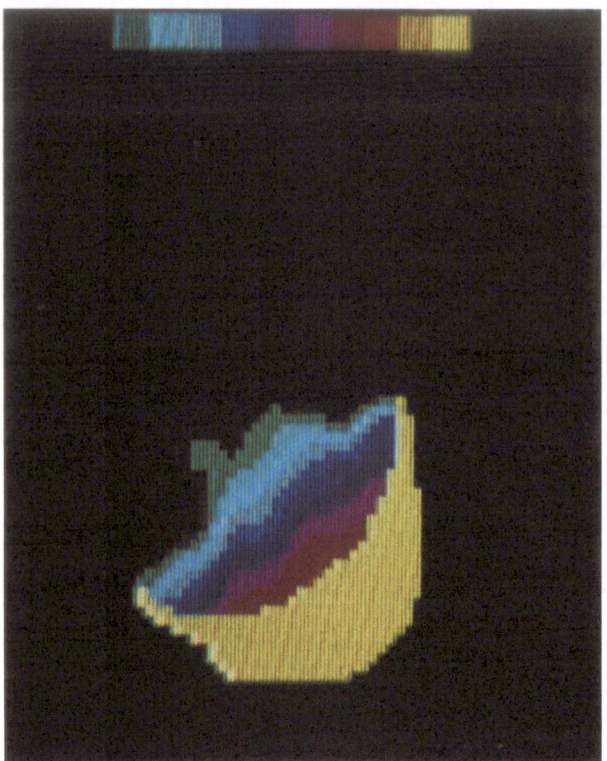

Figure 2.18 *Regional ejection fraction image: Right ventricle*, RAO view, at rest. In analogy to the left ventricle (Figure 2.8) symmetric semiannular EF bands, which decrease in value toward the outflow tract. Wall motion corresponds to 100% EF (yellow band).

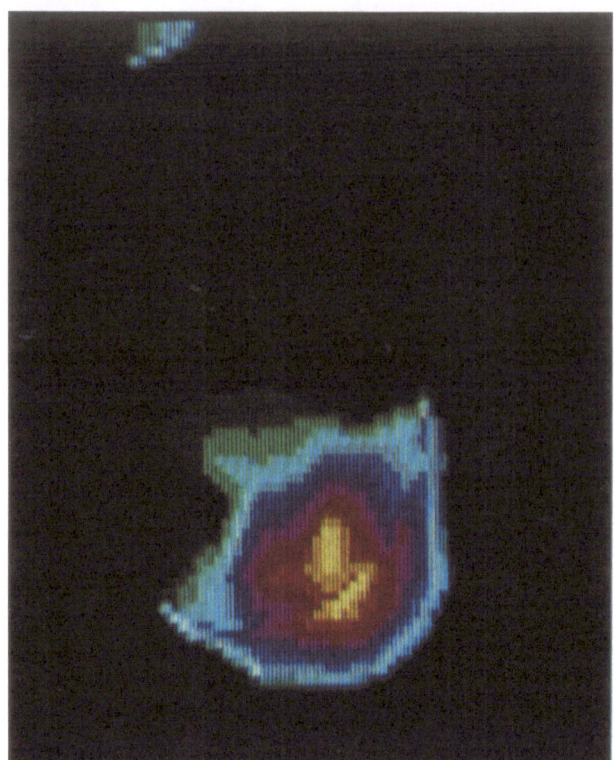

Figure 2.19 *Regional ejection rate image: right ventricle*, RAO view, at rest. In analogy to the left ventricle (Figure 2.11) functional symmetry along the long axis with maximum rates where the largest volume is completely displaced (crescent-shaped yellow zone).

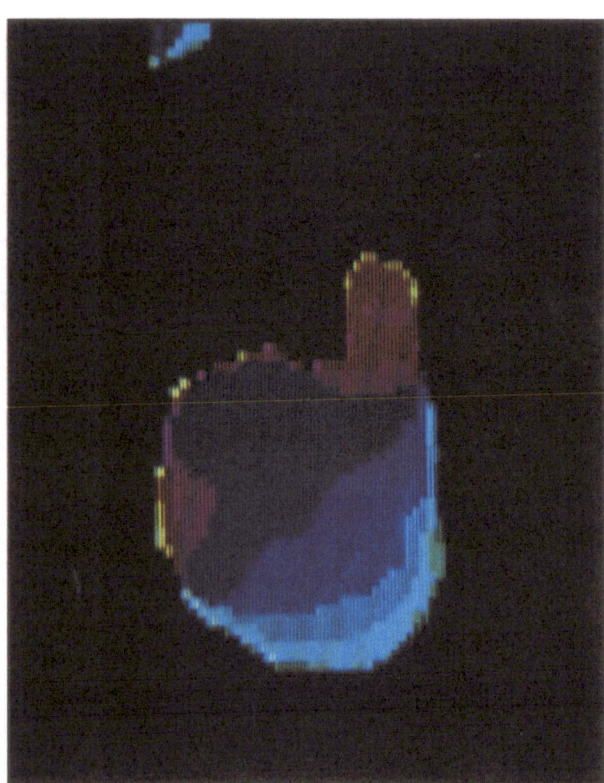

Figure 2.20 *Regional mean (transit) time image: right ventricle*, RAO view, at rest. In analogy to the left ventricle (Figure 2.14) low values at the ventricular periphery because of short persistence of activity or blood in the region of wall motion. Increase in persistence and time values toward the outflow tract. Longest times immediately below the pulmonary valve and in the pulmonary artery where blood and activity remain at the end of contraction.

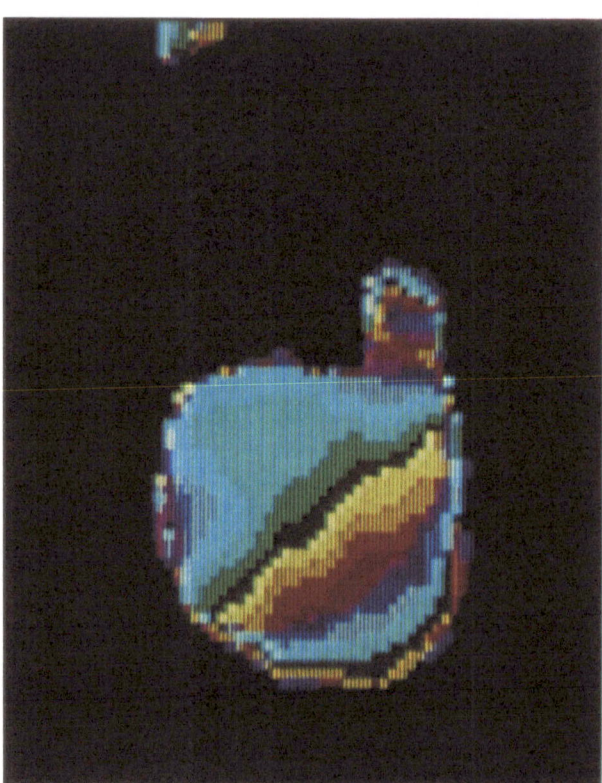

Figure 2.21 *Regional mean (transit) time image: right ventricle*, RAO view, at rest. Same image as Figure 2.20, but with better discrimination of value-levels or colours: each colour-level is further subdivided in 8 distinct colours. For findings see under Figure 2.20.

14

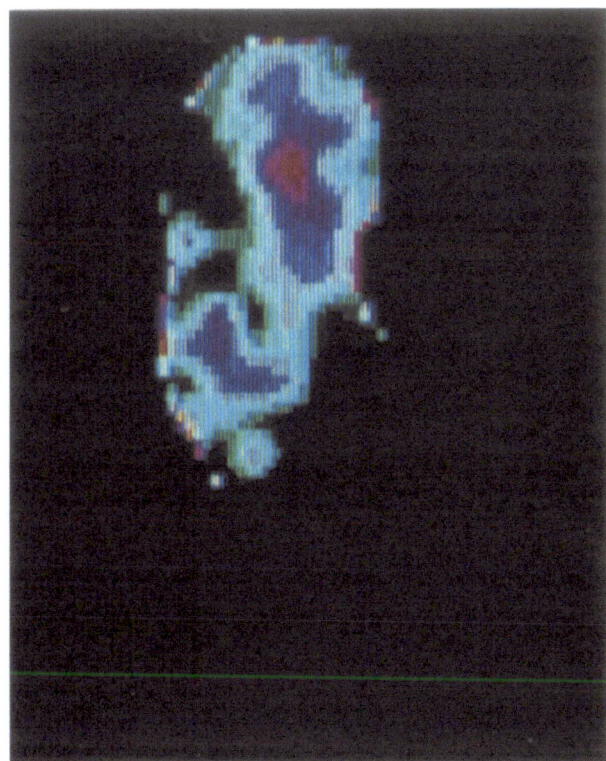

Figure 2.22 *Regional systolic increase image: left ventricle,* RAO view, at rest. During systole there is normally increase of activity and blood at the ascending aorta. Some increase may also appear at the entrance of pulmonary veins into the left atrium due to residual lung activity flowing into the heart.

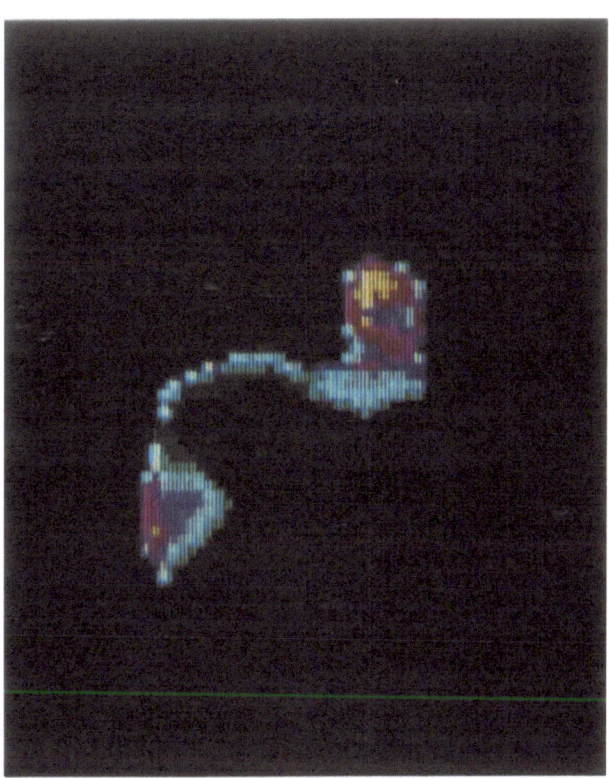

Figure 2.23 *Regional systolic increase image: right ventricle,* RAO view, at rest. During systole there is normally increase of activity and blood in the pulmonary outflow tract and main pulmonary artery. Some increase may appear at the right atrium due to inflow of residual activity from the superior vena cava.

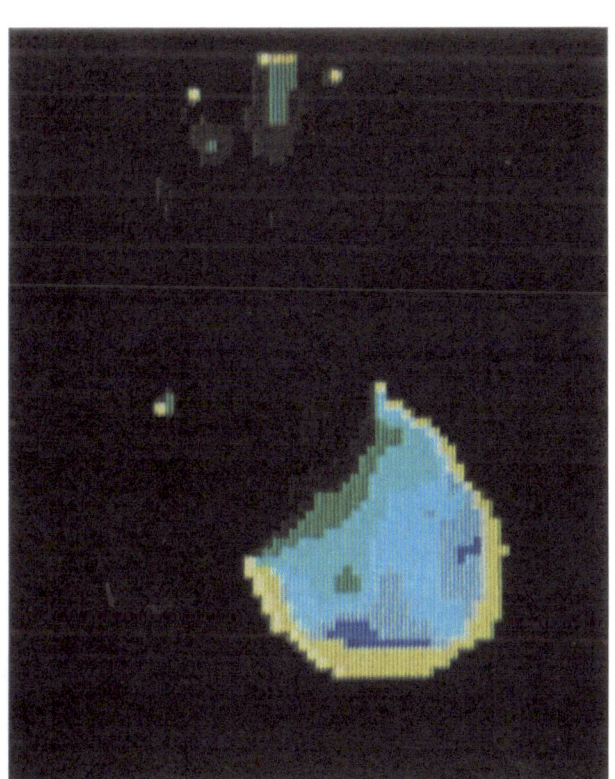

Figure 2.24 *Regional ejection fraction image: first half systole,* left ventricle, RAO view, at rest. This image usually shows significant random fluctuations that make diagnosis uncertain. Only defects (no EF) or severe dysfunctions can be related to pathology with certainty.

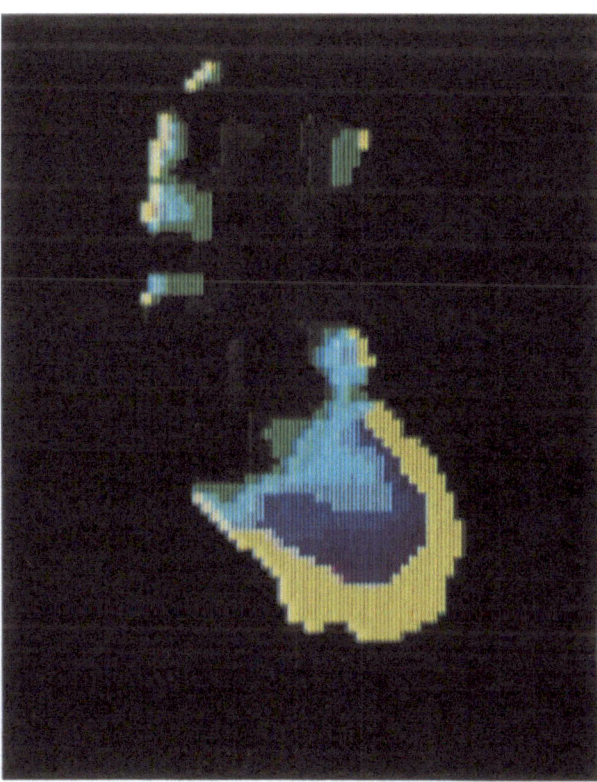

Figure 2.25 *Regional ejection fraction image: second half systole,* left ventricle, RAO-view, at rest. This image usually presents wall contraction (yellow band) except in the segment of mitral valve prolapse.

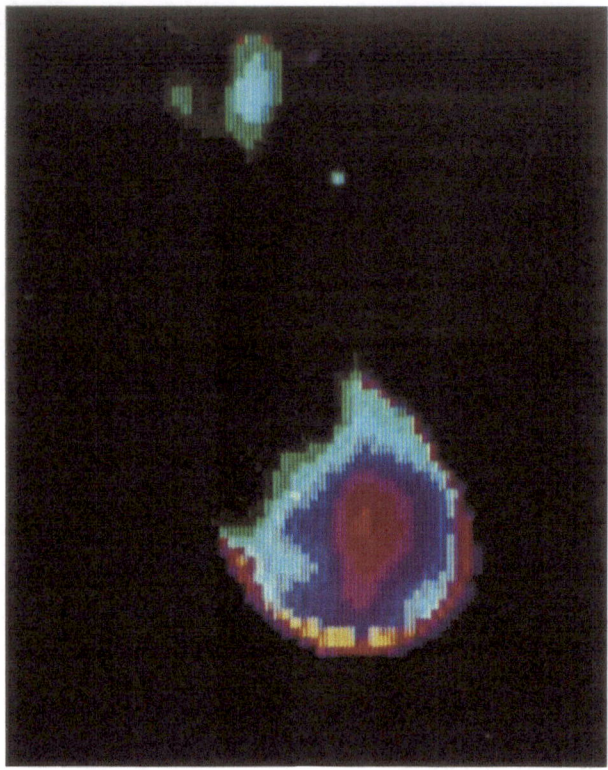

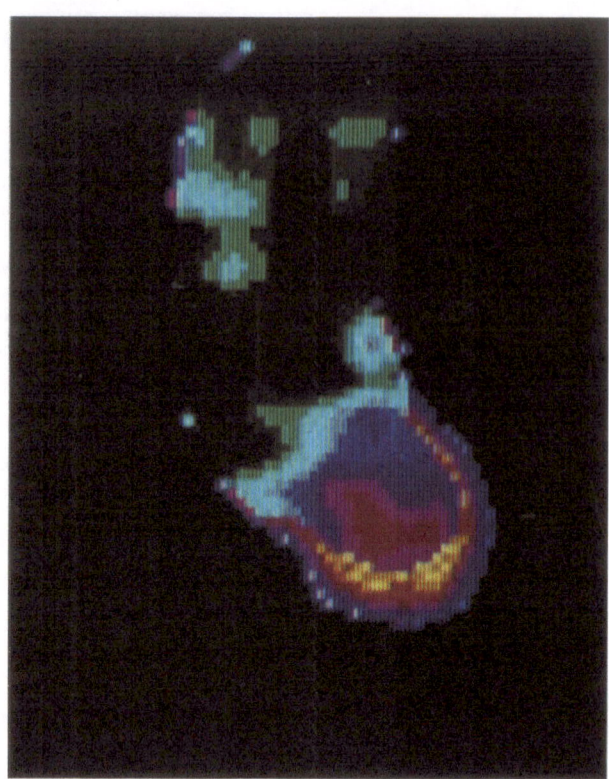

Figure 2.26 *Regional ejection rate image: first half systole,* left ventricle, RAO-view, at rest. The image presents fewer random fluctuations than the corresponding REFI image. Maximum rates are usually situated at the centre of the ventricle. Defects (no rates) or very low rates at the periphery are diagnostic.

Figure 2.27 *Regional ejection rate image: second half systole,* left ventricle, RAO view, at rest. In contrast to the first half systole this image normally shows maximum rates at a peripheral shell. Loss of these rates is diagnostic.

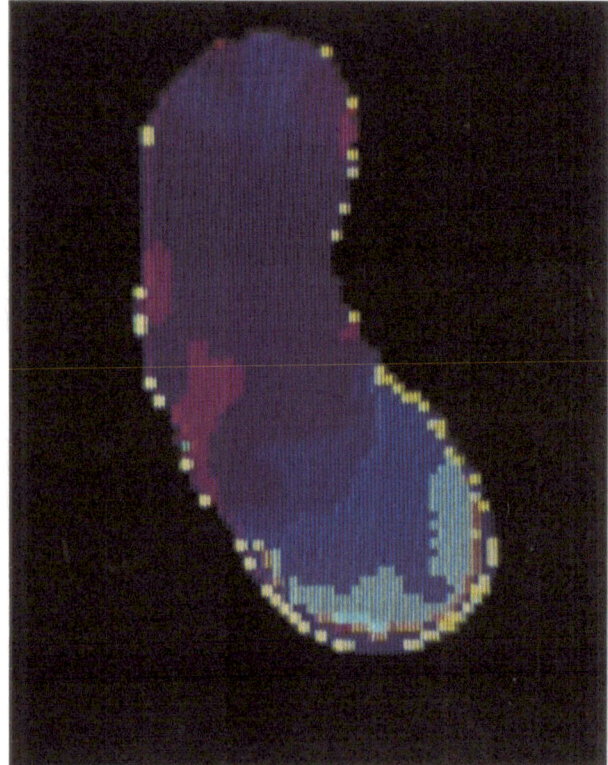

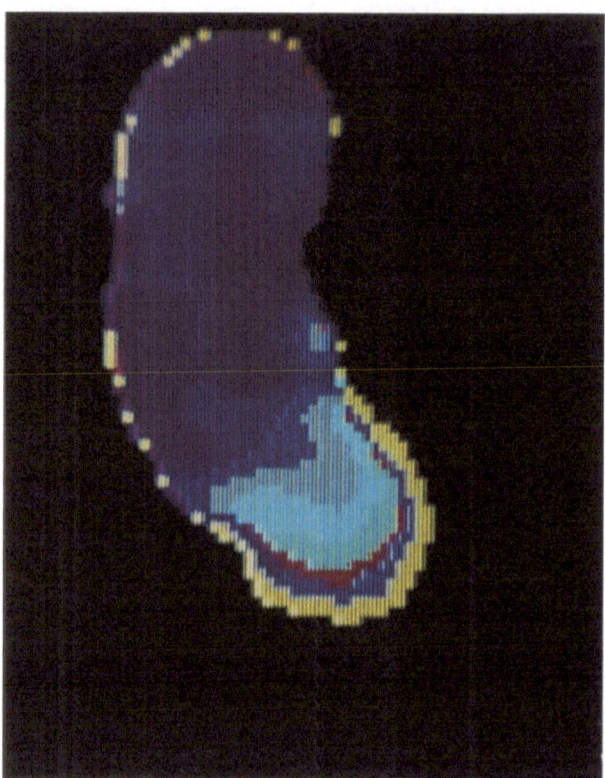

Figure 2.28 *Regional mean (transit) time image: first half systole,* left ventricle, RAO view, at rest. The image contains fewer random fluctuations than the corresponding REFI image. Long times as seen in the subvalvular region or the ascending aorta encountered in the ventricular periphery can be related to pathology.

Figure 2.29 *Regional mean (transit) time image: second half systole,* left ventricle, RAO view, at rest. Several symmetrical levels of short times normally appear in the periphery. For pathological findings see under Figure 2.28.

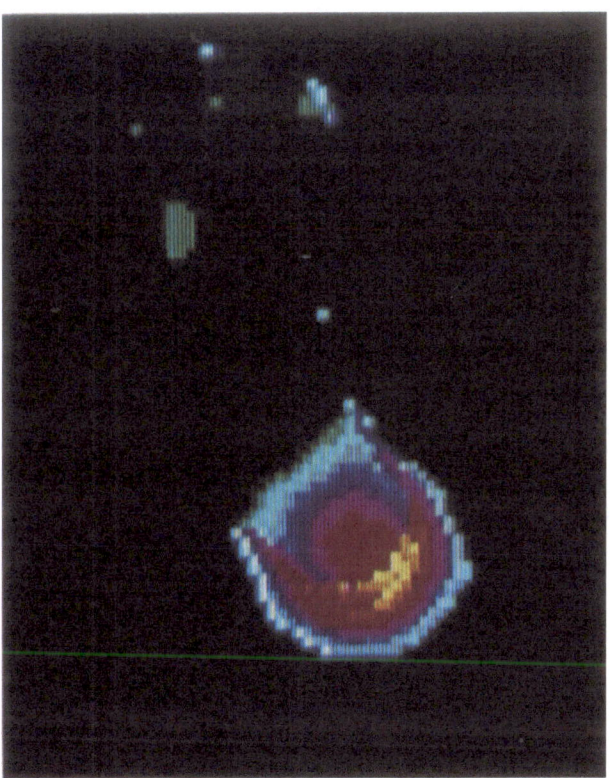

Figure 2.30 *Regional rapid filling rate image: left ventricle,* RAO view, at rest. Symmetrical inflow directed to the apex where maximum rates are normally situated. Deviations of rates are seen with reduced regional compliance and/or distortion of inflow through mitral valve prostheses.

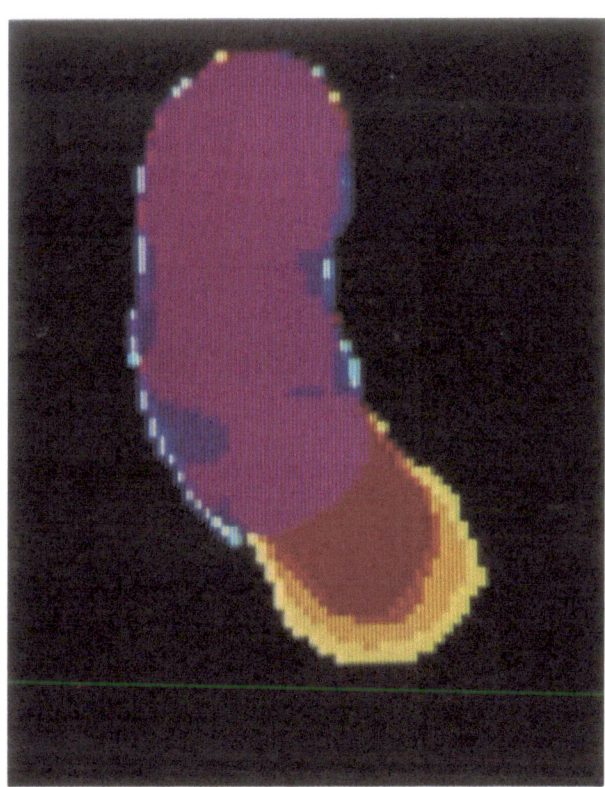

Figure 2.31 *Regional rapid filling mean time image: left ventricle,* RAO view, at rest. Contrary to systolic contraction longest mean times result at the periphery as a symmetrical shell as long inflow and compliance are normal. With disturbed filling function interruption of the longest peripheral time-values are observed.

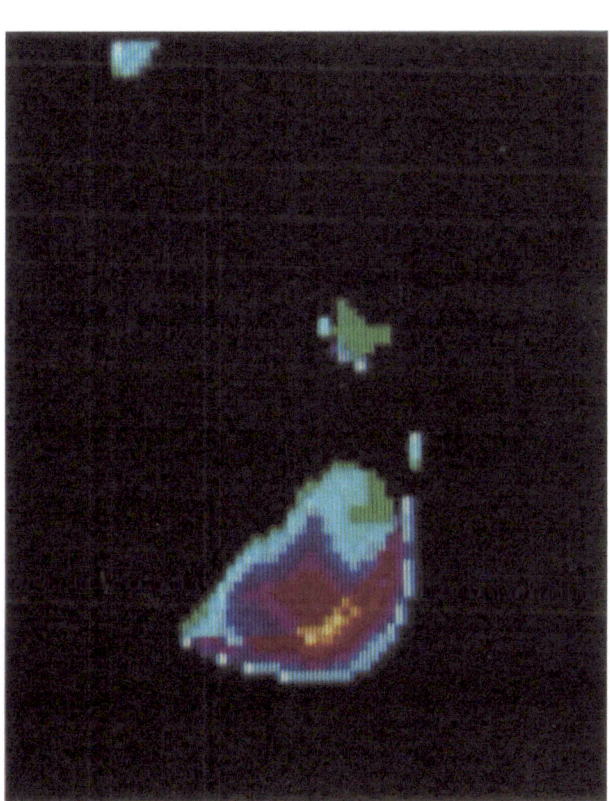

Figure 2.32 *Regional rapid filling rate image: right ventricle,* RAO view, at rest. In analogy to the left ventricle (Figure 2.30) symmetrical inflow directed to the apex where normally maximum rates are situated.

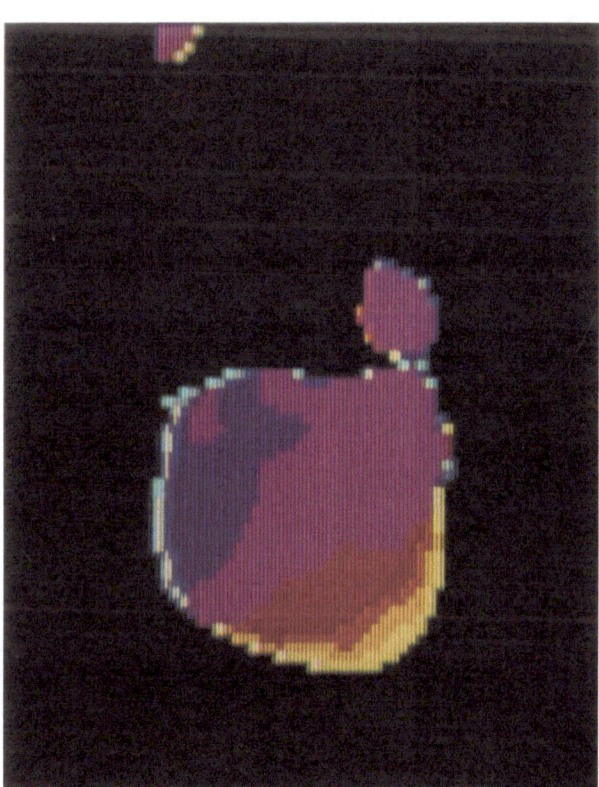

Figure 2.33 *Regional rapid filling mean time image: Right ventricle.* RAO-view, at rest. In analogy to the left ventricle (Figure 2.31) longest mean times result at the periphery as a symmetrical shell (yellow).

17

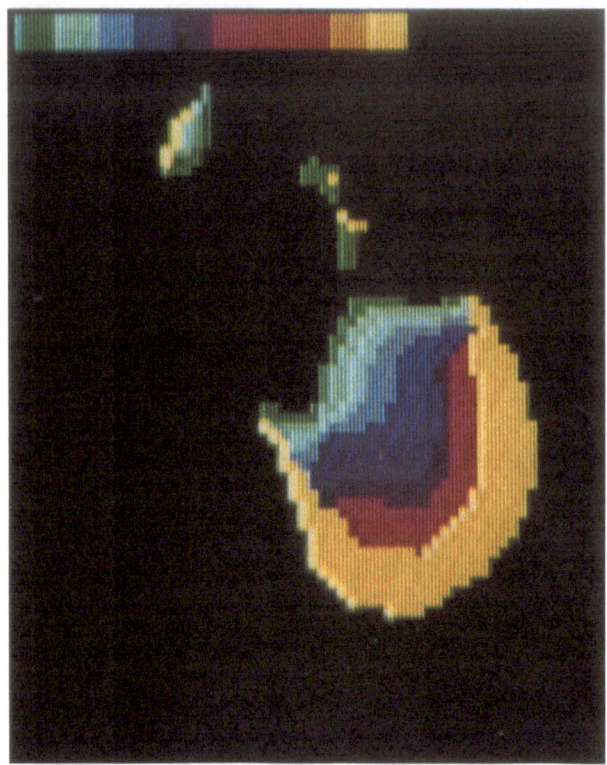

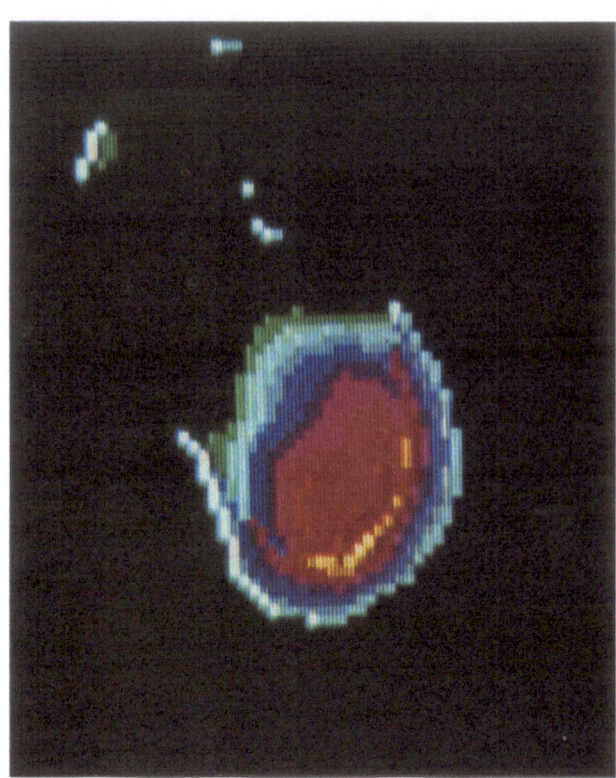

Figure 2.34 *Regional ejection fraction image: LAO view,* left ventricle, at rest. Slight asymmetry of EF bands at the septal side where less contraction occurs than on the lateral side. Residual volume mainly remains in the subaortic region. Colour scale 10% EF; wall motion 100% EF (yellow).

Figure 2.35 *Regional ejection rate image: LAO view,* left ventricle, at rest. In analogy to the RAO view the highest rates are located at the inner part of the 100% EF band. Slight asmmetry at the septal side.

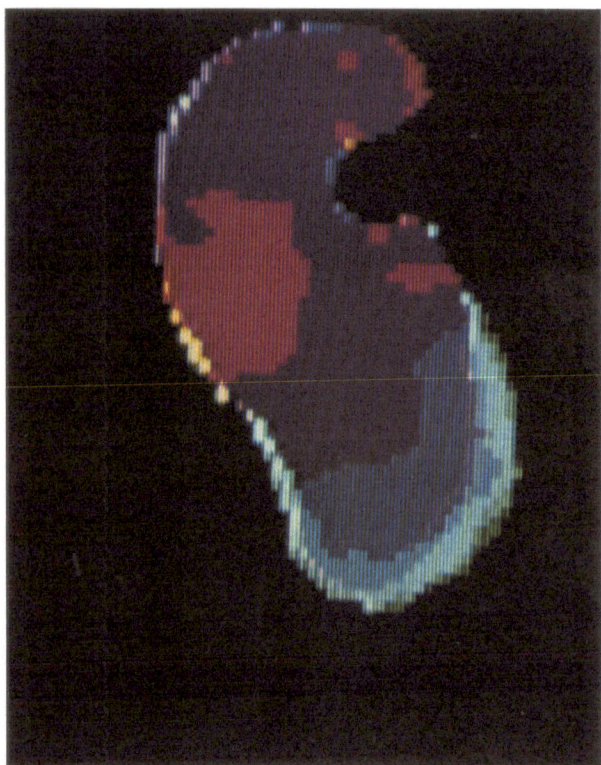

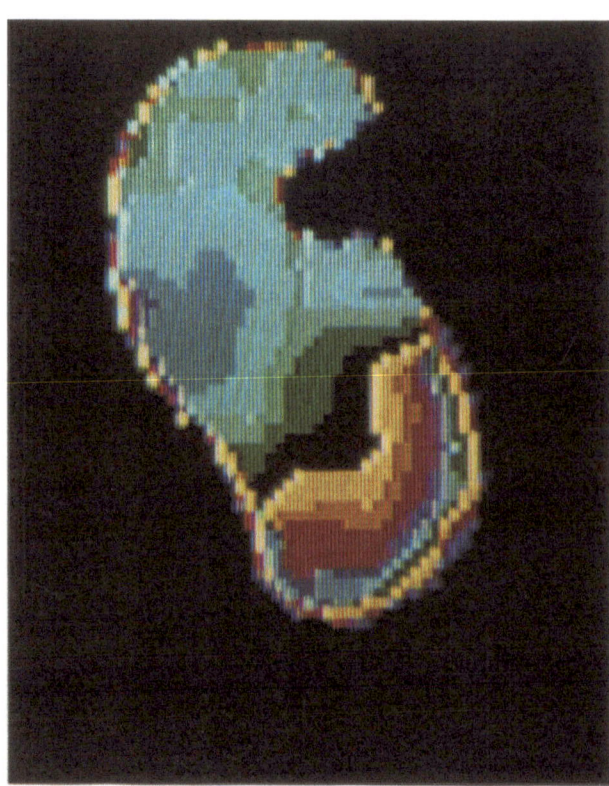

Figure 2.36 *Regional mean (transit) time image: LAO view,* left ventricle, at rest. As in the RAO view the shortest times result in the ventricular periphery from where blood is rapidly displaced. Slight asymmetry at the septal side.

Figure 2.37 *Regional mean (transit) time image: LAO view,* left ventricle, at rest. Same image as Figure 2.36, but with better discrimination of value-levels or colours: each colour-level is further subdivided in 8 distinct colours. For findings see under Figure 2.36.

3

Technical Details of Functional Imaging Involving Patients, Protocols and Equipment

J. W. FLEMING, E. J. ANDREWS JR. AND M. M. MELLO

Accurate, reproducible, radionuclide ventriculographic (RNV) studies are dependent upon careful attention to details in all parameters when acquiring and processing data. Each aspect of these details is like a link of a chain – the weakest link can cause a breakdown of accuracy of the measurement of global function and affect the quality of functional images.

Fundamentally, RNV studies are based upon the premise that radionuclide (RN) counts in the ventricles are directly proportional to volume; changes in volume during ventricular contraction (i.e., change in counts) reflect function of the overlying myocardium. Thus, RNV 'wall motion' is a reflection of regional volume changes and ejection fractions reflect global volume changes. Any factor which may limit the availability of recorded counts below a critical level can invalidate the study, whether it be a prolonged slow injection, an inappropriate recording time, or choice in processing of background subtraction and representative cycles (RC).

Since functional imaging described here (Schad, 1978a, 1979a) always includes imaging of the first half of systole, reducing counts for processing by one-half, the importance of the critical number of counts available for recording is obvious (*see below*).

PATIENTS

Haemodynamic status

A rest study should be done at a reasonably basal state. For comparable studies the patient should be in the same position, upright or supine. Patients in the supine position may have left ventricular (LV) ejection fractions (EF) at variance with those obtained when the patient is in the upright position (Upton *et al.*, 1980).

Protocols for exercise on the bicycle should be standardized. The exercise protocol should include a period of warmup and gradual increase of Mets required. Foster *et al.* (1981) have shown clearly that sudden, strenuous exercise without warmup can produce ischaemia-like electrocardiographic (e.c.g.) abnormalities in 60–70% of healthy subjects. Likewise, exercise protocols have a significant influence on LV function and radionuclide angiography (Foster *et al.*, 1983). Our standard protocol for bicycle exercise follows Foster *et al.* (1983):

graded exercise (25 W increased every 2 minutes to fatigue, or to a heart rate (HR) of 85% of age-predicted maximum), with injection of radionuclide during the peak of exercise. If the patient gets significant chest pain or ST abnormalities, the radionuclide injection is completed before discontinuing exercise. If a patient cannot reach a target heart rate of 85% of maximum HR the e.c.g. test should be labelled 'non-diagnostic'; however, RNV functional imaging later may show true abnormalities at HR of less than 100 beats per minute, in some cases (*see* comments on cardiac anaerobic metabolism at HR 120 in Chapter 5). Omission of propranolol for 3 days prior to a study can improve the accuracy of the test by allowing the patient to reach a target heart rate but, often, physicians are unwilling to subject the patient to a risk of sudden withdrawal of this drug.

Some patients who are deconditioned may reach a target HR in 1–2 minutes. This may be associated with e.c.g.–RNV abnormalities similar to those with sudden, strenuous exertion, without a period of warmup, as described above. Thus, if the radionuclide injection should be given to a deconditioned patient the moment a target heart rate is achieved, before the patient has a true period of sufficient exercise, inaccuracies may result.

For practical reasons, the Florida Heart Center exercise protocol was changed from the usual rest–exercise sequence to: (1) establishing basal HR and blood pressure, (2) exercise with RNV injection at peak of exercise, (3) resting for 15–30 min until the patient has returned to basal status and then (4) repeat, at rest, the RNV study. This sequence has helped to eliminate occasional difficulties of excessive background activity during the shorter recording time of exercise (*see below*). Elimination of excessive RN background during exercise is especially important in larger or heavier patients where the chest wall attenuates recording of radionuclide photon activity and further lowers count rate, while increasing background scatter.

Site of intravenous injection

Jones *et al.* (1972) for years have advocated the use of the right external jugular vein as a practical intravenous site of least resistance to flow of injected radionuclides. In our experience, the right antecubital site of injection is sufficient for reliable studies in most patients. Our total experience with injections in veins distal to the antecubital veins indicates that a potential increased resistance to injection can produce a prolonged bolus and result in inaccurate functional imaging in about 20–30% of exercise studies. Furthermore, our studies of injections into the superior vena cava or pulmonary artery (PA) via flow-directed catheters indicate that superior imaging can be obtained by injections as close to the ventricle as possible. If PA injection studies are done, certain techniques in processing should be considered (Dymond *et al.*, 1984).

It has been shown that a standard radiographic injector can be used for the injection of the radio-isotope with timing related to the e.c.g. This allows the injection (6–10 ml/s with 15–20 ml/s of saline to flush the system) to be timed so that the bolus arrives in the superior vena cava during ventricular diastole. This technique helps keep the bolus compact by accelerating the venous flow to the superior vena cava and reducing local diffusion of the radioactivity (Schad, 1984).

Recording of simultaneous electrocardiograms

It is very important to establish, precisely, the cardiac rhythm at the estimated time of peak distribution of the radionuclide counts in the left ventricle. One should delineate transient ectopic beats, atrial fibrillation or ventricular pacing. For instance, the study may need to be repeated at the same sitting if it is demonstrated that a series of premature ventricular beats occurred at the exact moment of recording the RNV. Also cardiac pacing often produces characteristic inferior and apical wall motion abnormalities which may be confused with ischaemia in functional imaging. For example, a pacemaker patient with a resting study and a normal sinus rhythm at a rate slightly higher than the pacing rate may have a normal RNV image. Later, that same patient may present with a history of chest pain; if the patient is in a pacing rhythm, the inferior wall motion abnormality (WMA) may be misinterpreted as ischaemia or interval infarction (*see* Chapter 18).

Patient's position in relationship to the gamma-camera

From the view point of correlating RNV findings with cine contrast ventriculographic studies and delineating the inferior and free walls of the left ventricle, the right anterior oblique (RAO) view is the most desirable projection (Bodenheimer *et al.*, 1978). However, many laboratories use the anterior (ANT) position because maximum counts can be obtained from this view. The further a patient rotates laterally from the anterior view the greater is the distance from the camera as well as increased attenuation. Thus fewer total counts are available to the camera. The Passau laboratory uses a 30° RAO view. The Florida laboratory used an ANT view routinely until our change in sequence to exercise first, followed by the rest study allowed us to use the 30°

RAO view, routinely. Figures 3.1–3.4 illustrate clearly that in the ANT and RAO projections, there are major differences in LV contours and regional wall motion, especially in the inferior wall (*also see* Chapter 12).

The RAO projection also eliminates overlap of the inferior wall and the descending aorta (Figures 3.5 and 3.6). We have demonstrated that, after one to three heartbeats, counts appear in the descending aorta which lies immediately behind the heart and its inferobasalar border (Fleming, 1982). The fixed, unchanging counts in the aorta may be averaged by the camera-computer system with inferior ventricular counts. Thus, the inferior wall may be depicted as having little or no motion (Figure 3.7). This may result in a spurious decrease in EF and misinterpretation of inferior 'wall motion abnormality' (Figure 3.8). An evaluation of 34 patients during cardiac catheterization showed that an RAO projection of 20° separated the aorta from the right heart border in all but eight patients. Only two required greater than 30° for separation of the inferior heart border and aorta (Fleming, 1982).

Dymond *et al.* (1982) reported their observations of the influence on RNV of the site of radionuclide injection (right or left arm) and projection (RAO or LAO). They stressed the need for quality control of the bolus of injected radionuclide.

EQUIPMENT

Acquisition of data

Collimator

A collimator measuring 1½ inches (38 mm) thick can improve depth of resolution of a radionuclide study but this can reduce the total number of counts available to the camera-computer system. Our two centres have continued to use a 1 inch (25 mm) collimator in order to improve counts available with a reasonable control of scatter. Our limited experience with the 1½ inch collimator suggests that there may be image degradation from the decreased countrate.

Camera-computer system

A multicrystal gamma-camera and computer system* is the basic unit used in the studies reported here. Schad and Nickel (1978a, 1979a) devised the use of a microcomputer with special software in conjunction with the basic unit in order to obtain additional imaging. The Florida Heart Center, in cooperation with the Passau group, developed a modification of the original Schad–Nickel program utilizing an IBM microcomputer and Forth language. Later, an addition of a program which allows subtraction of counts in the region of the right ventricle was added in cases where there is a delayed emptying of the right ventricular counts. There are minor differences in the results of the two laboratories.

* Baird System–77, Bedford, Massachusetts, USA.

Recording times

Boyer et al (1978) reported the importance of correlating recording time with heart rate, illustrating that slower heart rates should be correlated with a more prolonged recording time (40 ms) and faster heart rates require a shorter recording time (20 ms). We have demonstrated, using a Vanderbilt phantom (Fleming, 1982) that not only the global ejection fraction but the images (Figure 3.9) will be changed drastically if a fixed recording time (30 milliseconds) is maintained while varying the rate from 60 to 160 cycles/minute. Table 3.1 summarizes the changes in

Table 3.1 Phantom study

Recording times ms	Rate beats/min	EF %
30	60	61
30	130	52
30	160	47

'ejection fractions' when the recording time remains fixed at 30 ms and the rate is variable. In another phantom study, similar variations occurred when a fast rate was fixed and the recording times were variable (Table 3.2). These studies help to confirm

Table 3.2 Phantom study

Recording times ms	Rate beats/min	EF %
50	150	48
40	150	53
30	150	61
20	150	76

our clinical practice of varying recording times with different heart rates. The recommended recording times for various heart rates, as used in our laboratory, are listed in Table 3.3.

Processing of data

Frames of data

There must be an adequate number of frames of recorded data in order to process a specifically significant representative cycle (RC). Our experience has indicated that 10–12 frames (RC) must be available for accurate processing. This can be checked by counting the number of steps on the downslope of the volume curve.

Total counts

After all of the links in the chain of technical details described above are lined up and brought together, in the final analysis, the computer records the number of counts during systole and diastole. We concluded in the past that 30 000–40 000 total counts were needed for accurate functional imaging. We

Table 3.3 Recommendations for recording times for System 77

Heart rates beats/min	Recording times ms
50– 69	40
70–109	30
110–129	25
130–170	20

recommend now that the total ventricular count during *systole* should be 8000 or more for adequate data. Counts from 5000 to 8000 are borderline but may give adequate images in some cases.

Schad (1984) has indicated that additional technical considerations are helpful. Of particular importance is the proper handling of background activity. For a second injection using ^{99m}Tc, background subtraction of the activity remaining from the first injection is required. The corresponding background matrix should be recorded as close as possible in time to the second injection. For this reason, the first 100 frames of data collected immediately before the second injection are used to create the background matrix.

SUMMARY

Reliable and diagnostic radionuclide ventriculography is dependent upon multiple factors including precise exercise protocols, properly delivered bolus of the radionuclide (injections), position of the patients, correlation with simultaneous e.c.g. recordings, and many aspects of acquisition and processing of data, especially varying the recording times with the heart rate. In the final analysis, many of these details will determine whether or not there are adequate counts for processing reliable data.

Adequate total counts are essential for functional imaging, especially for images of the first and second half of systole which are created by dividing LV systolic counts in half. It is precisely these images which have proven to be the most helpful in the diagnosis of ischaemia.

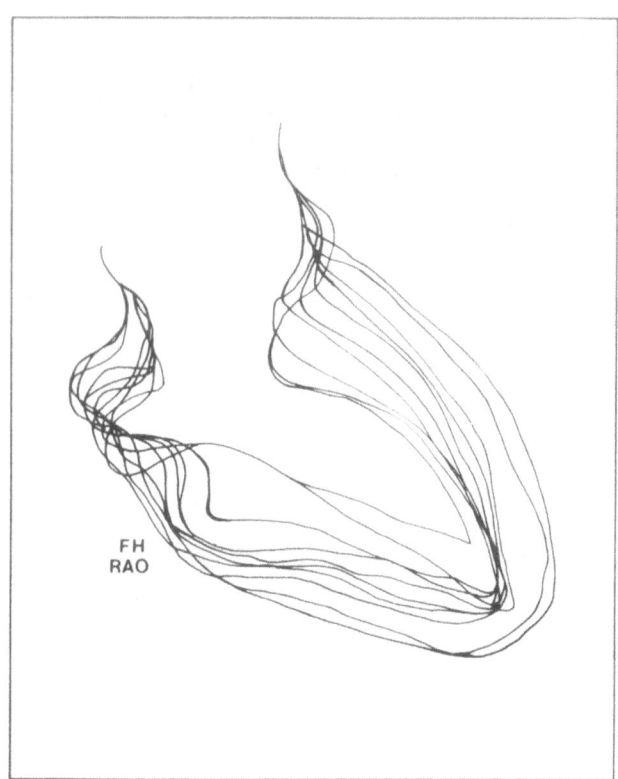

Figure 3.1 *RAO projection, contrast left ventriculogram*, frame by frame contour drawings. Systole begins at outer perimeter. Patient with mitral valve prolapse. This contour drawing shows marked excursion of the inferior wall, mostly in late systole when inferior bulging of the mitral valve is more pronounced.

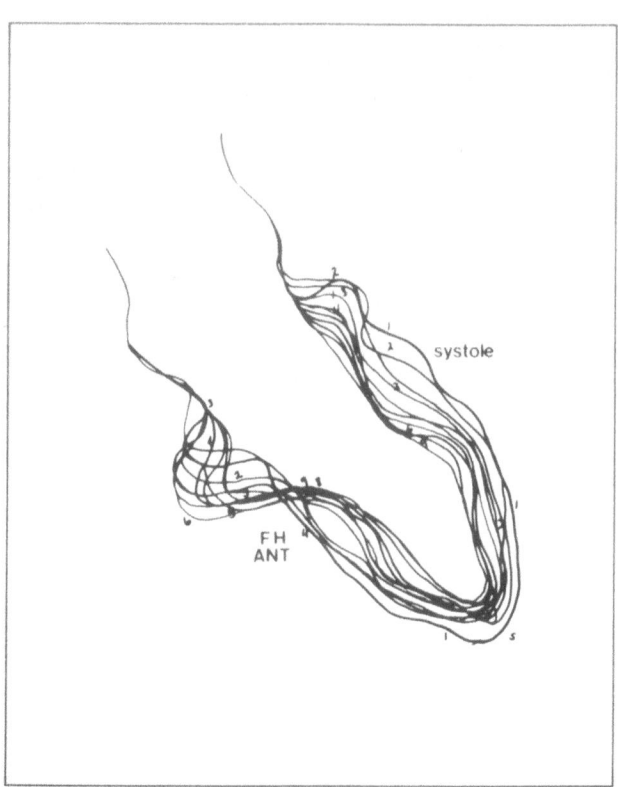

Figure 3.2 *Anterior projection, contrast left ventriculogram*, frame by frame contour drawings. Systole begins at outer perimeter. *Same patient with mitral valve prolapse as illustrated in Figure 3.1.* Note the marked difference in contour and diminished inferior wall motion in this projection. The mitral valve bulging and contour of decreased inferior wall motion account for the notched inferior border in the RNV in the anterior projection.

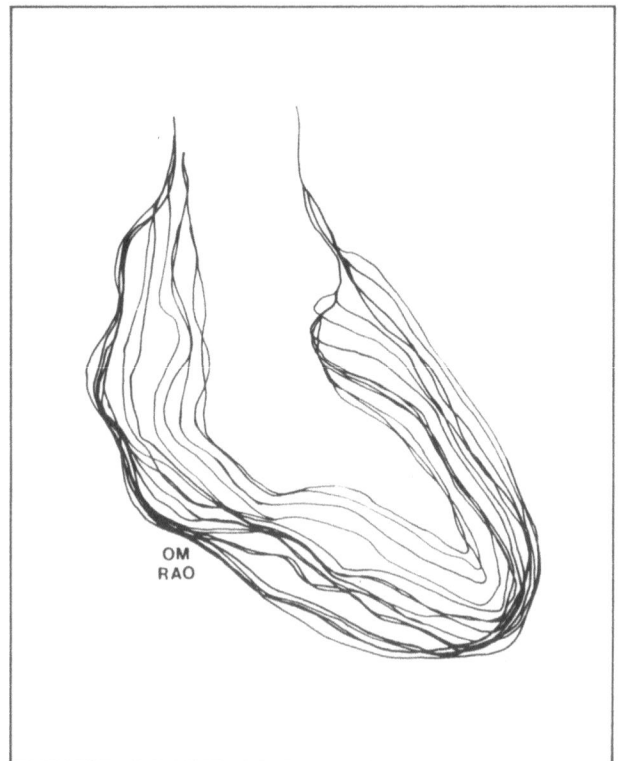

Figure 3.3 *RAO projection, contrast left ventriculogram*, frame by frame contour drawings. Systole begins at outer perimeter. Patient with mitral valve prolapse and mild pectus excavatum. This drawing shows marked excursion of the ventricular inferior wall as compared with the same patient illustrated in Figure 3.4.

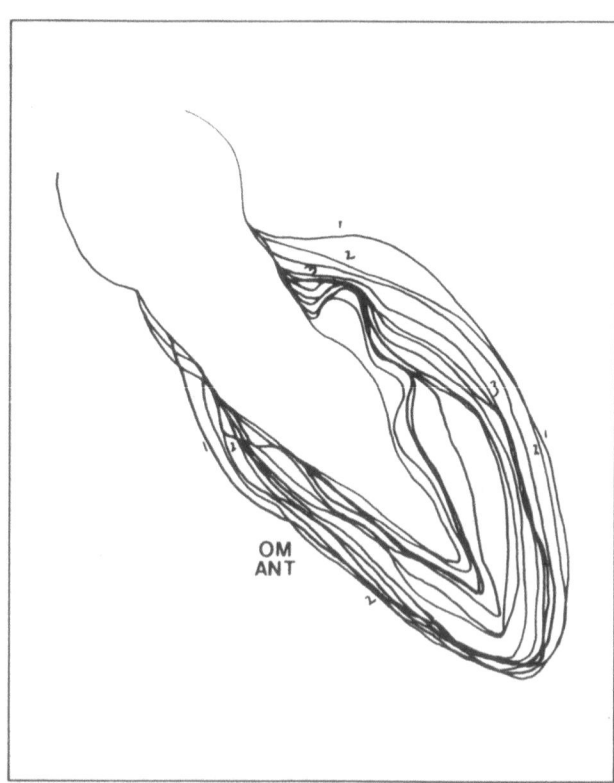

Figure 3.4 *Anterior projection, contrast left ventriculogram*, frame by frame contour drawings. Systole begins at outer perimeter. *Same patient with mitral valve prolapse as illustrated in Figure 3.3.* Notice the marked change in contour and decreased inferior wall motion as compared with the same patient in Figure 3.3.

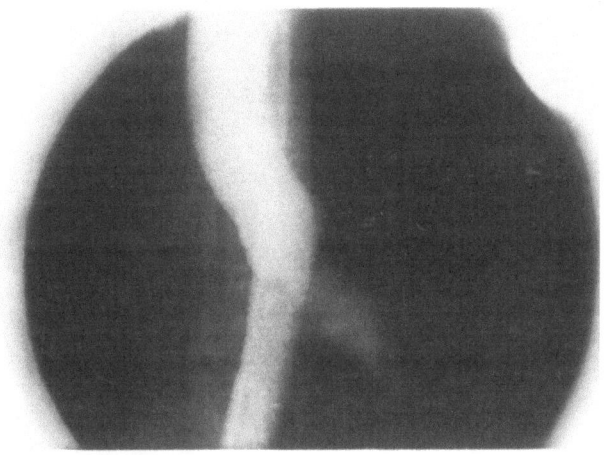

Figure 3.5 *Anterior projection, contrast ventriculogram.* The opacified aorta overlies the base and inferior margin of the left ventricle in this anterior projection.

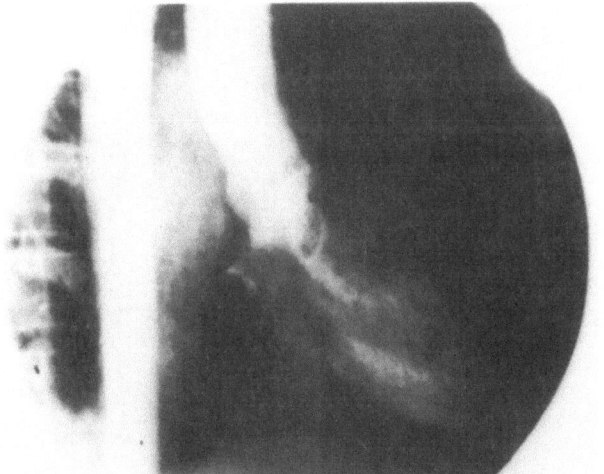

Figure 3.6 *The RAO projection, contrast ventriculogram.* The opacified aorta clearly is removed from the area of the left ventriculogram by rotation of the patient 30° in the RAO projection.

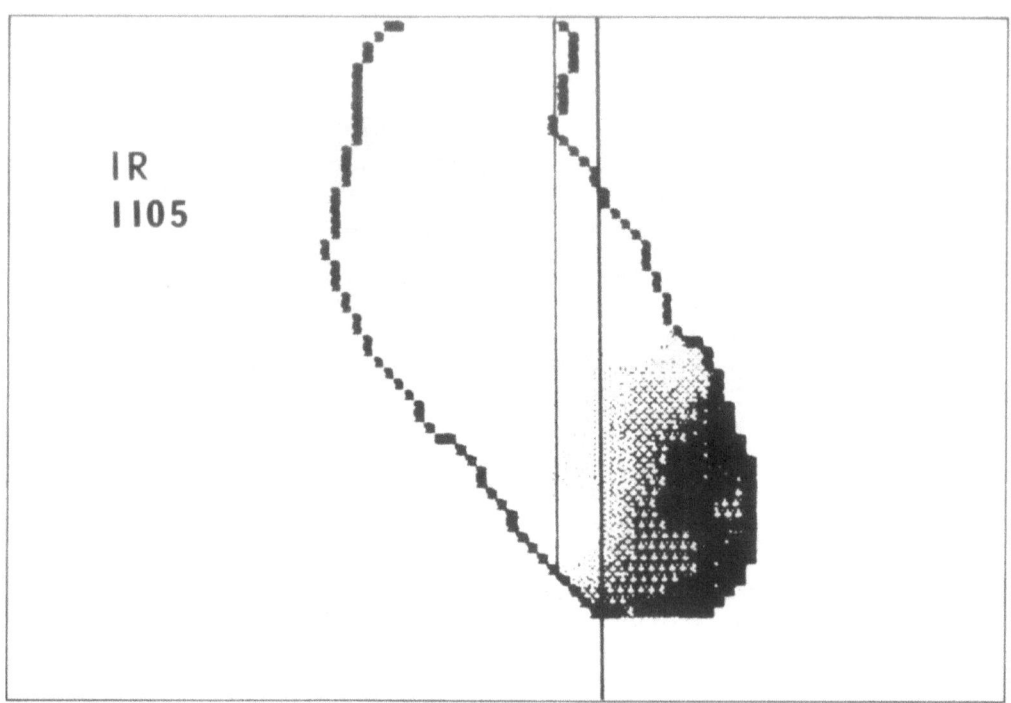

Figure 3.7 *First pass radionuclide ventriculogram in anterior projection.* This regional ejection fraction image shows marked diminution in 'wall motion' or changes in count inferiorly. This is the same patient pictured in Figures 3.5 and 3.6. This suggests that unchanging counts in the aorta may interfere with computerized interpretation of wall motion changes when the aorta overlies the base and inferior border of the left ventricle in the anterior position. See Figure 3.8 for further confirmation.

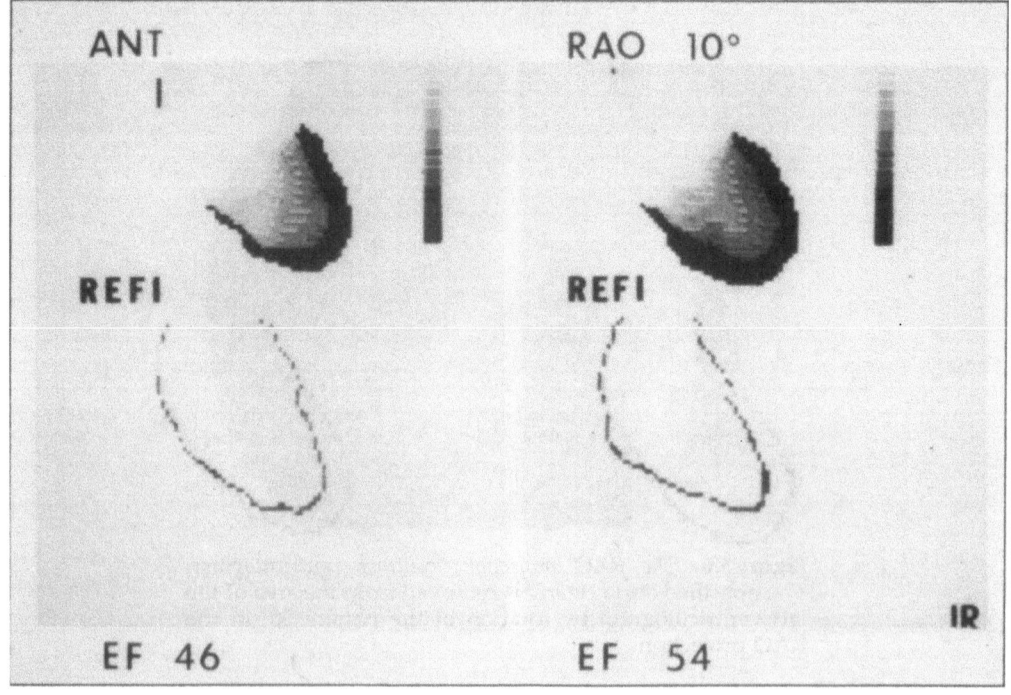

Figure 3.8 *Radionuclide ventriculograms compared in the anterior and RAO projections.* The study on the left, in the anterior projection, shows definite 'wall motion abnormality' with an ejection fraction of 46%; the study on the right, in the RAO projection was done a few minutes after the first study and shows a marked variation with normal wall motion and ejection fraction (54%). These two studies are on the same patient represented in Figures 3.5, 3.6 and 3.7, indicating the significant influence of fixed counts in the aorta in the RNV.

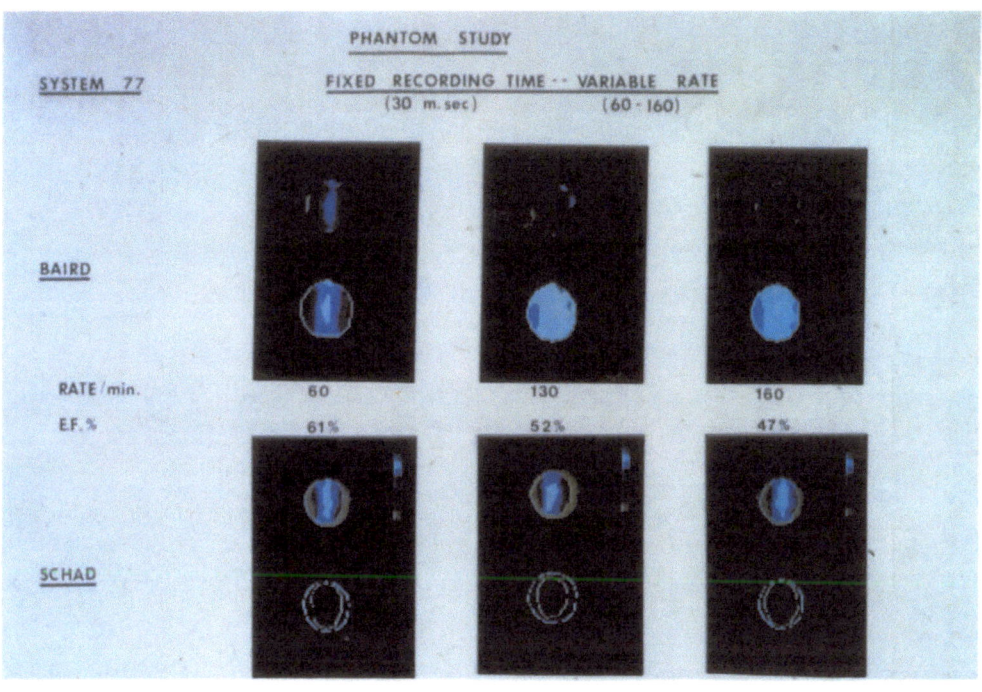

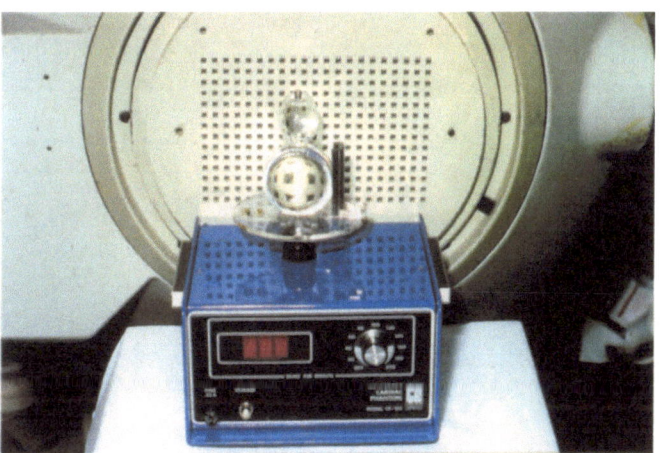

Figure 3.9 *Phantom study with fixed volume and radionuclide content.* Rotation of the Vanderbilt phantom chamber with intermittent display of nuclear radiation simulates an 'ejection fraction' or changes in counts. When the recording time remains fixed (30 ms) a variable rotation rate (equivalent to heart rate) from 60 to 160 resulted in marked differences in 'ejection fractions' and imaging (see summary in Table 3.1).

25

4

Systolic and Diastolic Functional Imaging in Evaluation of Ischaemic Heart Disease

N. SCHAD, F. BRUZZONE AND F. ROMEO

The rapid deterioration in contractility in myocardial territories with inadequate coronary blood flow leads to abnormalities of regional ventricular wall contraction and to diminished regional ejection of blood. Maximal flow through equivalent coronary narrowings, however, may vary significantly from patient to patient (Wright et al., 1980). Therefore, left ventricular regional function in jeopardized coronary vascular territories may become the determinant of functional significance of coronary narrowings. Consequently, analysis of regional function at the major coronary vascular territories may be indispensable for clinical decision making.

Although the coronary arteriogram can determine the location of obstruction in all major coronary vessels, conventional analysis of the arteriogram does not yield a precise assessment of the physiological significance of coronary obstructions of intermediate severity (Marcus, 1983). Various methods of assessing left ventricular wall motion, such as contrast or radionuclide ventriculograms and echocardiograms, have been used to determine the functional significance of coronary narrowings. High correlation between non-invasive radionuclide and invasive angiographic segmental wall motion has been found for normal and abnormal contracting segments (Schad et al., 1979a). The sensitivity of wall motion studies in determining the functional significance of coronary narrowings is, however, limited mainly because they reflect two-dimensional measurements and, moreover, are frequently done at rest or in one projection only.

At present, *functional imaging* of regional left ventricular events with radionuclide first pass angiocardiography at rest and exercise is probably the most promising, fastest and easiest technique to non-invasively assess regional ventricular function at the coronary vascular territories. The functional images (regional ejection fractions, rates and mean times) reflect three-dimensional regional changes during the preselected time-interval, i.e. *left ventricular contraction*.

Functional images showing normal function have been presented and illustrated in Chapter 2. One of the inherent properties of ventricular function is a certain *degree of symmetry of volume changes* with respect to the ventricular long axis. On the functional image recorded in a given projection the regionally measured volume changes at the centre result from function of two well-separated wall regions. At the periphery, however, volume changes are derived from function of one wall segment only whose extension is determined by the curvature of the heart. The degree of regional volume change relates to the amount of residual volume remaining in the cylinders measured through the heart, for example at the end of contraction. Thus, the 'lowest' regional function occurs at the ventricular base where most residual volume is located. In contrast, in the zones of wall motion where all blood is removed during contraction, the 'highest' regional function will be measured.

Although closer observation of any functional image generally leads to the discovery of an irregular structure, we can with advantage approximate its main property, i.e. functional symmetry. Minor deviations from symmetry of volume changes are common, particularly at the posterior wall (mitral valve prolapse) and at the upper septal wall or pulmonary infundibulum. Generally, however, regional partial loss or lack of functional symmetry indicates dysfunction. The degree of regional dysfunction may vary considerably. Very low regional function or functional defects point to extension of malfunction in depth, i.e. compromising a large area of ventricular wall at the centre, and a smaller one at the ventricular periphery. Changes occurring at two instances very close in time are usually found to vary irregularly as the time between the two instances decreases. But, the more irregularities and random fluctuations contained in functional images, the less reliable become minor regional alterations for diagnosis. More severe and significant changes are provoked by stressing the patient. With these inherent properties of functional images in mind, one can proceed to evaluation (Figures 4.9–4.16).

In regional ejection fraction images, wall motion disorders characteristically produce the bands of regional EFs which are smaller than in segments with normal wall function (Figure 4.9). Lower regional EFs appear to 'advance' from the base to the periphery. At the periphery a very small sized 100% band (yellow: one pixel only) can be considered as akinesia, a functional defect may be due to akinesia or dyskinesia (paradoxical motion). Toward the centre very low regional EFs or defects point to a larger compromised area of ventricular wall motion. Since first and second half systolic REFI images contain many more random fluctuations than the REFI images reflecting the entire systole, only defects or very low regional EFs can be used for diagnosis with certainty.

Regional ejection rate image reflecting entire systole normally presents the crescent-shaped shell of highest rates at the inner side of the 100% EF band or wall motion (p. 8). Loss of part of the peripheral crescent-shaped high rate yellow band and central shifting of highest rates is a very sensitive sign of dysfunction. The peripherally lost high rates are substituted by lower ones (blue or lighter coded). Only exceptionally does one find the highest yellow-coded rates at the centre of the ventricle in addition to high peripheral values when the ventricle is dilated and contracts well (aortic insufficiency), or without peripheral high rates when the ventricular cavity is very small and wall motion strong (severe hypertrophy). The main diagnostic value of regional ejection rate images certainly lies in the observation of the site of regional highest rates. Very low rates or defects point to akinesia, the latter eventually to dyskinesia. During first half of systole maximum rates are usually located at the centre of the ventricle, during the second half, however, at the periphery. Therefore, in regional ejection rate images reflecting the first half of contraction only defects or very low rates can be considered with certainty to be the result of pathological function.

Dyskinesia or systolic outward motion is best seen on the so-called *regional systolic rate of increase image* that exhibits all regions where blood increases during systole. Since by the mathematical process only regions with a predominant increase of blood during contraction are visualized, very short-lasting paradoxical motion (vibrations) is not presented. Thus, even small zones of dyskinesia in this image are diagnostically relevant. An increase immediately behind the location of the mitral valve indicates mitral reflux, or occasionally severe mitral valve prolapse.

The *regional mean transit image* visualizes the regional mean times elapsing from end-diastole to the centre of gravity of every single pixel-curve (regional histograms), thus reflecting regional persistence of blood during systole (p. 9). With regional wall dysfunction the contribution from the corresponding wall segment to outflow is reduced with the result that regional persistence of blood is prolonged from the corresponding peripheral segment toward the centre and ventricular outflow tract. In the image, long subvalvular mean times 'advance' toward the periphery, pointing to wall dysfunction in that zone. Thus, the regional mean (transit) time image reveals differences in degree of flow contribution from distinct wall segments during contraction. The larger and the more severe the wall dysfunction is, the lower the flow-contribution from that area resulting in longer mean times manifest underneath the malfunctioning wall segment. In fact, very long mean times as normally only encountered at the outflow tract or the ascending aorta become visible under infarcted segments with the patient at rest, indicating poor function and long systolic persistence of blood in these regions. Analogous images have been recently observed with

nuclear magnetic resonance examinations where low flow underneath infarcts can produce intracavitary signals. With ischaemia only, such long peripheral mean times usually are not observed at rest. Under stress, however, they can be observed if function severely deteriorates, for example in ischaemic areas where collateral flow at exercise becomes inadequate (Figure 4.11). Exceptionally, long mean times as normally seen at the outflow tract may be seen at rest in cases with severe preinfarction angina. Drawing information from all systolic images the mean time image is much less subject to random fluctuations than the subtraction image or the REFI image. Consequently, first and second half systolic mean time images are also more reliable than the corresponding REFI images. *Very long times in the periphery as normally seen only in the subvalvular area can be considered as the result of pathological function if encountered in first and second half systolic mean time images.* Thus, the regional mean time images provide information not only about the extent but also about the degree of severity of regional systolic dysfunction, i.e. about the functional significance of coronary obstructions and the adequacy of collateral flow.

To define the value and *accuracy* of single systolic functional images for non-invasive detection of coronary artery narrowings the function of 301 left ventricular vascular territories has been evaluated at rest and peak exercise in nine functional images in the RAO view, in 43 patients (Schad *et al.*, 1984c). Distinction was made between dysfunction located at the apical supra-apical segments corresponding to the terminal left anterior descending (LAD)-territory, at the proximal anterior region supplied by the first diagonal arteries and the entire LAD-territory. Similarly, the regions of the marginal, distal posterolateral and entire circumflex territory (CX) were separately evaluated. For the right coronary artery (RC) only one territory was considered, so that a total of seven different territories resulted per patient (Figure 4.1). Dysfunction in these territories at rest and peak exercise was compared to the status of the corresponding coronary arteries. A total of 103 coronary narrowings could be found in these patients, i.e. 103 territories were compromised, 198 were normal. Thus, statistically speaking, a mixed population of compromised and normal territories could be evaluated. This study included functional images covering the events during the entire systolic contraction as well as during the first and second half systole separately, at rest and exercise. Dysfunction limited to early systole, as frequently seen in myocardial ischaemia (tardokinesis) may be masked in functional images presenting entire systole, whereas it can be evaluated in the images of first half of systole. Moreover, the degree of regional recovery during the second half of systole provides additional important information about the functional reserve and viability of the specific vascular territory.

We also tried to discriminate dysfunction at the RC-territory from dysfunction produced by mitral valve prolapse. Regional evaluation was first done in the radionuclide functional images, then in the coronary angiograms paying attention to the latter,

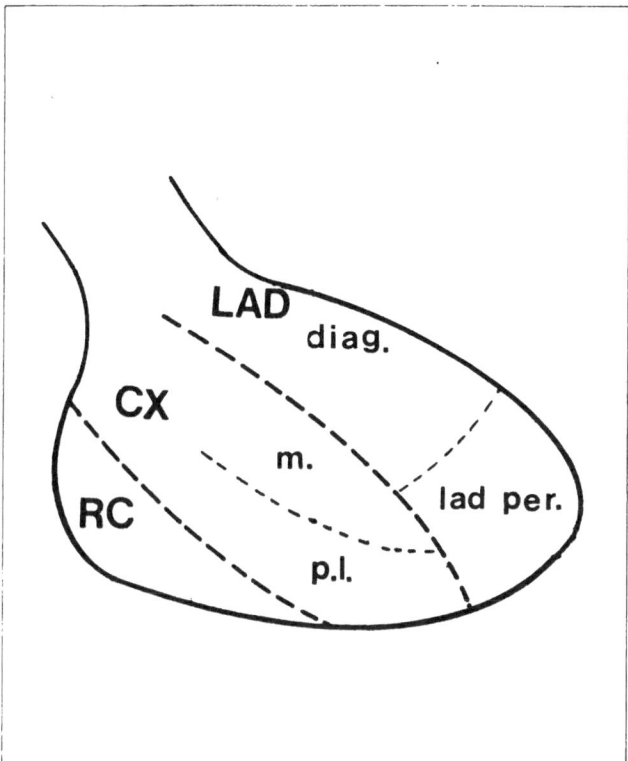

Figure 4.1 *The coronary vascular territories in the RAO view.* The left anterior descending territory (LAD) is subdivided into the upper zone perfused by diagonal arteries (diag.) and the apical–supra-apical zone supplied by the peripheral LAD (per.) and its branches. The circumflex territory (CX) comprises a zone attributed to the marginal artery (m.) and another zone perfused by the posterolateral branches (p.l.). Major variations are encountered for the circumflex and right coronary (RC) territories; one of these two territories may be dominant.

particularly to alterations at the origin of major secondary branches. In case of left or right coronary preponderance minor adjustments in the correspondence between the vascular territory and the feeding vessel were necessary. *Two functional images had to be positive to define the radionuclide study as positive.* For each patient a matrix of findings was prepared for the resting study and another for the exercise study and stored in a computer for further evaluation.

Sensitivities for every distinct functional image and for the radionuclide study as a whole at rest and peak exercise were computed. For calculation of sensitivities all functionally true positive territories were divided by all territories with coronary narrowings, i.e. a close local correlation was presumed between the territory with dysfunction and the coronary artery obstruction. Because of the considerable variations in the vascular distribution of the RC and CX arteries sensitivities for the entire inferoposterior wall combining the territories of both vessels were also included as well as overall sensitivities of all territories together.

Specificities for every functional image and for the entire radionuclide study were calculated for the three major coronary vascular territories considering each of the seven territories separately. All functionally true negative territories were divided by all territories without coronary narrowings. Since, however, dysfunction may occur distant from the

narrowing of the feeding vessel specificities were also computed for the anterior and inferoposterior wall on the basis that the LAD or CX/RC vascular tree respectively did not show any obstructions.

As expected, rest and exercise examinations generally lead to higher *sensitivities* than resting studies alone for detection of regional dysfunction due to coronary narrowings. For better comparison the two graphs (Figures 4.2 and 4.3) illustrate the single sensitivities found for the LAD and combined CX–RC territory respectively. Regional ejection fraction images almost consistently show the lowest sensitivities, first and second half systolic images included. The highest sensitivities are presented by the first and second half ejection rate and mean time images, the latter being at rest even somewhat more sensitive than the former. The large discrepancy in sensitivity between the mean time image of the entire systole and its first and second half systolic part is probably due to temporal masking of early peripheral dysfunction by tardokinesis. This temporal overlap of late normal function influences the mean time image more than the ejection rate image probably because, in the latter, loss of high ejection rates is seen at the periphery and therefore less subjected to spatial overlap by other adjacent regions, whereas in the mean time images diagnosis of dysfunction is based on the advance of longer times from the subvalvular area to the periphery. *High sensitivities of the radionuclide examination can be reached if all functional images are taken together for evaluation* (Figure 4.4). These sensitivities usually result lower than the highest sensitivities of a single image, since two positive images were required to judge the study as positive.

Eight territories were *false negative* at rest, four at exercise and only two at rest and/or exercise. In two cases of proximal LAD stenosis only a localized peripheral dysfunction at the apex and at the diagonal territory was seen so that on the basis of strict local correlation a false negative result for the entire territory was listed. Another reason for a peripheral false negative apical territory observed in two cases was a borderline narrowed peripheral LAD stenosis with apical tethering seen only at exercise. In contrast, dysfunction has been missed only at rest because of collateral flow around the apex and in the marginal territory (two instances), of a hypoplastic circumflex system (two cases) and with a borderline stenosis of the diagonal branch (one case). In two cases the inferoposterior territory was not related to the correct vessel (CX/PL and RC). The examination at rest and exercise resulted false negative in one instance of proximal LAD narrowing where only the diagonal and peripheral LAD territory was considered as positive and in another instance of proximal CX narrowing where only the posterolateral territory was evaluated as positive.

As usually observed, *specificities* are low if sensitivities are high and vice versa, particularly if territorial dysfunction is related to the coronary vessel at the same location, as it was done for determination of sensitivities. In fact, ejection fraction images and their first and second systolic parts show low sensitivities but relatively high specificities. In contrast, first and second half ejection rate and mean

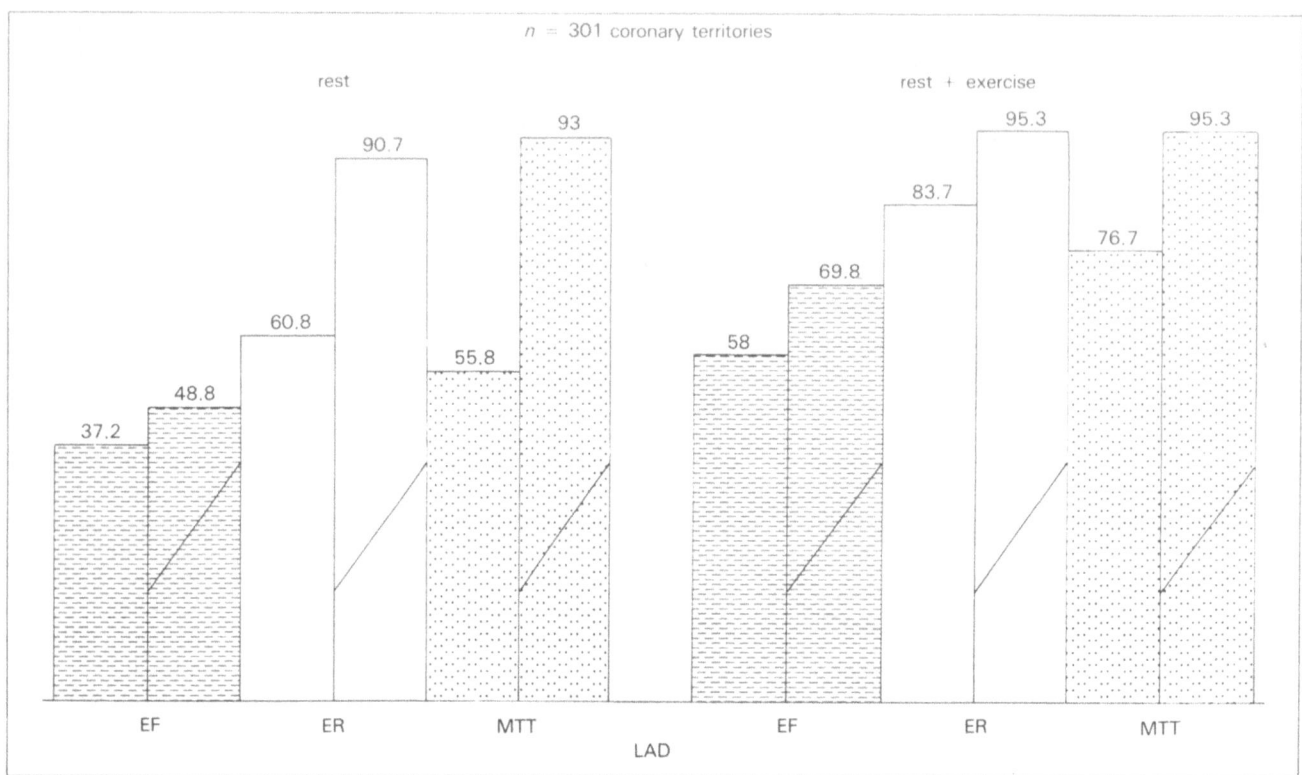

Figure 4.2 *Sensitivity of single functional images for detection of coronary narrowings at the anterior wall (LAD).* Functional images cover the entire systole, as well as the first and second half of systole separately (/), at rest and rest and exercise taken together. EF: regional ejection fraction image, ER: regional ejection rate image, MTT: regional mean (transit) time image (times of centre of gravity). Rest and exercise images together as well as half/half systolic images yield higher sensitivities than resting examinations alone or images covering the entire systole respectively. The highest sensitivities are obtained with ejection rate and mean transit time images.

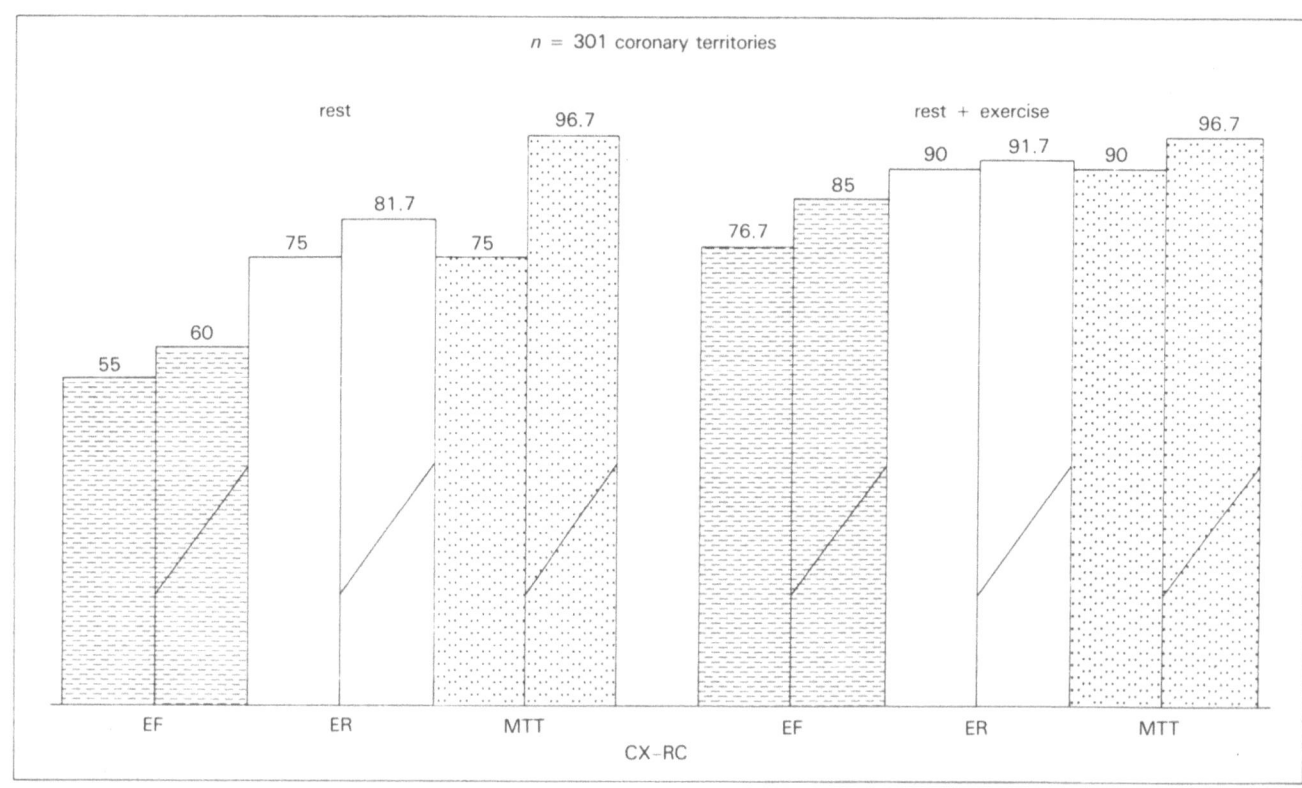

Figure 4.3 *Sensitivity of single functional images for detection of coronary narrowings at the inferoposterior wall (CX–RC).* Functional images cover the entire systole, as well as the first and second half of systole separately (/), at rest and rest and exercise taken together. EF: regional ejection fraction image, ER: regional ejection rate image, MTT: regional mean (transit) time image (times of centre of gravity). Rest and exercise images together as well as half/half systolic images yield higher sensitivities than resting examinations alone or images covering the entire systole respectively. The highest sensitivities are obtained with ejection rate and mean time images.

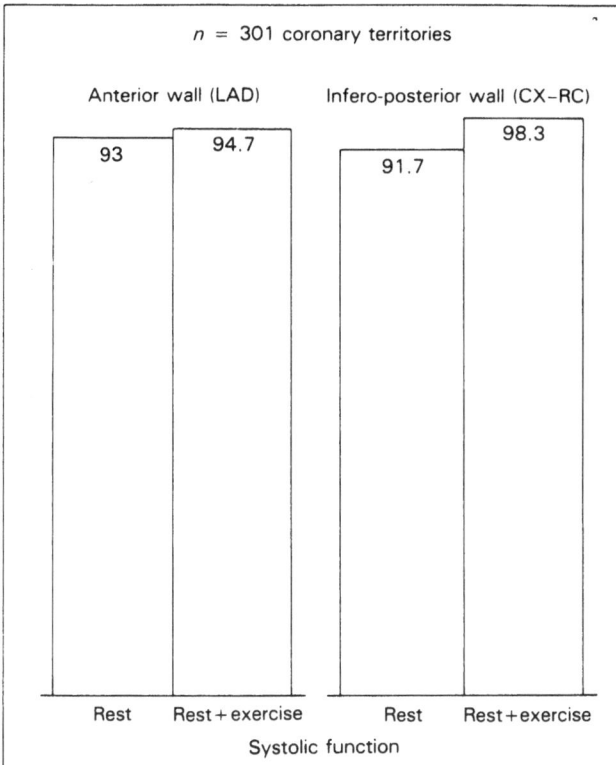

Figure 4.4 *Sensitivity of combined systolic functional images in detection of coronary narrowings* at the anterior (LAD) and inferoposterior wall (CX–RC), at rest and rest and exercise together. Two functional images had to show positive signs to judge the radionuclide examination as positive. Sensitivities of combined images exceed 90% so that the presented functional images can be used for screening patients for CHD.

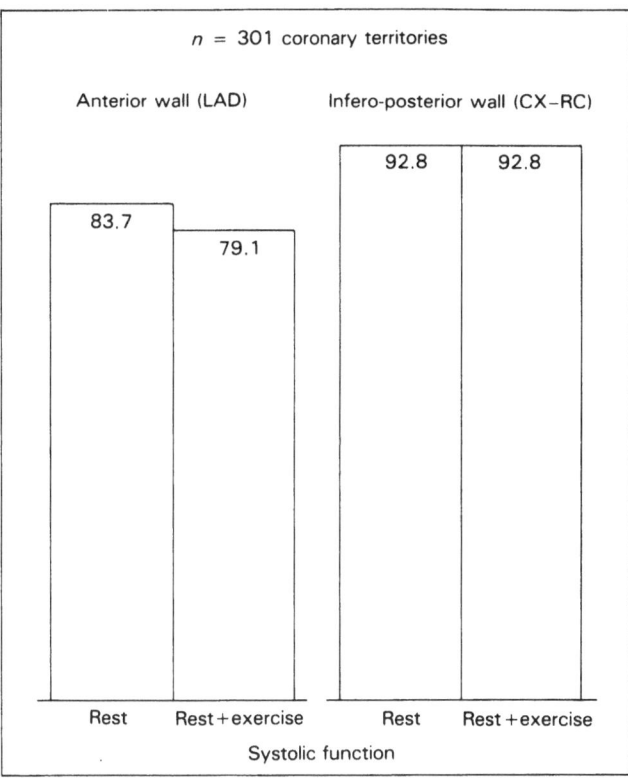

Figure 4.5 *Specificity of combined systolic functional images in detection of coronary narrowings* at the anterior (LAD) and inferoposterior wall (CX–RC), at rest and rest and exercise together. Two functional images had to show positive signs to judge the radionuclide examination as positive. Acceptable specificities of 80% and more can be obtained.

time images show high sensitivities and lower specificities. By analogy with the true positive findings, results are considered *false positive* only if two or more images show dysfunction whereas the corresponding vessel does not show any narrowing. By the use of the criterion of strict local correlation overall specificity of the radionuclide examination frequently was under 80%. Dysfunction in one evaluated territory may, however, be caused by a more centrally located obstruction, for example apical dysfunction by proximal LAD stenosis. Consequently, dysfunction at a territory may be false positive if only compared to the vessel at the same location but not if related to the feeding central vessel. Indeed, by computing specificities for the LAD territory or anterior wall and the CX/RC territory or the inferoposterior wall on the condition that only a dysfunction was considered as false positive when the entire vascular tree of the LAD or CX/RC did not present any narrowing one generally obtains specificities around 80% or higher (Figure 4.5). In 21 of the 198 normal territories false positive findings were observed if compared to the normal vascularization of the anterior (LAD) or inferoposterior wall (CX/RC). Comparison with the LV angiogram, however, revealed dysfunctions at the same territories, i.e. no false positives resulted by comparison with the LV ventriculogram. Causes other than coronary narrowings were responsible for these malfunctions.

Major discrepancies between sensitivities and specificities are found for the *ejection fraction images.* If these images are *excluded* from the study no changes in the number of true positives are observed for the LAD-territories at rest and for all territories at rest and exercise. Only minor reduction in sensitivity will result for the inferoposterior wall when one considers the resting or exercise study alone. The specificities improve because the number of false positives decrease in all territories. This can be explained by the significant random fluctuations observed in ejection fraction images. Thus, without losing any information, the REFI images could be omitted from the set of functional images. These images, however, are still the generally best understood functional images, their 100% yellow (black) band reflects wall motion, and their grey-shade printing is much easier evaluated than those of the ejection rate and mean time images. Therefore, for demonstration purposes, the REFI images are kept in the set of functional images.

Prolapse of the mitral valve with its bulging of the posterior wall is characterized by diminished regional function at the posteromedial segment of the LV. Difficulties in the differential diagnosis of right coronary ischaemia may arise if only functional images of the entire systole are evaluated. Since dysfunction due to mitral valve prolapse often becomes significant during the second half of ventricular systole while RC ischaemia with tardokinesis improves during that same time-interval, comparison of first and second half systolic function sometimes is helpful in discriminating these entities.

In fact, with the ejection rate and mean time first and second half systolic images only in three of 36 cases at rest and two of 36 cases at peak exercise it was not possible to make the differential diagnosis of the prolapse; only one false positive mitral valve prolapse was diagnosed in this group (for prolapse of mitral valve, *see* Chapter 12).

It is certainly also of interest to *compare* the sensitivity of changes of *global left ventricular ejection fraction* and *end-systolic volume* that occur under stress with the sensitivity of the functional images in the same patients. Figure 4.6 shows the sensitivities

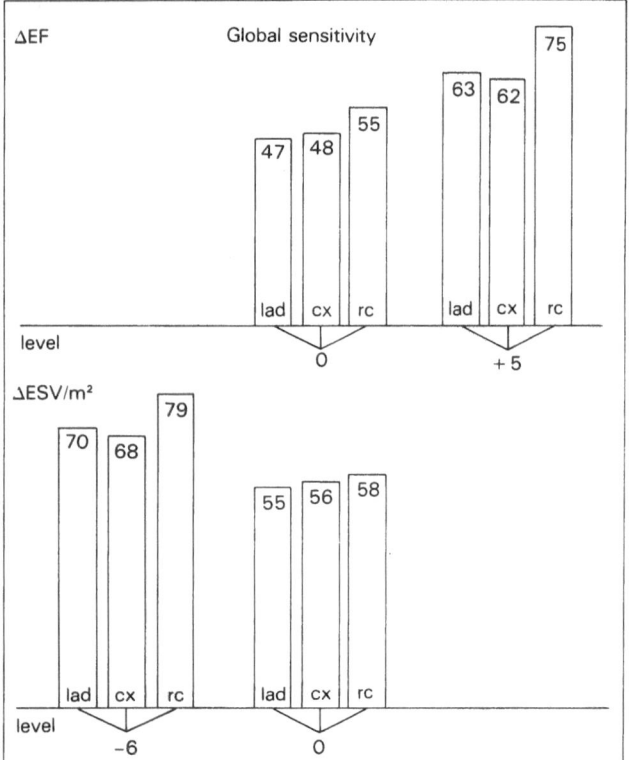

Figure 4.6 *Sensitivity of global LV-parameters for detection of coronary narrowings at the three major coronary territories.* Changes of ejection fraction (Δ EF) and end-systolic volume per square metre body surface area (ESV/M²). Two levels of separation between true positives and false negatives are shown. A true positive response is considered if global EF does not increase or does not increase more than 5 points with exercise, or end-systolic volume does not decrease or does not decrease more than 6 ml/m² respectively. All resulting sensitivities are lower than those obtained in the same patients from functional images (see Figure 4.4).

of global information at two levels of separation between true positives and false negatives. A true positive response would be considered if global ejection fraction does not increase by more than 5 points with exercise. In this case, global ejection fraction response always shows lower sensitivities than ejection rate and mean time images and their first and second half systolic parts. Similarly, if the criterion of endosystolic volume not decreasing more than 6 ml/m² with exercise is adopted, a lower sensitivity is obtained than with functional imaging. Generally speaking, global parameters such as global ejection fractions or endosystolic volumes must present lower sensitivities in detecting

regional dysfunction because they are a balance of all territories and therefore may mask regionally restricted dysfunction.

From this study it can be concluded that for screening patients for coronary artery disease sensitivity can be considerably improved by analysis of functional images reflecting regional ejection rates and mean times for the entire, first and second half of systole. Acceptable specificities can also be achieved if the entire vascular territory of major coronaries is considered. For practical purposes, any dysfunction at the anterior LAD-territory is an indication for coronary angiography, as any large dysfunction at the inferoposterior territory is.

For many years ventricular *diastolic function* has been recognized as being as informative as systolic contraction (Grossman and McLaurin, 1976; Gaasch *et al.*, 1976), particularly in ischaemic heart disease. Traditional diagnostic techniques, however, have limited clinical investigation of diastolic events. Alterations of isovolumic relaxation and the following rapid filling phase have been observed after myocardial infarction and also in patients with angina under stress (Papapietro *et al.*, 1979; Reduto *et al.*, 1981). With first pass technique it was demonstrated that global left ventricular rapid filling was altered even at rest in patients with ischaemic heart disease even without previous myocardial infarct and with normal systolic function (Bonow *et al.*, 1981). Today, there is general agreement that the diastolic phase may be the earliest indicator of left ventricular dysfunction due to ischaemic heart disease (Sutton *et al.*, 1978; Rousseau *et al.*, 1981).

There is a biochemical metabolic basis explaining early changes of diastolic function in ischaemic heart disease. Myocardial relaxation is the result of an interplay of active and passive phenomena. The first phase (manifested by the maximum velocity of relaxation) represents an active process dependent on energy and upon the dissociation of actin and myosin. Ischaemia not only provides less energy for this ATP-dependent dissociation (Weisfeldt *et al.*, 1974) but also leads to local acidosis that in turn increases affinity of calcium for the sarcoplasmic reticulum and therefore prolongs relaxation (Nakamaru *et al.*, 1970). It is also conceivable that repetitive episodes of ischaemia may cause irreversible alterations of diastolic function and that its restoration after an ischaemic attack may take longer than that of the systolic function.

Other cardiopathies, however, such as valve-disease or hypertrophic cardiomyopathy can also alter the rapid filling phase so that investigation of global rapid filling rates allows no discrimination between the different possible causes of reduced ventricular compliance. Ischaemic heart disease with its fundamental characteristic of segmental localization requires for discrimination regional analysis of function in the coronary vascular territories. Consequently, functional imaging of regional rapid filling rates provides an adequate instrument to study regional left ventricular compliance.

The *regional rapid filling rate image* normally exhibits maximum rates pointing to the ventricular apex (*see* Figure 2.30). Distribution of inflow rates is symmetrical in relationship to the long axis of the

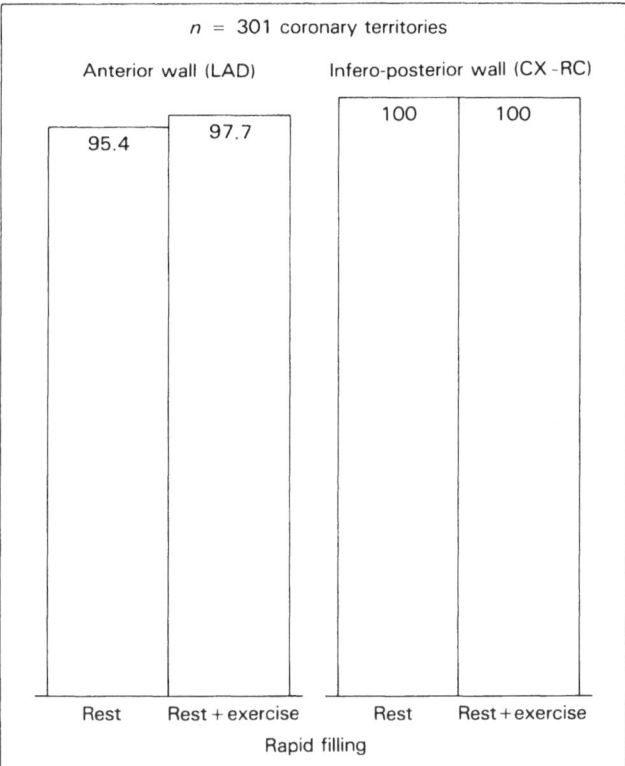

Figure 4.7 *Sensitivity of functional images of diastolic rapid filling in detection of coronary narrowings* at the anterior (LAD) and inferoposterior wall (CX–RC), at rest and rest and exercise together. Analysis is mainly based on the image of regional rapid filling rates. The observed sensitivities are higher than those obtained by the combined systolic functional images in the same patients (see Figure 4.4).

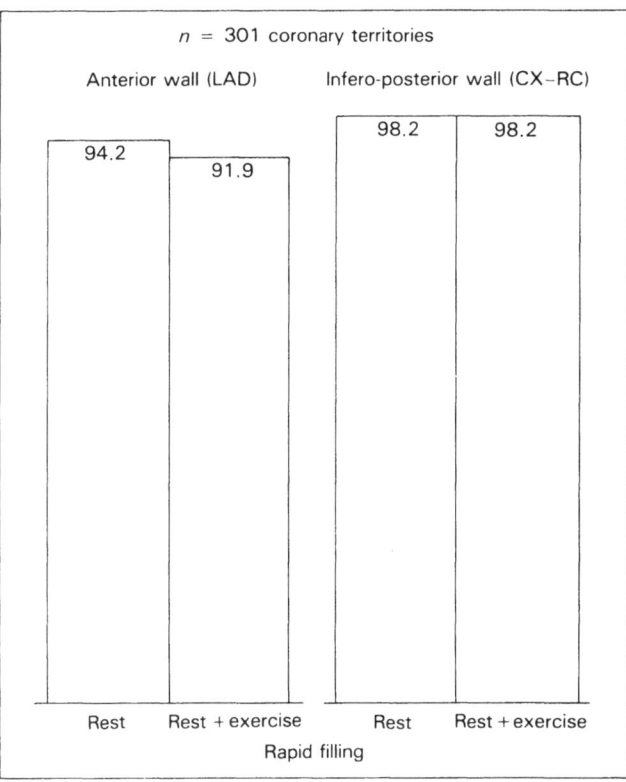

Figure 4.8 *Specificity of functional images of diastolic rapid filling in detection of coronary narrowings* at the anterior (LAD) and inferoposterior wall (CX–RC), at rest and rest and exercise together. Analysis is mainly based on the image of regional rapid filling rates. Specificities of regional rates of rapid filling are much higher than those obtained by the combined systolic functional images in the same patients.

ventricle. Contrary to the regional ejection rate image, this image corresponds to regional rates of increase of blood or activity during the rapid filling phase. One may also obtain an *image of regional decrease of activity* during the same diastolic time interval. Normally, the latter image shows decrease of activity in the ascending aorta and inward motion of its walls but nothing is seen in the ventricular zone.

In ischaemia, or after myocardial infarct, *inflow is deviated* to segments with preserved normal compliance. In the regional rapid filling rate image, high filling rates are correspondingly deviated to the normal segments so that segments with low or no rates of flow point to functionally compromised territories. Despite the short time-interval of rapid filling lasting only about 200 ms and the few images available for processing (*see above*), the areas with reduced compliance are very distinct and usually easier to delineate than on first and second half systolic functional images. Both systolic ejection rate images and diastolic rapid filling rate images frequently show alterations at rest which deteriorate during exercise. In areas lacking significant rapid inflow the rapid filling decrease image may even show predominant *'paradoxical' inward motion* or lack of any segmental motion during this initial diastolic time interval. This phenomenon can be explained by a pulling effect on the non-compliant segments during rapid relaxation of the compliant zones.

To define the value and *accuracy* of the regional

rapid filling rate image for non-invasive detection of coronary artery narrowings the regional diastolic function of 301 left ventricular vascular territories has been evaluated at rest and peak exercise in the above 43 patients where regional systolic function was also analysed (Schad *et al.*, 1984d). The same seven different vascular territories were distinguished. Diastolic reduced regional rapid filling rates at rest and peak exercise were compared to the status of the corresponding coronary arteries. 103 vascular territories were compromised by coronary narrowings; 198 were normal. The same evaluation process was adopted as for the systolic functional images. The findings in the regional rapid filling rate image were added to the matrix of results of systolic functional images prepared for every patient. In addition, all territories presenting 'paradoxical' inward motion during rapid filling were noted.

The two graphs (Figures 4.7 and 4.8) report the *sensitivities* and specificities obtained from the regional rapid filling rate image at rest and exercise for the anterior LAD territory and the combined inferoposterior territory respectively. As expected, and also observed with *systolic* functional images, rest and exercise examinations together generally yield higher sensitivities than resting studies alone. But, even at rest, high sensitivities result. All observed sensitivities are higher than those obtained from the corresponding systolic functional images (Figure 4.7 vs Figure 4.4). Most remarkable, however, *specificities* are significantly higher than those yielded by systolic functional images, particularly for the anterior LAD territory (Figure 4.8 vs Figure 4.5). This appears to be the result of a stronger contrast between normal and abnormal areas of function in the rapid filling phase as compared to systole. Thus, the low or missing rates of rapid filling correlate well with the areas of coronary artery narrowing and decreased ventricular compliance.

At the anterior wall, two territories were *false negative* at rest. One case with LAD stenosis presented with significant apical collateral flow. Consequently, only the diagonal territory was positive at rest. However, with exercise the entire LAD territory became abnormal. A second case with borderline proximal LAD stenosis had a false negative rest study but became positive for the diagonal and peripheral LAD territory under stress. By the use of the criterion of strict local but not functional correlation this exercise result could also be considered as a false negative for the entire LAD territory. The cumulative sensitivities represented in the above graph are based on these three false negative territories for the anterior wall. At the inferoposterior territory three false negatives were noted for the entire CX territory and one for the posterolateral territory, but all on the stress study only. No false negative resulted at rest or at the RC territory so that sensitivities for rest examinations alone and rest and/or exercise studies were the same. This may be explained by the many different varieties of CX distribution and their more central location that makes it difficult or even impossible to distinguish from the RC territory particularly when the heart becomes small during exercise.

In nine of the 168 normal territories *false positive* findings were observed, i.e., no narrowing at the topographically correlated vessel or its major feeding artery could be seen. On the rest and exercise study the diagonal territory was found false positive four times, the LAD, posterolateral and RC territory only once each. Two false positives of the diagonal and LAD territory resulted as false positive only during exercise. Comparison with the LV angiogram, however, revealed systolic dysfunction at the same territories, i.e. no false positives resulted by comparison with the LV ventriculogram. Other causes than coronary narrowings were responsible for these local malfunctions. The graph (Figure 4.8) reports the specificities for rest and exercise studies based on false positives seen at rest and/or exercise.

The rapid filling phase lasted on the average 209 ms (range 200–280 ms) at rest and 172 ms (range 125–200 ms) at exercise examinations. During this short-lasting initial diastolic phase some *paradoxical inward motion* of the non-compliant ischaemic or infarcted territories was frequently observed in the image that exhibits the regions where activity or blood predominantly decreases. Precisely, paradoxical inward motion was seen at the anterior wall in 40% of the territories compromised by coronary narrowings at rest as well as at exercise; at the inferoposterior territories the frequency amounted to 45% at rest and 28% during exercise respectively. This paradoxical inward motion is the result of a pulling-effect of the adjacent rapidly relaxing normal territories. It mostly involved only part of the less compliant territory, the remaining zones showing lack of any motion or minimal outward motion. The degree and extent of paradoxical inward motion certainly indicates the severity of dysfunction; if seen in ischaemia during exercise it points to the myocardium in jeopardy (Figure 4.11).

The same image that eventually demonstrates some paradoxical diastolic inward motion can also show the zone of the *mitral valve prolapse* which, during initial diastole, does not present outward, but rather some inward, motion. The degree and extent of this phenomenon obviously may vary in correspondence to the severity of the prolapse. In the rapid filling rate image a defect most often results instead of the increase rates seen normally. On the basis of these criteria on both images only one case resulted as false negative for the diagnosis of coexisting prolapse of the mitral valve.

In summary, functional images visualizing regional systolic or diastolic events can be routinely used for screening patients for coronary artery disease provided their sensitivity surpasses 90%. Regional ejection rate, mean (transit) time and rapid filling rate images yield such high sensitivities with acceptable specificities. In addition, from these images one obtains information about the degree and severity of dysfunction allowing determination of functional significance of single coronary narrowings at rest and during stress (Figures 4.9–4.16).

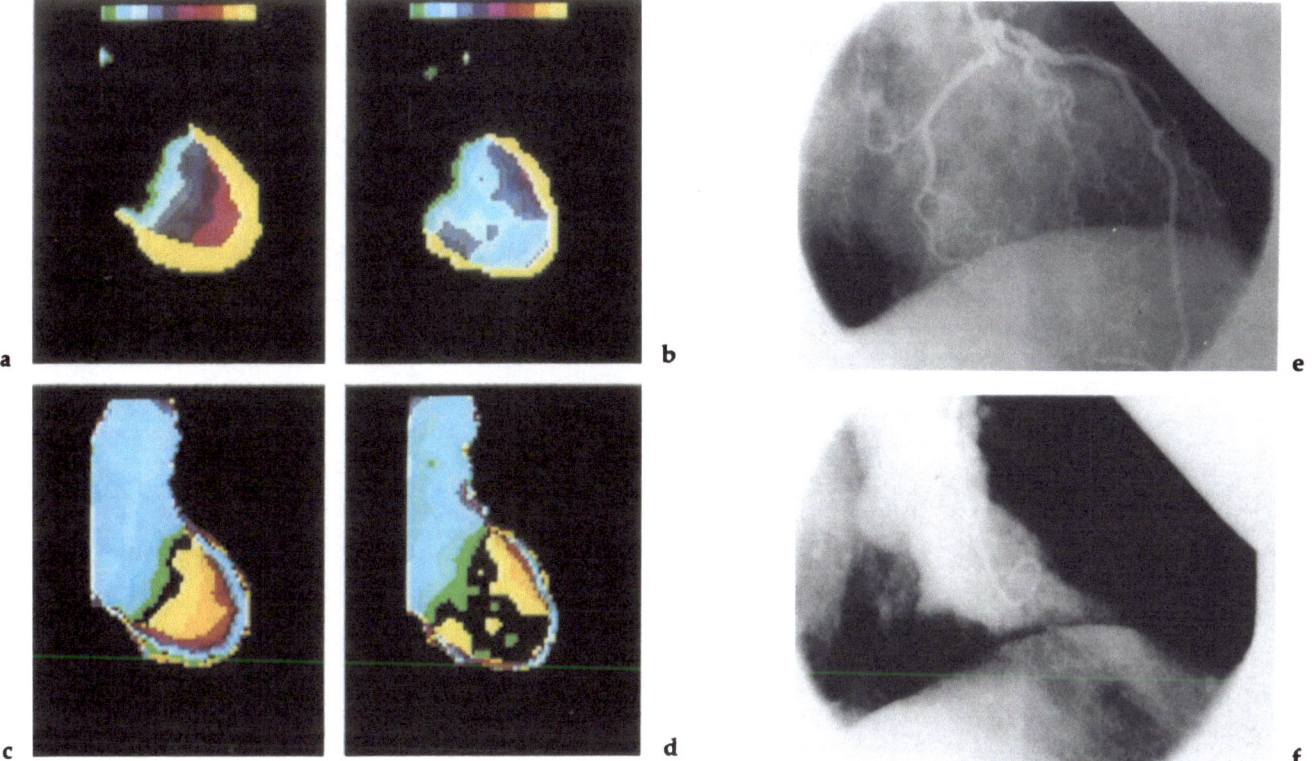

Figure 4.9 *Angina pectoris: proximal stenosis of the LAD supplying the retroapical region, narrowing of D_1, hypoplastic RC.* **a,b,c,d,** REFI and regional MTT at rest and exercise: At rest (**a,c**) minor changes posteriorly. Under stress (**b,d**) deterioration of EFs at the apex and long mean times advancing toward the retroapical region suggesting functionally significant LAD stenosis.

e,f, Coronary angiogram in RAO view: significant proximal stenosis of the LAD supplying the retroapical region (**e**). Levogram at end-systole (**f**) hypokinesia at the apex and posterior wall with mild mitral valve prolapse.

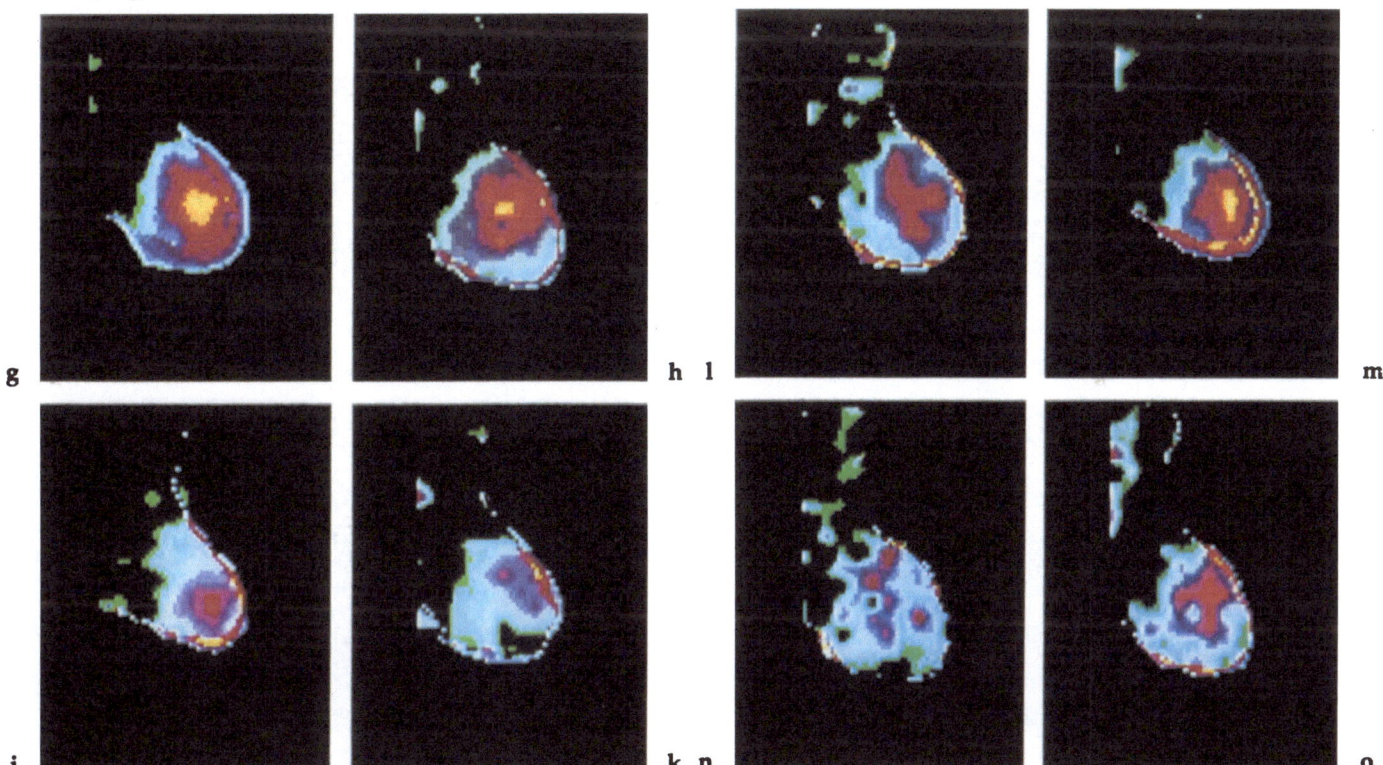

g,h,i,k, Regional ERs and RF-rates at rest and exercise: At rest (**g,i**) reduced ejection and rapid filling rates at the anterior and posterior wall suggesting ischaemia. Under stress (**h,k**) deterioration of ERs at the apex and retroapical region. Defects, i.e. no RF-rates, at the apex and posteriorly pointing to significant reduction of compliance.

l–o, Regional ERs of first and second half systole: at rest first half systole (**l**) reduced rates along the anterior wall and postero-inferiorly recovering during the second half of systole (**m**), except posteriorly. Under stress (**n,o**) fragmented rates recovering during the second half systole at the middle anterior wall only.

35

Figure 4.9 *(continued)*

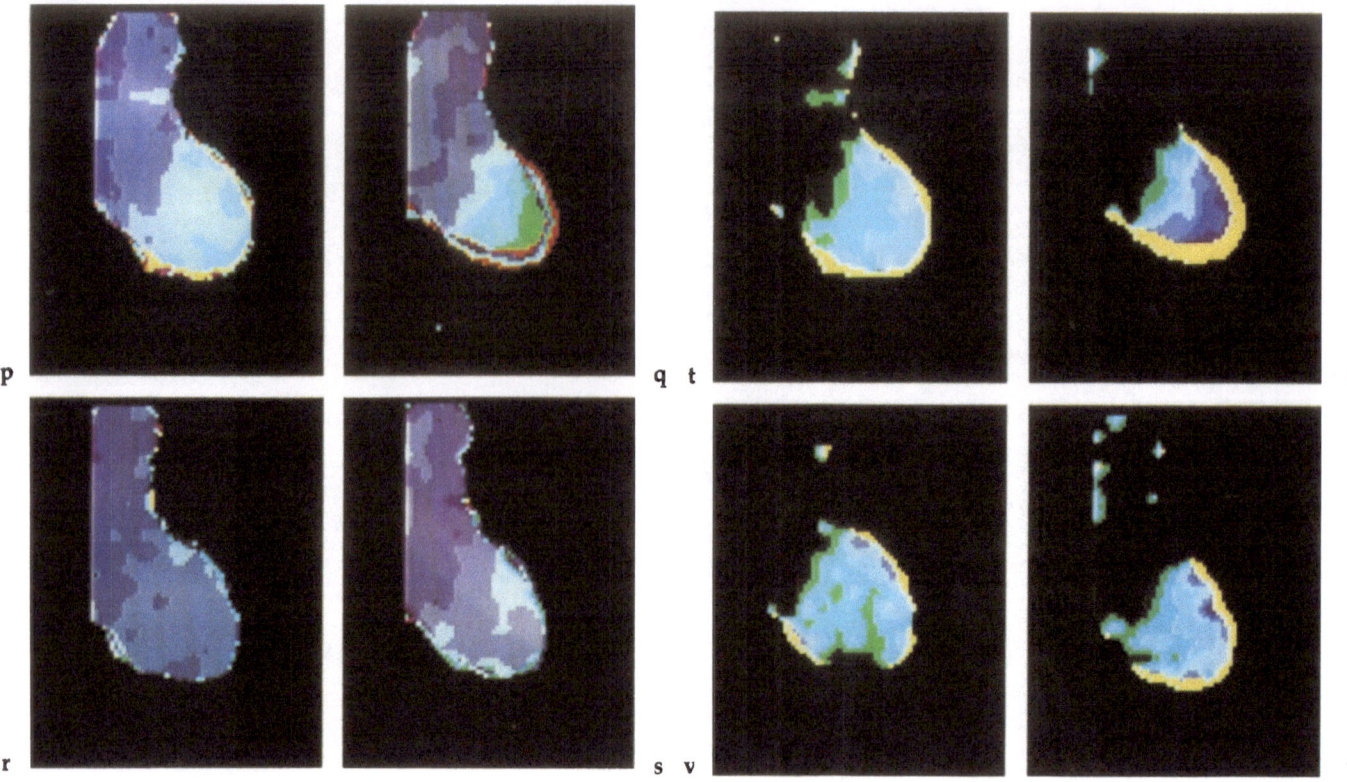

p

q

r

s

p–s, Regional MTTs of first and second half systole: at rest first half systole (**p**) long mean times pointing to the jeopardized territories: LAD,D,RC recovering during second half systole. Under stress first half systole long mean times over the entire left ventricle partially recovering during second half and pointing to the most severe dysfunction at the end of LAD and RC territory.

t

u

v

w

t–w, Regional EFs of first and second half systole: at rest first (**t**) and second half (**u**) systole dysfunction cannot be clearly localized, except posteriorly. Under stress first half systole (**v**) functional defects at the end of the LAD and RC territories somewhat recovering during second half systole (**w**), i.e. indicating ischaemia, whereas posterior defect points to MVP.

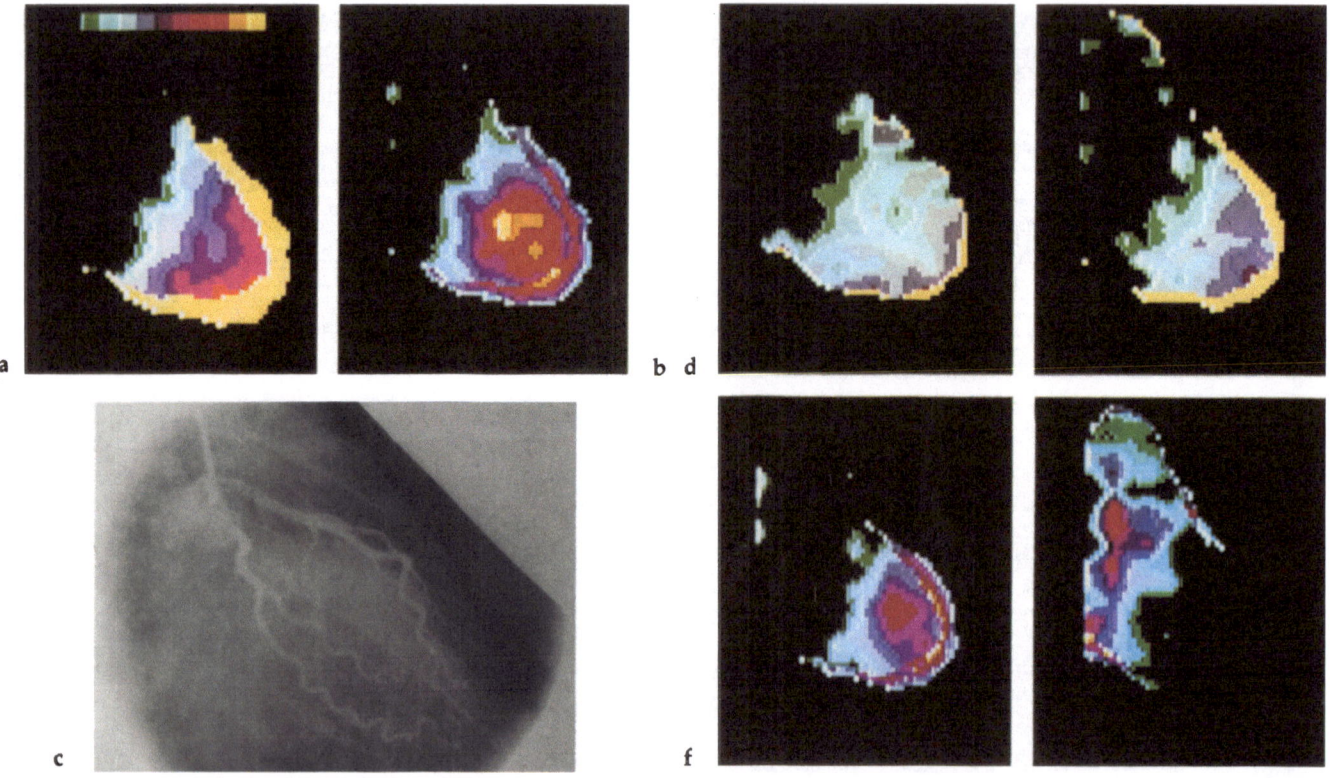

a

b

c

d

e

f

g

Figure 4.10 *Precordial chest pain. Narrowing of the first and second diagonal branch, mitral valve prolapse (rest).*

a, REFI at rest: central irregularities, dysfunction at the posterior wall.

b, Regional ERs at rest: reduced ERs at the upper anterior wall with central shifting of high rates. Defect at the most posterior wall segment.

c, Coronary angiogram in RAO view: narrowing of the diagonal branch.

d,e, Regional EFs of first and second half systole: during first half systole defects at the upper anterior wall, some motion at the posterior wall. Conversely to first half, during second half systole some motion at the upper anterior wall pointing to ischaemia (tardokinesis) and defect posteriorly indicating MVP.

f,g, Regional RF rates (**f**) reduced along the anterior wall and posteriorly, regional inward motion during RF at the upper anterior and posterior wall (**g**).

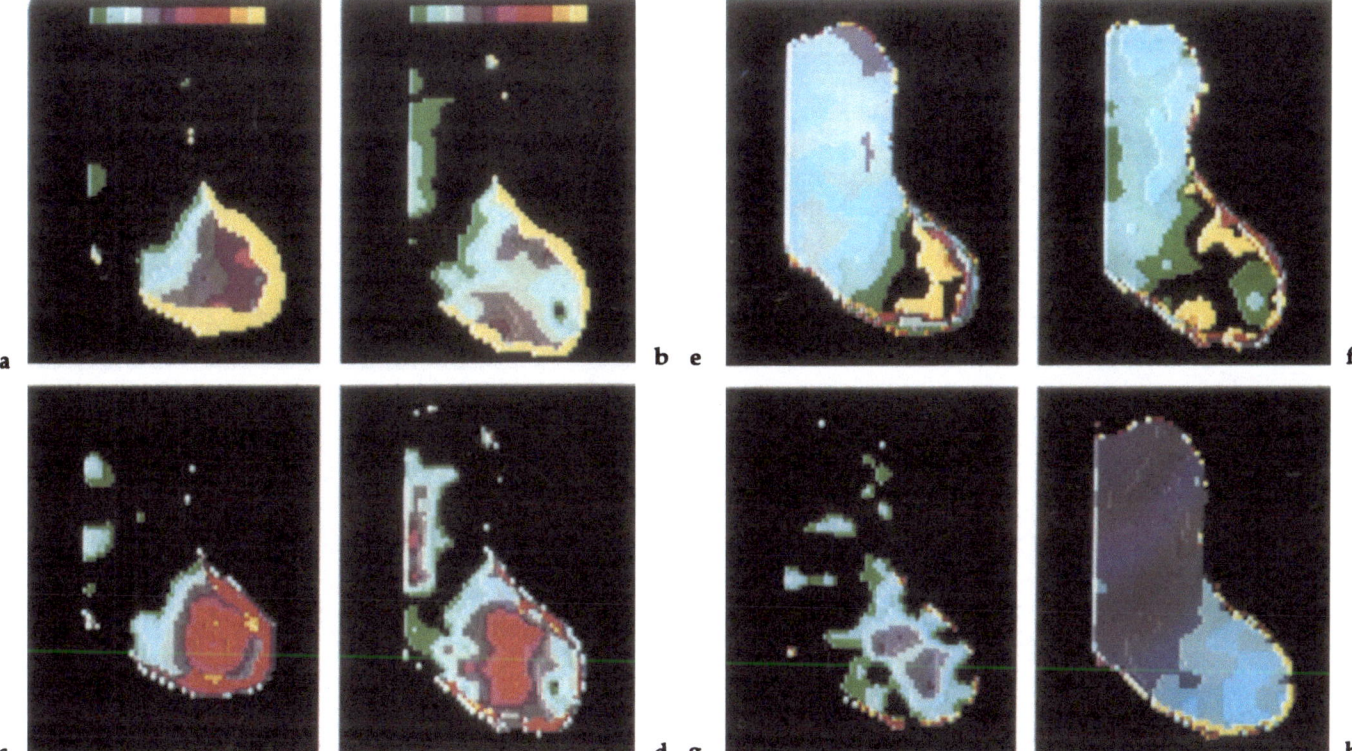

a   b   c   d   e   f   g   h

Figure 4.11 *Angina pectoris, no history of MI: proximal LAD occlusion, collateral flow from RC and D, multiple CX stenosis, peripheral RC narrowing.* **a,b,c,d,** REFI and regional ERs at rest and exercise: already at rest (**c**) loss of high rates at anterior wall (LAD territory narrowing); deterioration under stress (**b,d**) at apical and supra-apical segments (LAD stenosis. Inadequate collateral flow). Partial loss of rates or low EFs and ERs posteriorly.

e,f,g,h, Regional MTTs at rest and exercise, first half systole ERs and MTTs: at rest (**e**) long mean times (black) pointing to the anterior and posterior territories. With stress (**f**) very long subaortic mean times advanced toward the apex suggesting the anterior wall being in jeopardy: angiography and therapy are urgent. First half systole (**g,h**): defects and long mean times pointing to the three compromised territories.

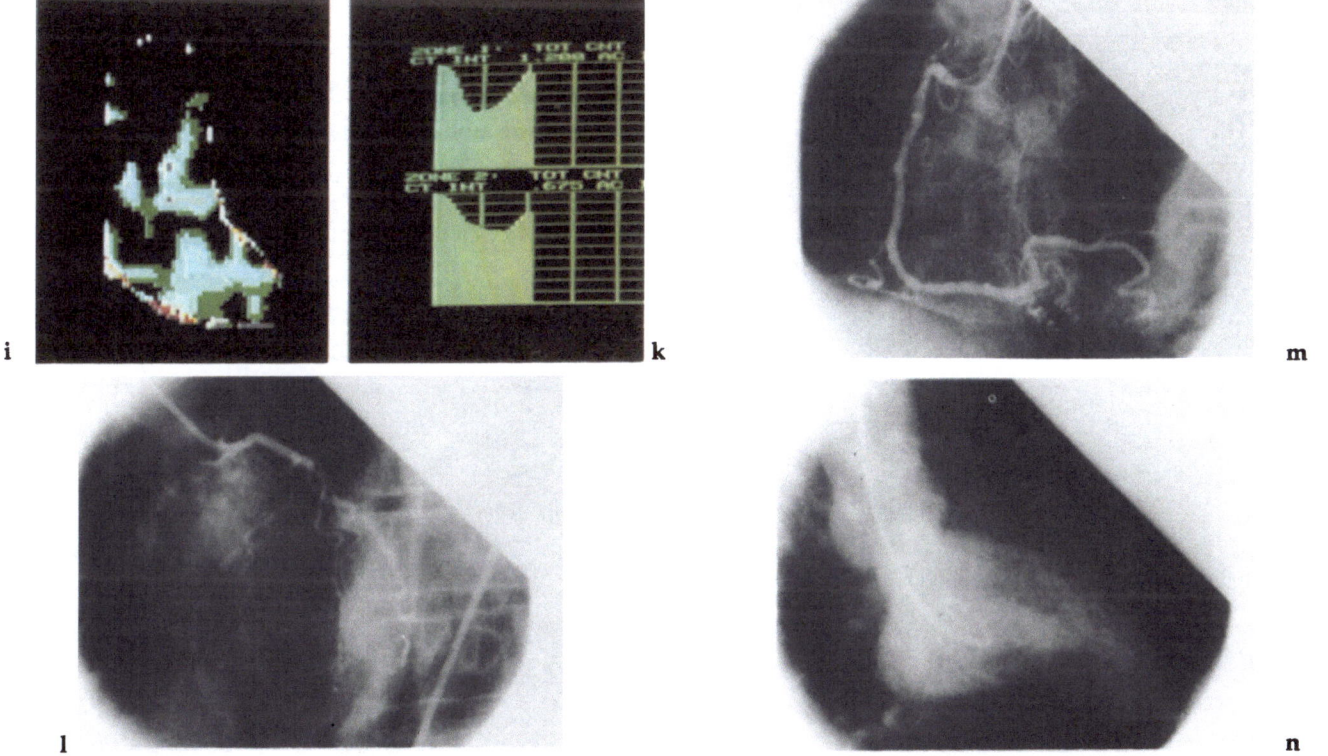

i   k   m   l   n

i,k, Regional RF rates at rest (**i**) show defects along the anterior wall, at the retroapical zone and posteriorly pointing to the territories at risk. Global LV volume curve (**k**) presents flattening of the RF part at rest (upper curve) and significant deterioration under stress (lower curve).

l–n, Coronary angiogram in LAO view: proximal LAD occlusion (**l**) with collateral flow from diagonal branch and RC (**m**). Levogram (**n**) shows hypokinesia at the apical and supra-apical segments and posteriorly.

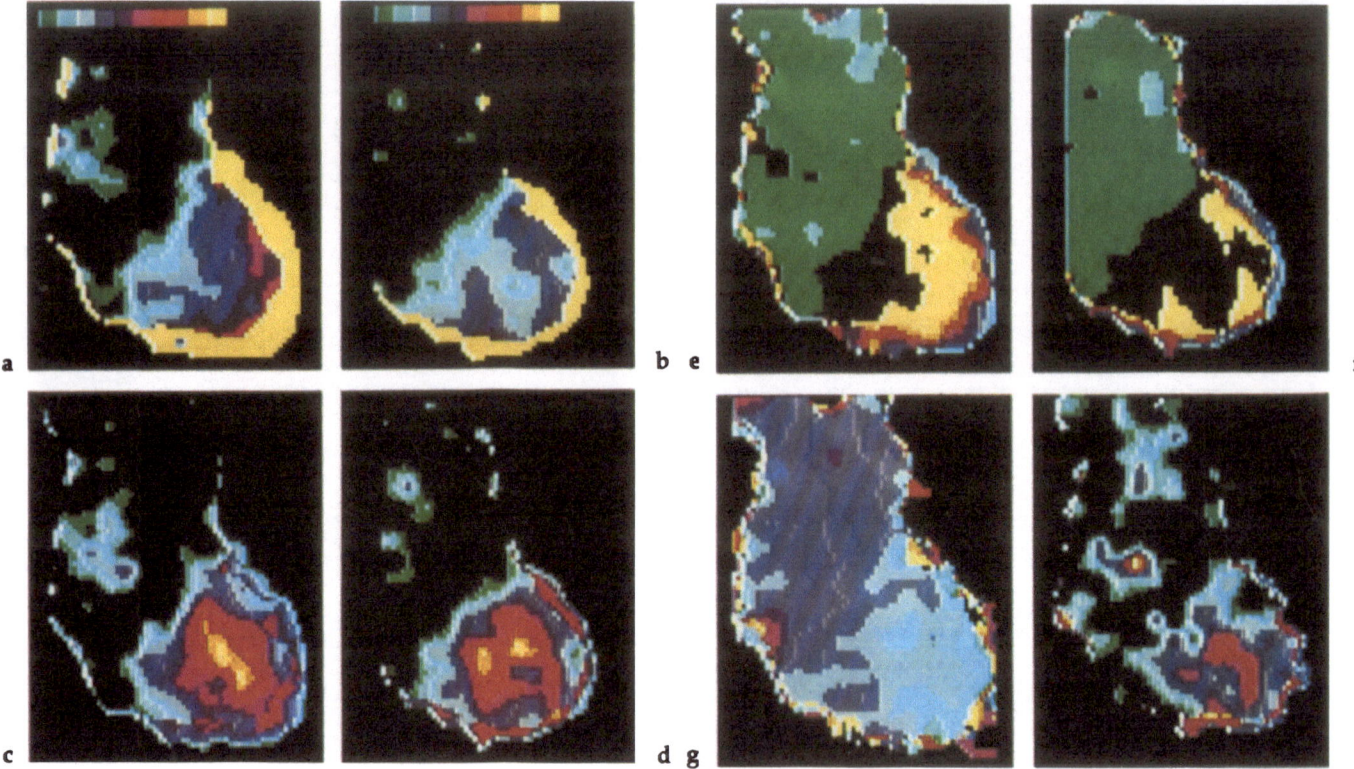

Figure 4.12 *Angina pectoris, no history of MI: central LC stenosis, peripheral LAD stenosis, narrowings of D_1 and D_2, CX and RC stenosis*
a,b,c,d, REFI and regional ERs: at rest 'noisy' EFs (**a,c**), reduced ERs at the anterior and inferior wall pointing to some narrowing of the corresponding vessels. Under stress (**b,d**) low EFs at the three territories, anterior deterioration of ERs indicates functionally significant stenosis.

e,f, Regional MTTs at rest and exercise: at rest (**e**) long times (yellow, black) advancing toward the periphery. Under stress (**f**) long times (black) reaching the periphery of the three territories in jeopardy, indicating functional significance of narrowings.
g,h, Regional MTTs and ERs during first half of systole: long mean times (**g**) and defects (**h**) pointing to the territories at risk.

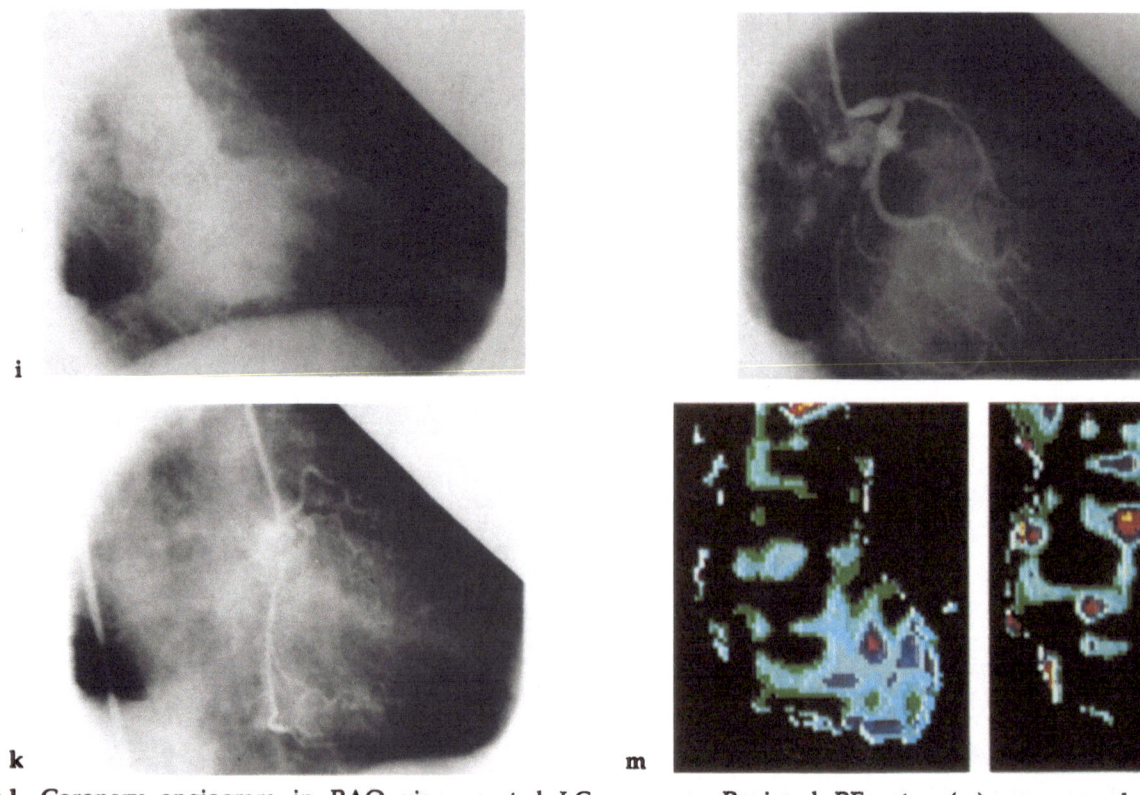

i,k,l, Coronary angiogram in RAO view: central LC stenosis, peripheral LAD and CX stenosis (**i**), RC stenosis (**k**). Levogram (**l**) presents hypokinesia at the upper anterior and posterior wall.

m,n, Regional RF rates (**m**) are severely reduced or missing at the upper anterior, apical and posterior wall, already at rest. The image of decrease during RF shows paradoxical inward motion along the anterior wall and posteriorly indicating the less compliant segments in danger: coronary angiography and therapy are urgent.

38

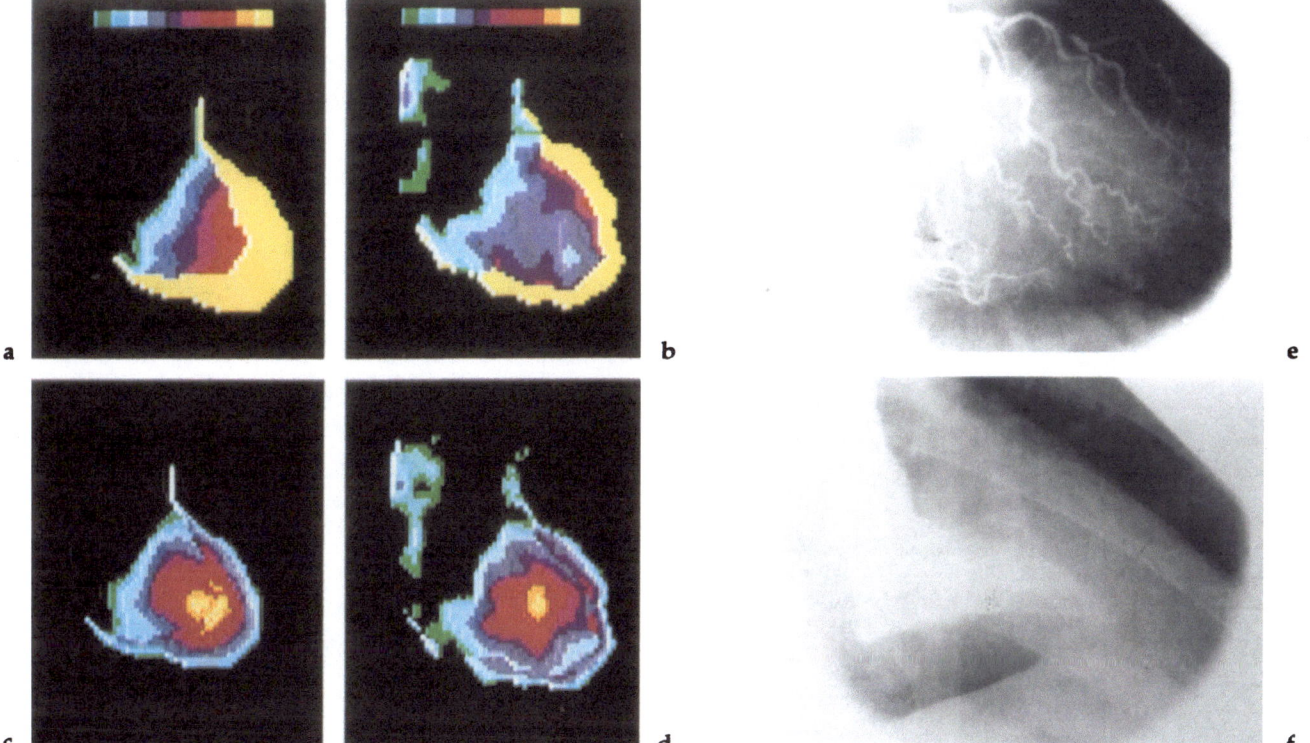

Figure 4.13 *Three vessel disease without prior MI: total occlusion with retrograde filling from the marginal branch, narrowing at the posterolateral branch, hypoplastic RC with diffuse irregularities.*
a,b,c,d, REFI and regional ERs at rest and exercise: at rest (**c**) loss of high ERs at the upper anterior wall, under stress (**b,d**) significant deterioration at the apex, anteriorly, posteriorly and inferiorly indicating three vessel disease.

e,f, Coronary angiogram in the RAO view: total occlusion of the LAD with retrograde filling from the marginal branch, narrowing at the posterolateral branch, hypoplastic RC with irregularities (**e**). The levogram shows slight hypokinesia at the apex with preserved global contraction (**f**).

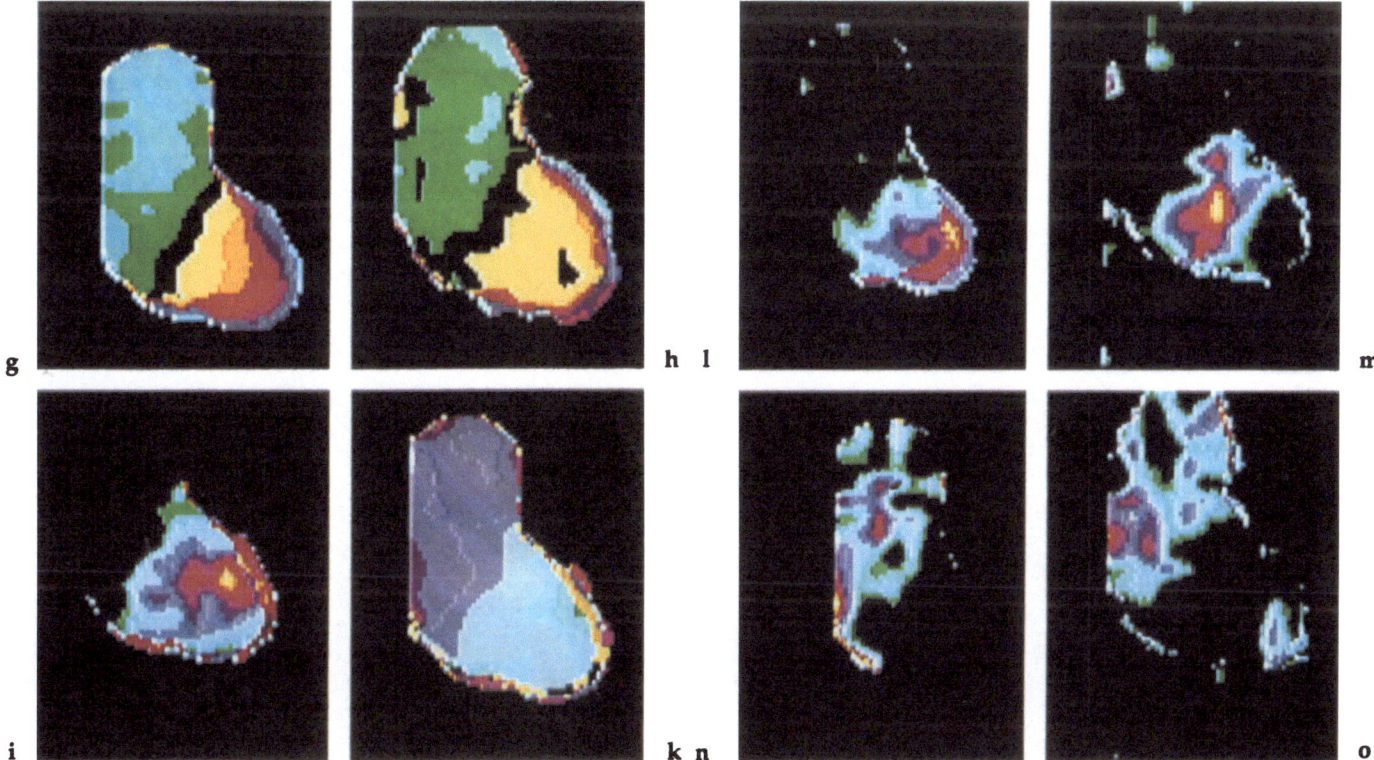

g,h, Regional MTTs at rest and exercise: at rest (**a**) no significant changes except at a small posterior segment, under stress advancing long times (yellow, black) toward the parietal zone.
i,k, Regional ERs and MTTs during first half of systole: low rates (**i**) at the apex, upper anterior wall and posteriorly, and long mean times (**k**) pointing to the three compromised territories.

l,m,n,o, Regional RF rates and decrease at rest and exercise: at rest (**l**) RF defects and inward motion (**n**) at the RC territory. Diffusely reduced RF rates at the upper anterior and posterolateral territories. Under stress (**m**) RF defects with inward motion and displacement of blood (**o**) at the diagonal and entire apical region extending in depth, indicating severe LAD obstruction with inadequate collateral flow: angiography is urgent.

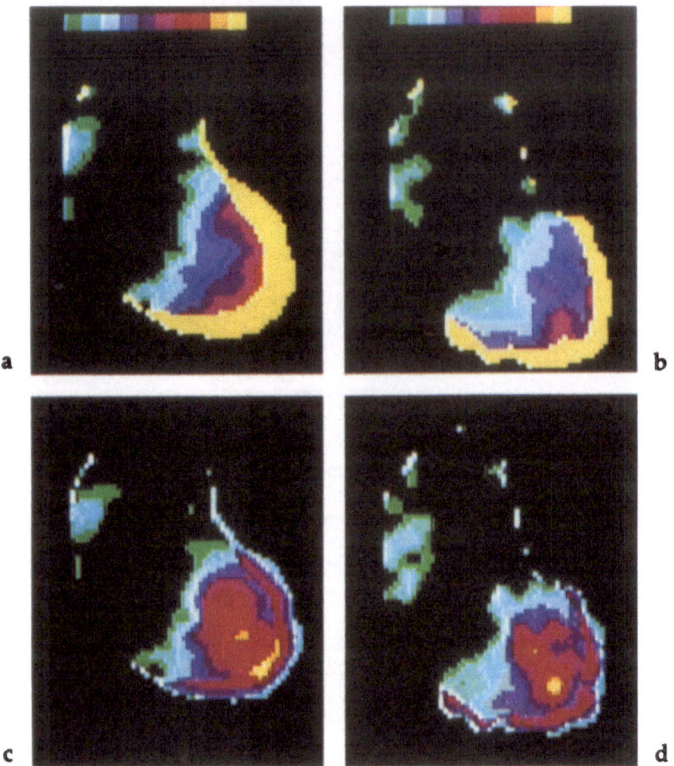

a

b

c

d

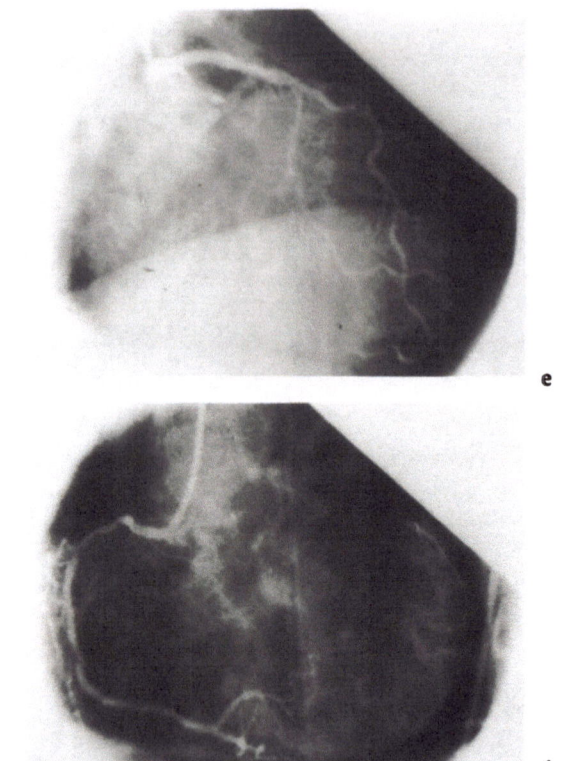

e

f

Figure 4.14 *Three vessel disease without prior MI: total CX occlusion with collateral flow from the RC, narrowings at the diagonal, peripheral LAD and RC.*

a,b,c,d, REFI and regional ERs at rest and exercise: at rest (**a,c**) only posteriorly reduced EFs but loss of high ERs at the upper anterior wall. Under stress (**b,d**) dysfunction at the entire anterior wall (LAD/D narrowings) and signifi-

cant deterioration at the posterior and posterolateral zone pointing to the most severe obstruction at the CX.

e,f, Coronary angiogram: in RAO view total occlusion of the CX (**e**), narrowings at the diagonal and peripheral LAD; in LAO view (**f**) narrowing of the RC at the initial third, collateral flow to the marginal and CX.

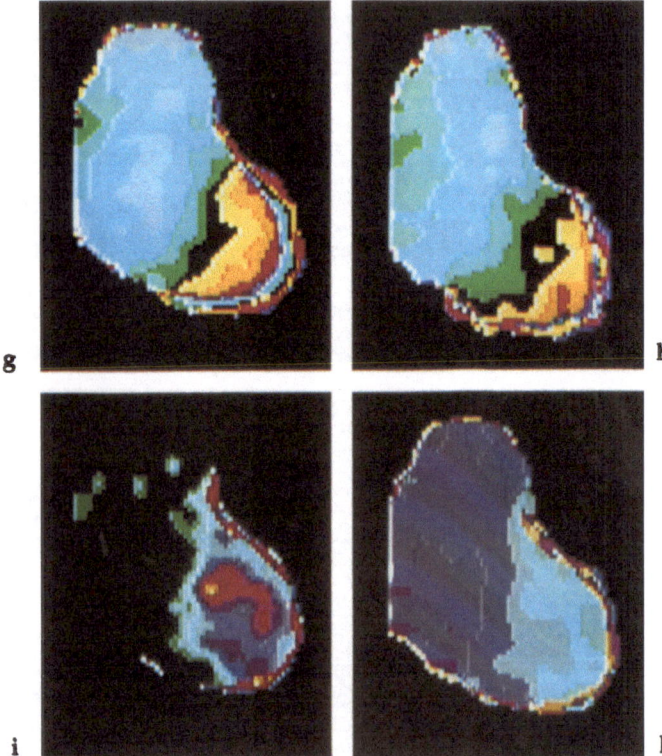

g

h

i

k

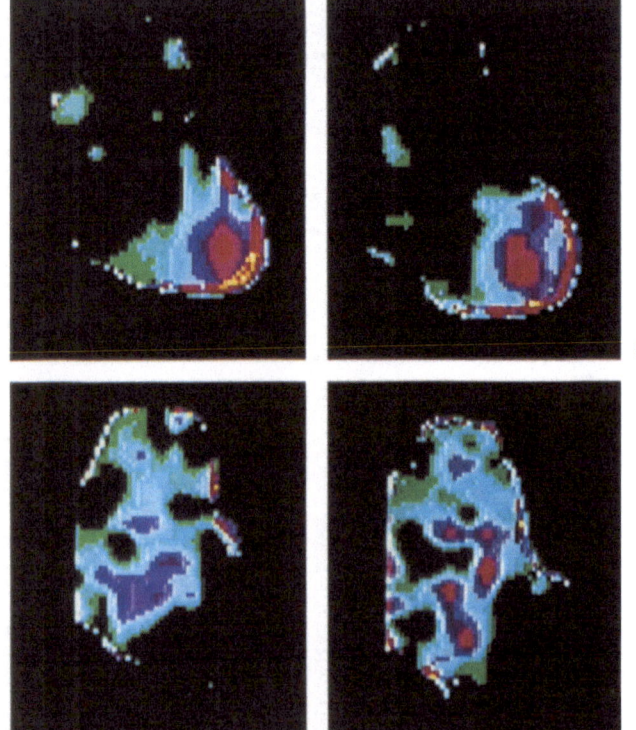

l

m

n

o

g,h, Regional MTTs at rest and exercise: at rest (**g**) slight advancing of long times anteriorly and somewhat expanded long times posteriorly; under stress (**h**) the advanced long times (black, green) point to the three compromised territories.

i,k, Regional ERs and MTTs during first half of systole: defects posteriorly (**i**), reduced ERs along the anterior wall; very long MTTs posteriorly (**k**) extending laterally pointing to the most severe obstruction

l,m,n,o, Regional RF rates and decrease at rest and exercise: at rest (**l**) RF defect and paradoxical inward motion (**n**) at the diagonal territory; reduced RF rates at the middle anterior wall and posteriorly extending centrally (posterolateral) pointing to the peripheral LAD, CX and RC narrowings. Under stress (**m**) RF defects posterolaterally with inward displacement of blood (**o**); expansion of lower RF rates to the apex.

40

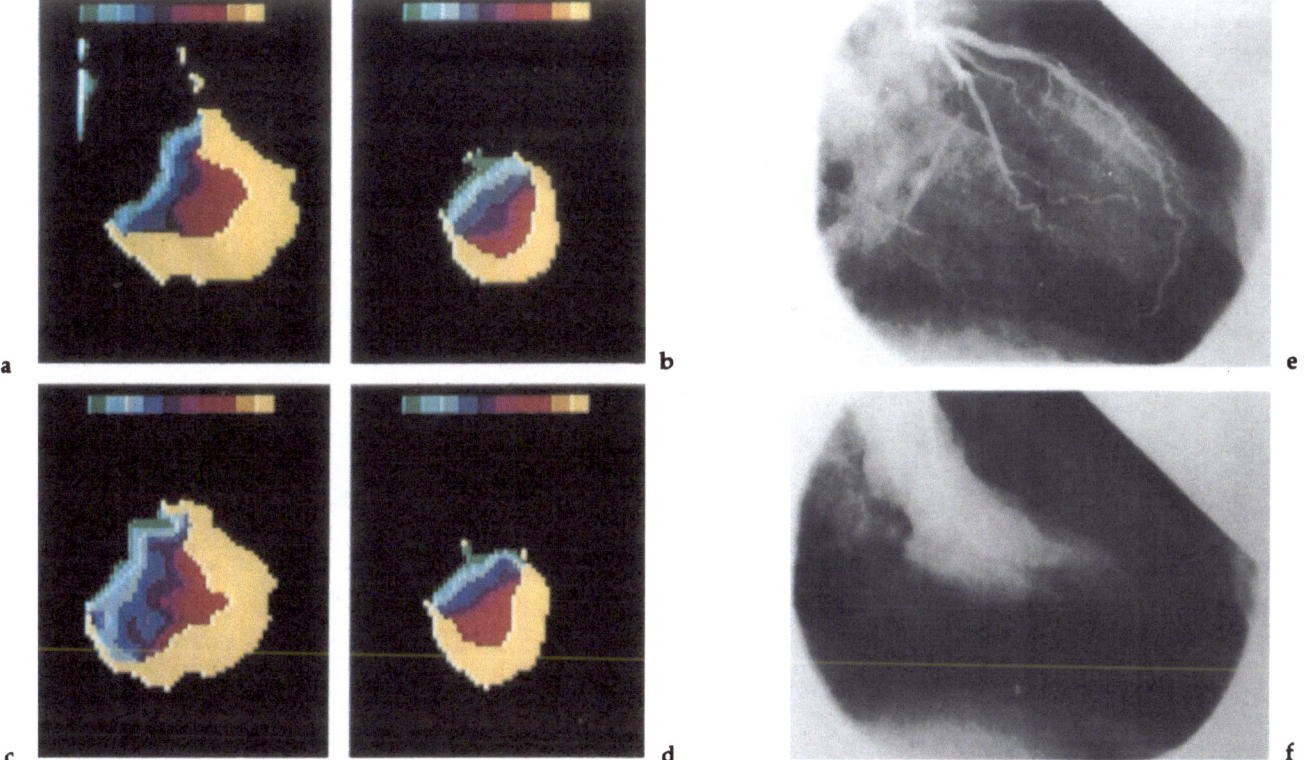

a   b

c   d

e

f

Figure 4.15 *Angina pectoris, significant CX-obstruction and narrowing of the first diagonal.*

a–d, REFI at rest and exercise RAO and LAO view: at rest (**a,b**) only slight loss of higher EFs (red) posteriorly, LAO (**b**) nearly normal. Under stress (**c,d**) bulging of the posterior wall with significant loss of higher EFs extending posterolaterally in RAO view (**c**), LAO normal EFs.

e,f, Coronary angiogram and levogram in RAO view: subtotal occlusion of the CX after origin of marginal branch providing some homocollateral flow (**e**). Left ventricular end-systole shows hypokinesia of the postero-inferior wall, mitral valve prolapse.

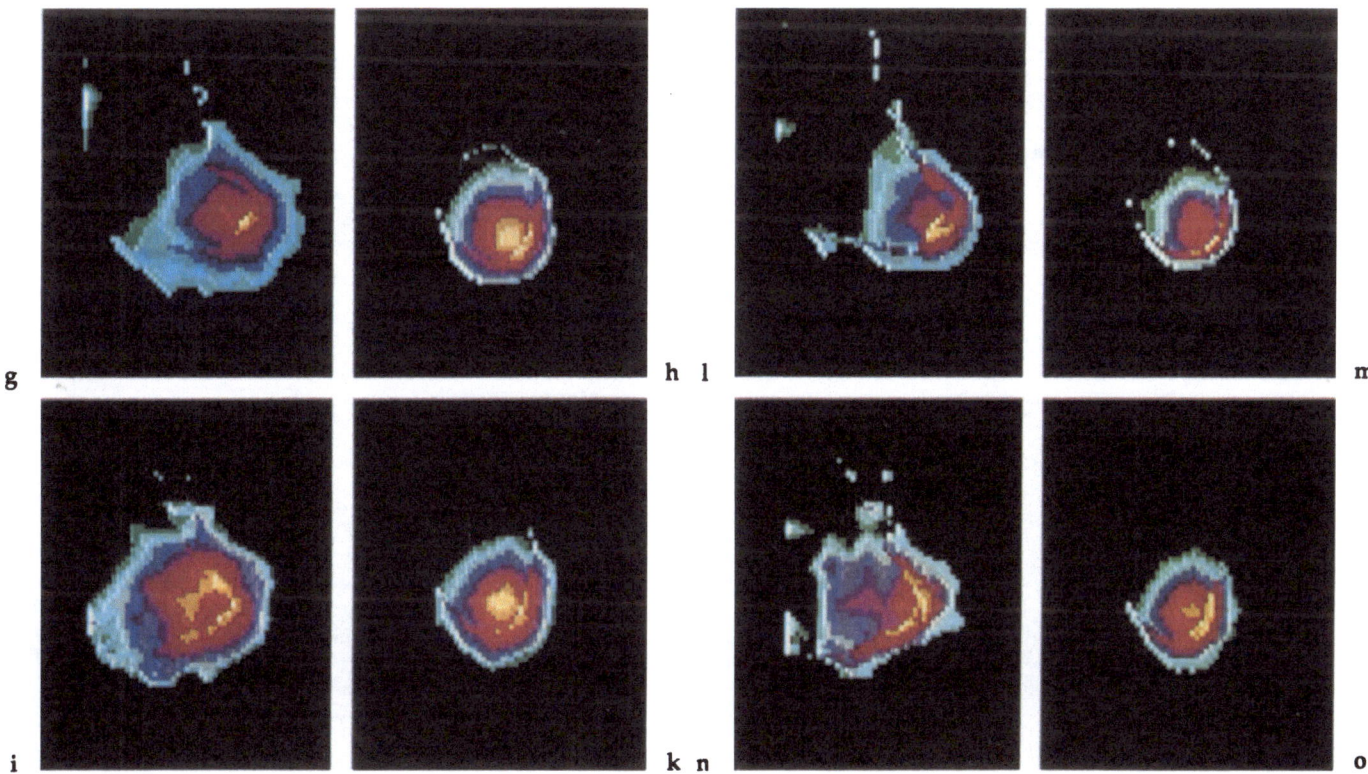

g   h   l   m

i   k   n   o

g,h,i,k, Regional ERs at rest and exercise RAO and LAO view: at rest (**g,h**) loss of high rates (yellow) at the upper anterior segment (**g**) posteriorly (**g**) and posterolaterally (**h**) with central shifting of high ERs. Under stress (**i,k**) same findings as at rest but deterioration in RAO view (**i**).

l–o, Regional RF rates at rest and exercise RAO and LAO view: at rest (**l,m**) already clearly reduced rates (compliance) at the upper anterior and posterolateral zone (**m**) with deterioration during stress (**n,o**).

41

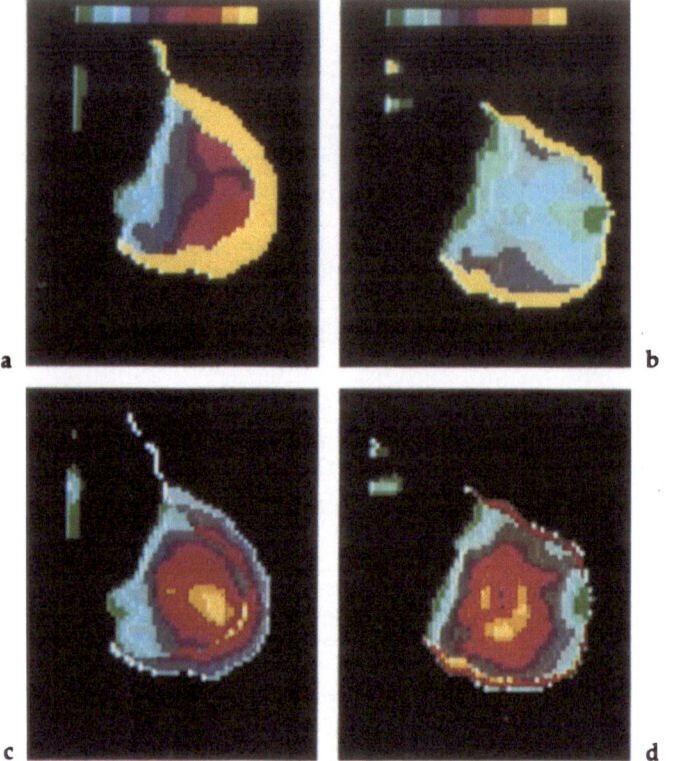

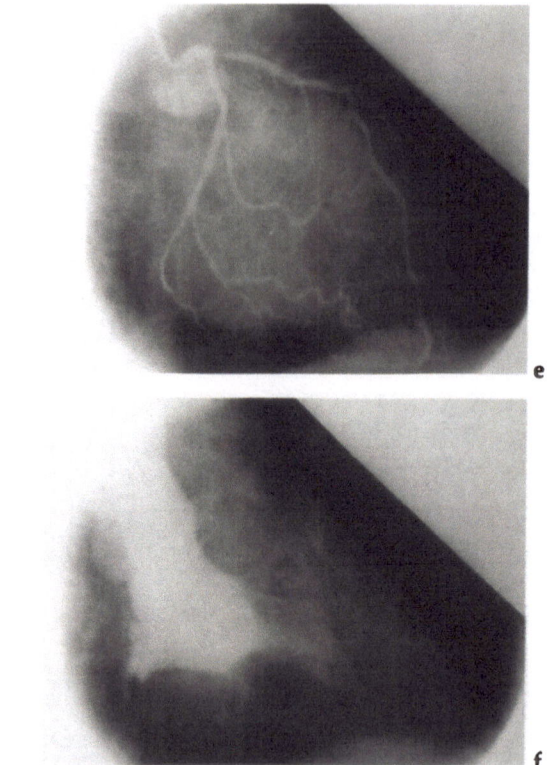

Figure 4.16 *Angina pectoris, anterior MI 5 days after carotid surgery, significant proximal LAD stenosis, prolapse of the mitral valve.*
a,b, REFI at rest before and after anterior MI: before MI (**a**) only mild reduction of EFs (purple) pointing to the anterior wall, after MI (**b**) severe reduction of anterior EFs with minimum (green) at the supra-apical zone and bulging. Defect posteriorly (MVP).

c,d, Regional ERs at rest before and after anterior MI: before MI (**c**) loss of high rates at the upper anterior wall and posteriorly, after MI (**d**) significant deterioration along the anterior wall with minimum (green) at the supra-apical region. Central shifting of high ERs.
e,f, Coronary angiogram and levogram in RAO view: significant proximal LAD stenosis (**e**), prolapse of the mitral valve (**f**).

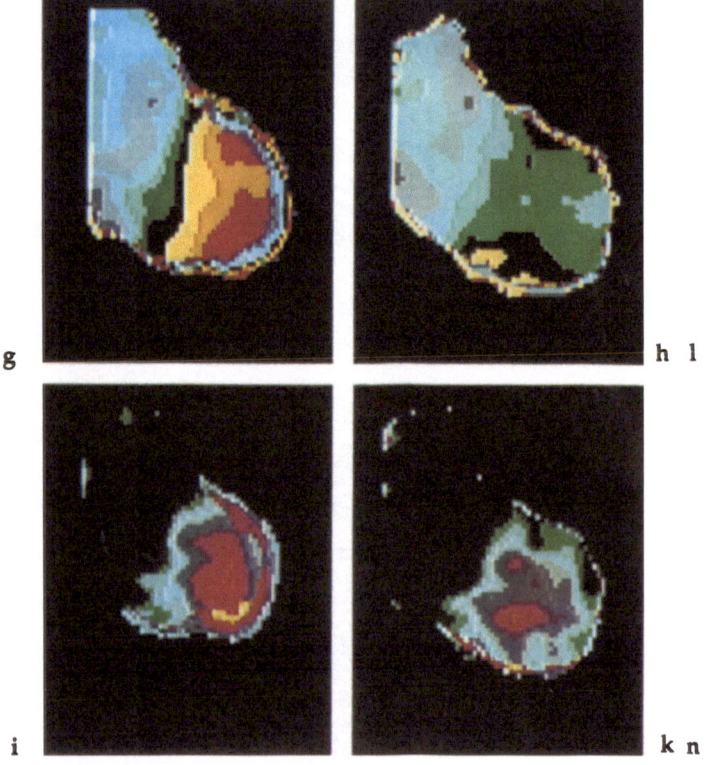

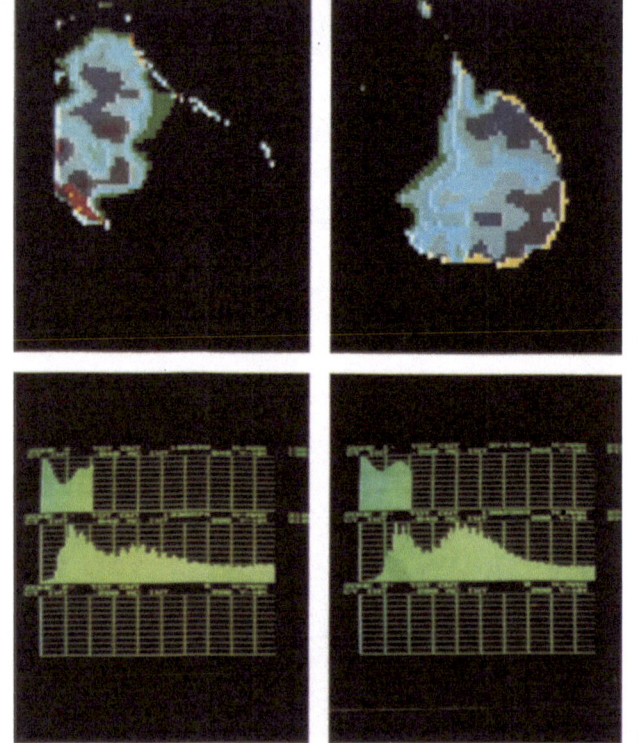

g,h,i,k, Regional MTTs and RF rates at rest before and after MI; before MI (**g**) long times (orange) point exactly to the zone where longest times (scar formation) appear after MI (**h**, light green). Parietal very long times (green) indicate infarction when seen at rest. Before MI (**i**) significant reduction of RF rates (compliance) at the anterior wall already at rest pointing to LAD territory at risk. Deterioration after MI (**k**).

l, Regional decrease during rapid filling at rest after MI: paradoxical inward motion at the anterior wall and at the zone of mitral valve prolapse.

m, REFI at rest first half of systole before MI: questionable reduction of EFs pointing to anterior wall.

n,o, Volume and washout curves of the LV at rest before and after MI: after MI (**o**) flattened volume curve and delayed washout and lung transit.

5

Functional Imaging in Ischaemic Heart Disease

E. J. ANDREWS JR. AND J. W. FLEMING

Initial experience with radionuclide ventriculography (RNV) in selected patient populations suggested that, at last, the diagnostic screening test for coronary artery disease (CAD) had been found which approached 100% in both sensitivity and specificity (Borer *et al.*, 1977). However, in the asymptomatic outpatient population RNV studies are only approximately 56% sensitive and 62% specific for detecting significant CAD when global parameters and cine wall motion evaluation are used for diagnosis (Osbakken *et al.*, 1983; Rozanski *et al.*, 1983). This number improves when peak systolic pressure/end systolic volume ratios, and pulmonary blood volume ratios, are used in addition to the ejection fraction response to exercise. Even with these additional evaluations, accuracy falls short of what is considered acceptable for an optimal diagnostic screening test. Because patients evaluated at the Florida Heart Center are often relatively asymptomatic outpatients, there was need for an improved non-invasive screening test for CAD. Experience with radionuclide functional imaging has now been gained in nearly 20 000 studies at the

Florida and Passau laboratories. Evaluation of 162 consecutive cases undergoing RNV and cardiac catheterization proved this method to be highly sensitive (96%) and specific (88%) for diagnosis of myocardial ischaemia even in the outpatient population (see Tables 5.1 and 5.2). This chapter will discuss this experience and present illustrations regarding the use of functional radionuclide imaging in ischaemic heart disease.

Gated as well as first pass RNV studies initially were used to evaluate patients at the Florida Heart Center. Global response to exercise was used as the major parameter for diagnosis. Cine wall motion images were also evaluated. It was found that approximately 30% of patients with significant CAD had a normal ejection fraction (EF) response to exercise (increase of 0.05 or greater). The number of false negatives was even greater when patients with typical angina or previous infarction were excluded. Cine wall motion evaluation did not improve significantly diagnostic accuracy and was subject to interobserver error. Functional images proved to be more quantitative than cine evaluation. Each colour

Table 5.1 Wall motion abnormalities – 163 patients

Diagnosis	Total number	REFI		First half REFI		Second half REFI		Mean transit time		Ejection rate	
		Rest	Exercise	Rest	Exercise	Rest	Exercise	Rest	Exercise	Rest	Exercise
CAD	95	30	38	73	90	35	30	53	70	56	73
Normal	37	0	0	3	3	3	4	2	5	3	5
Cardiomyopathy	7	3	3	6	6	4	5	6	7	7	7
Mitral valve prolapse	22	1	4	6	7	2	2	5	6	5	7
Aortic and mitral valve disease	2	1	1	2	1	1	1	1	1	1	2

Table 5.2 163 consecutive patients with cardiac catheterization and RNV study

Diagnosis	Total patients	Correct diagnosis RNV	False negative	False positive	Sensitivity	Specificity
CAD	95	91	4	—	96%	—
Normal	37	34	—	3	—	92%
CM, MVP, Valve disease	31	26	—	5	—	84%
Total patients	163	151	4	8	—	88%

Overall sensitivity for diagnosis of CAD = 96%
Overall specificity for diagnosis of ischaemia = 88%

(or grey scale) represents a number (counts) and there was greater interobserver agreement regarding abnormality. Because of improved diagnostic accuracy functional imaging has become the principle radionuclide screening test for CAD at the Florida Heart Center. Thallium studies are used only occasionally in our laboratory for patients with arrythmias and to separate myocardial scar (post-myocardial infarction) from potentially viable muscle prior to bypass surgery.

The various functional images have been described in Chapter 2. All of the images have proven to be useful, but in ischaemia the first half systolic images are the most reliable and specific (*see* Table 5.1). Slutsky *et al.* (1980) suggested that the first third ejection fraction (%) was a reliable indicator of ischaemia, and Johnson *et al.* (1975) felt that the volume ejected during early systole was a sensitive index of CAD. Ventricular dysfunction associated with ischaemia usually occurs early in the systolic cycle, but when only a number (EF) is used for diagnosis there appears to be considerable overlap between normal and abnormal. In addition, the low counts taken in only one third of the systolic cycle often introduce statistical error. This is eliminated by extending the early systolic image to the first half of systole. In our method, the functional image of the first half of systole is usually abnormal in patients with ischaemia even when global function (EF) is normal (*see* Table 5.1). The first half transit image appears to be slightly more sensitive than the first half regional ejection fraction image (REFI) or rate image, but all three are quite sensitive in detecting ischaemia. Several case examples have been selected to illustrate the value of systolic functional imaging in patient evaluation for CAD. Diastolic imaging may also prove useful in the future and has been discussed in Chapter 2 and Chapter 4.

CASE EXAMPLES

Case 1: Figures 5.1 and 5.2 (first diagonal and circumflex marginal)

This 43-year-old female had a strong family history of premature death due to CAD. Radionuclide study was obtained for screening and revealed a focal abnormality involving the anterolateral wall most pronounced during early systole. The first half images show the abnormality extending to the anteriolateral wall. Cardiac catheterization several days later confirmed narrowing of the origin of the diagonal branch of the left anterior descending artery of approximately 60% and a second lesion involving the first marginal branch of the circumflex artery. Ventricular function was excellent and ejection fraction on radionuclide study was normal as well.

Case 2: Figures 5.3 and 5.4 (LAD)

This 40-year-old male had an anterior infarction 1 month prior to the radionuclide study. The functional images in this case are typical of severe ischaemia

with early and late abnormalities near the apex related to infarction. A severe septal abnormality is also present which is best demonstrated in the LAO projection. This projection has also proven useful for evaluation of the posterior wall as well as the septum and is helpful in cases where evaluation is desired before and after angioplasty. Cardiac catheterization revealed a 95% lesion of the LAD artery.

Case 3: Figure 5.5 (LAD and circumflex with hypoplastic RCA)

This 56-year-old female had e.c.g abnormalities suggesting remote anterior infarction with a more recent episode of chest pain. The functional images are abnormal even at rest showing a wall motion abnormality extending to the apex. In this situation all images are abnormal. A late systolic abnormality is also present indicative of previous infarction. Cardiac catheterization showed good ventricular contractility except for akinesis of the apex and there was subtotal occlusion of the LAD artery with a hypoplastic right coronary artery and total occlusion of the second marginal branch of the circumflex artery.

Case 4: Figure 5.6 (triple vessel disease)

This 50-year-old male was admitted to the Internal Medicine service with history of oesophagitis and/or ulcer disease. A rest radionuclide study was obtained on Friday afternoon as part of the initial workup and the severe abnormalities easily seen on the functional images are typical of severe ischaemia. The patient was taken immediately to cardiac catheterization where severe triple vessel disease was found and coronary bypass was performed that evening. Postoperative study, not shown here, was normal. The patient has remained asymptomatic. This case points out the value of only a rest study with functional imaging. Rest studies show wall motion abnormalities in 77% of cases with CAD.

Case 5: Figure 5.7 (LAD and mild RCA)

This 59-year-old male obtained a radionuclide study as part of a 'checkup'. He denied cardiac symptoms but developed severe wall motion changes with exercise which are quite typical of ischaemia. In addition, rather severe e.c.g changes also developed and cardiac catheterization revealed a 99% lesion of the LAD artery and mild disease in the right coronary system. Coronary bypass was undertaken with function returning to normal.

Case 6: Figure 5.8 (triple vessel disease)

This 47-year-old male jogged 2 miles a day and was asymptomatic. Exercise study shows abnormality early in systole in the region of the anterolateral wall. Global function, however, is relatively well preserved. Cardiac catheterization revealed severe triple vessel disease and after coronary bypass, function and wall motion returned to normal.

Case 7: Figure 5.9 (LAD and circumflex)

This 36-year-old nurse was seen because of a strong family history of coronary artery disease. The initial study in 1980 was suspicious for ischaemia but cardiac catheterization at that time was considered to reveal only minor arteriosclerotic changes. She subsequently developed an acute myocardial infarction and repeat catheterization revealed total occlusion of the right coronary artery and progression of disease in the left anterior descending artery to 60%. Fifty per cent narrowing was also now seen in the circumflex artery and coronary bypass was recommended. She has subsequently done well but this case does point out the sensitivity of the early study in detecting ischaemic change even before this was considered significant by angiography.

Case 8: Figure 5.10 (LAD)

This 26-year-old male was seen for evaluation because of chest pain. Functional images are typical of ischaemia in the LAD distribution and subtotal occlusion of his LAD artery was found at catheterization. This case is interesting because of the relatively young age of the patient.

Case 9: Figure 5.11 (RCA and circumflex)

This 50-year-old male was evaluated because of a history of shortness of breath with exertion. Images show a more posterior and inferior early systolic abnormality and at cardiac catheterization he was found to have a 65% lesion of his right coronary artery and a 90% lesion of the circumflex artery with a relatively normal LAD system. It was felt that he should be followed medically but because of persistence of systems, he subsequently underwent angioplasty with good result, and he has remained asymptomatic.

Case 10: Figure 5.12 (diagonal branch LAD)

This 43-year-old male had a history of chest pain following a probable previous infarction. Functional images show a very high lateral abnormality which appears in early systole and persists through late systole consistent with high lateral infarction. Coronary catheterization revealed complete occlusion of the first diagonal branch of the LAD with the remainder of the coronary arteries appearing normal. He is being followed medically.

CONCLUSION

These cases were selected to give a cross-section of abnormalities seen with functional imaging in patients with myocardial ischaemia. Abnormalities are usually detected even when coronary disease is localized. It is also of interest to note that global function is often preserved in spite of rather significant coronary artery disease (Weisfeldt, 1984) and conversely some patients show severe ventricular dysfunction with only a "single" coronary lesion. In the series of patients listed in Table 5.2 of 95 patients with CAD 32 (33%) had normal ejection fractions, and eight of 37 normal patients (22%) had abnormal EF values with exercise. Although the effect of coronary artery disease upon global function is variable, wall motion changes found with functional imaging are usually quite consistent and extremely helpful in the diagnosis of coronary artery disease.

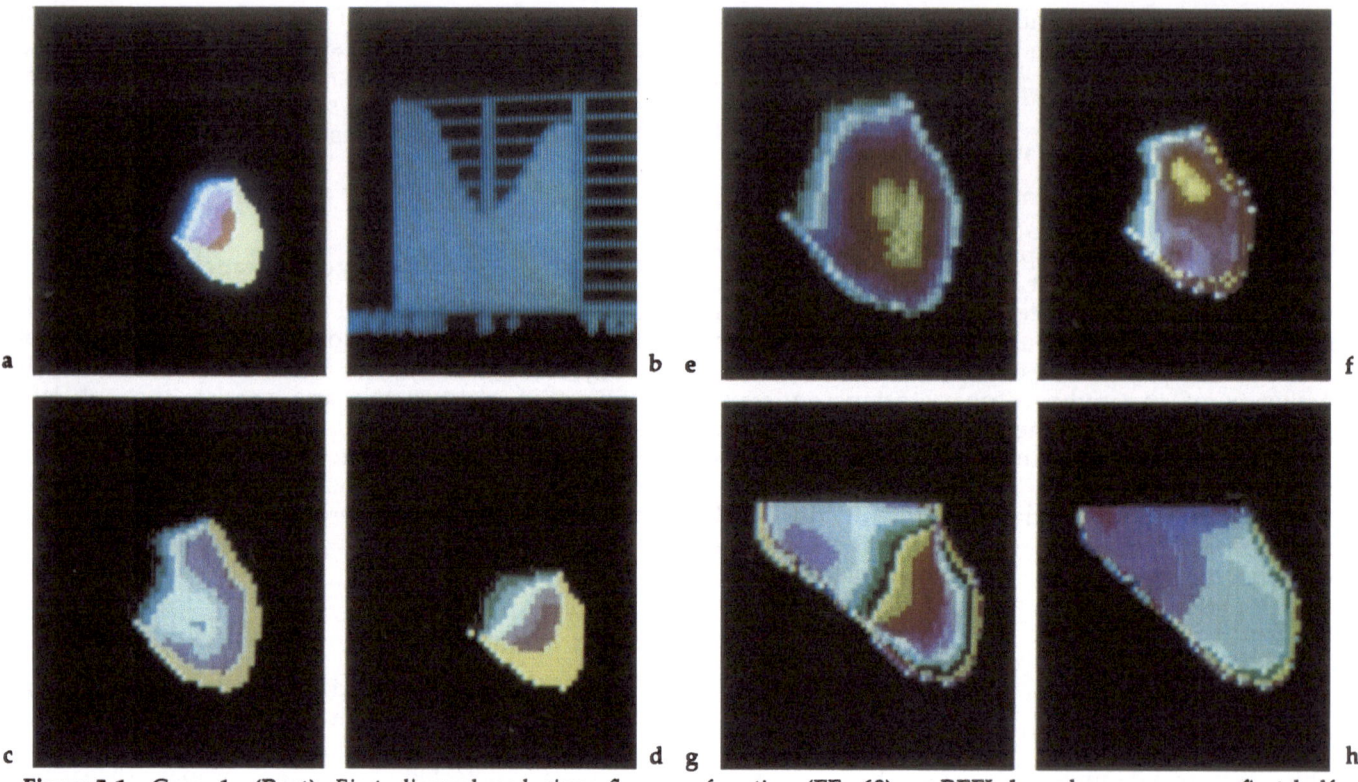

Figure 5.1 Case 1: (Rest) *First diagonal and circumflex marginal*. 43-year-old female with family history of CAD. Early systolic images are abnormal in spite of good global function (EF=60). **a**, REFI; **b**, volume curve; **c**, first half REFI; **d**, second half REFI; **e**, ejection rate; **f**, first half ER; **g**, transit; **h**, first half transit.

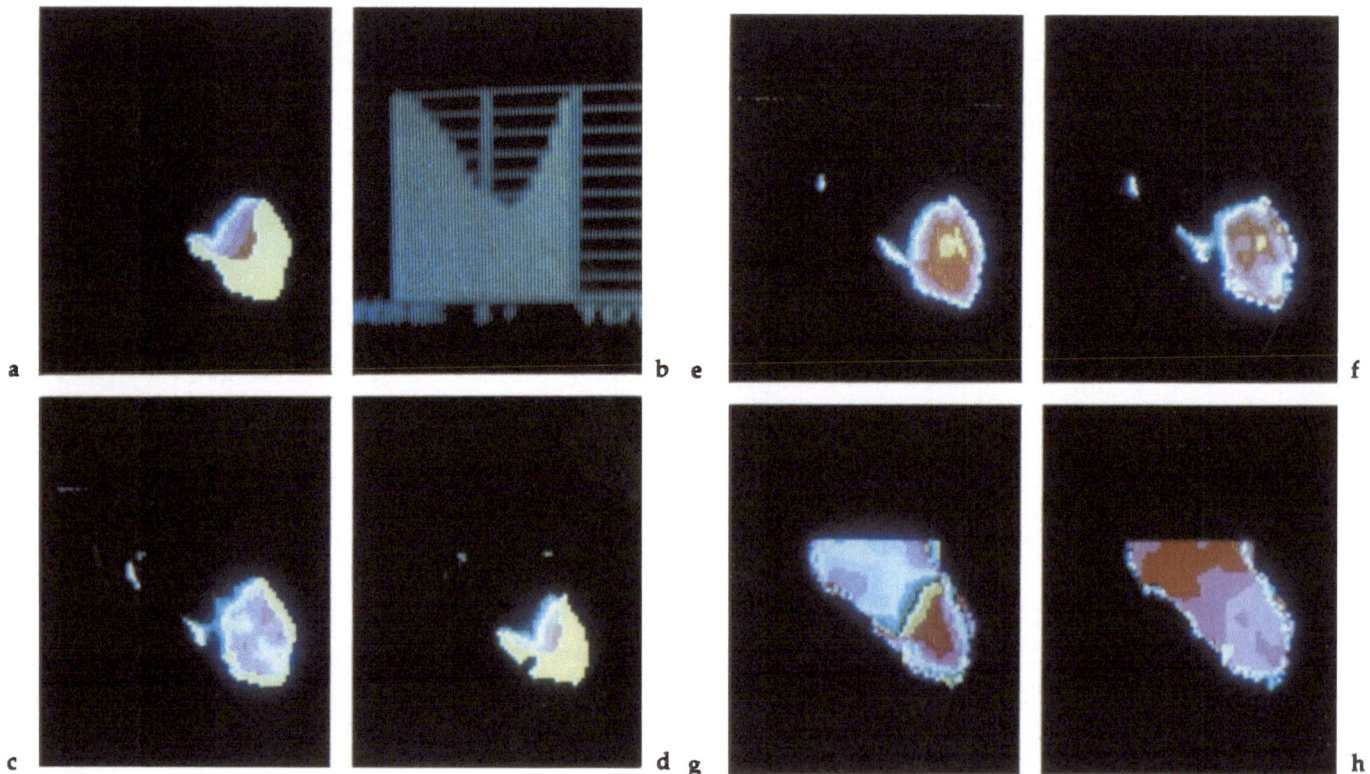

Figure 5.2 Case 1: (Exercise) Note accentuation of early systolic abnormalities but preservation of global function (EF=70). **a**, REFI; **b**, volume curve; **c**, first half REFI: **d**, second half REFI; **e**, ejection rate; **f**, first half ER; **g**, transit; **h**, first half transit.

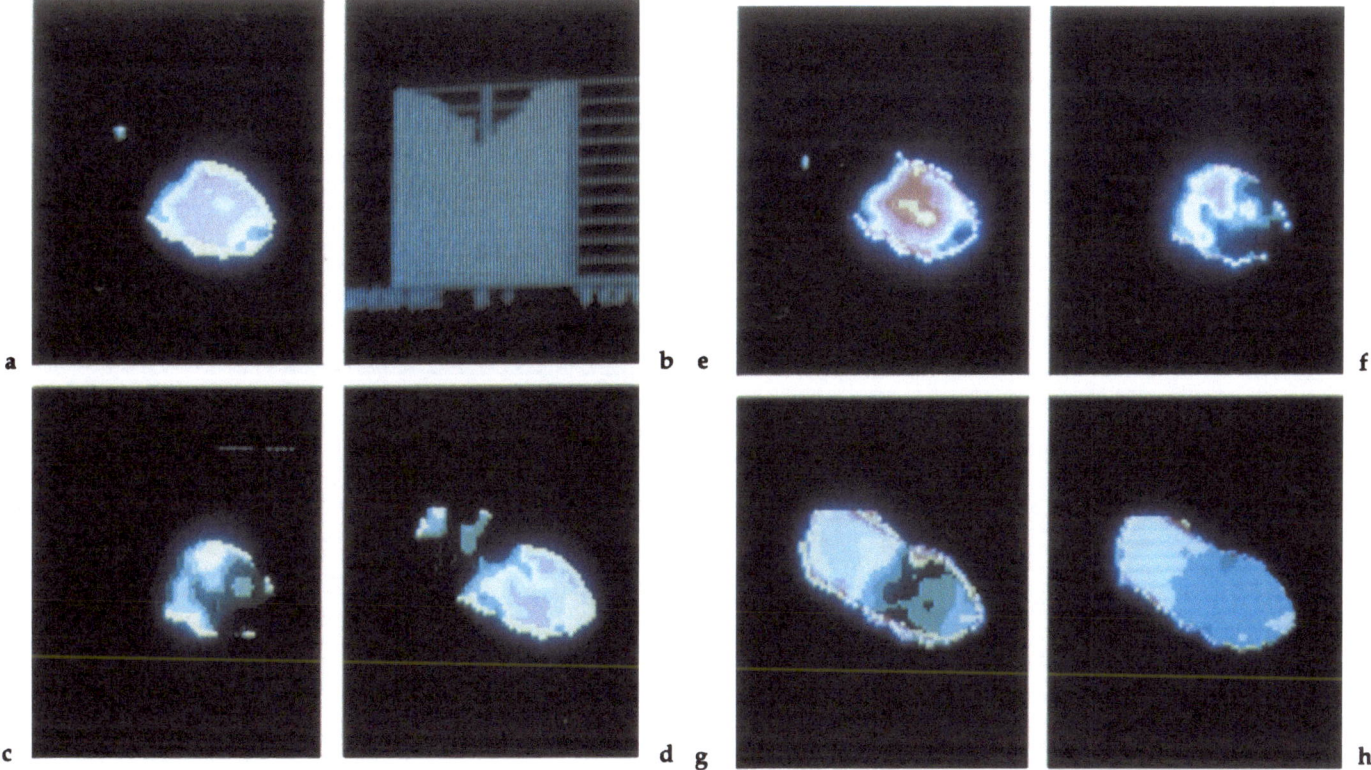

Figure 5.3 Case 2: (Rest) Anterior projection; *LAD*. 40-year-old male 1 month post anterior infarction. Early systolic abnormalities typical of ischaemia. **a**, REFI; **b**, volume curve; **c**, first half REFI; **d**, second half REFI; **e**, ejection rate; **f**, first half ER; **g**, transit; **h**, first half transit.

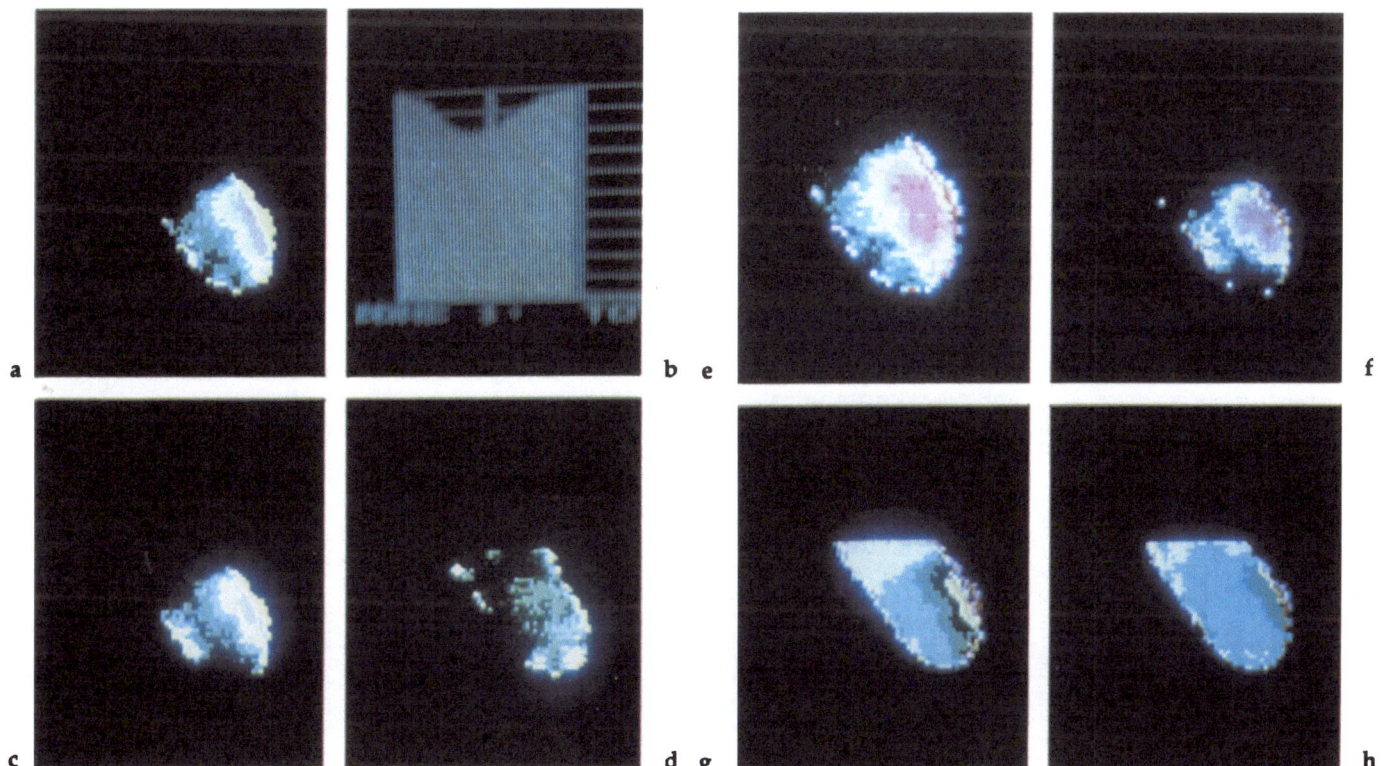

Figure 5.4 Case 2: (Rest) LAO projection. The septum is well seen in this projection (left) with early and late systolic changes typical of infarction. **a**, REFI; **b**, volume curve; **c**, first half REFI; **d**, second half REFI; **e**, ejection rate; **f**, first half ER; **g**, transit; **h**, first half transit.

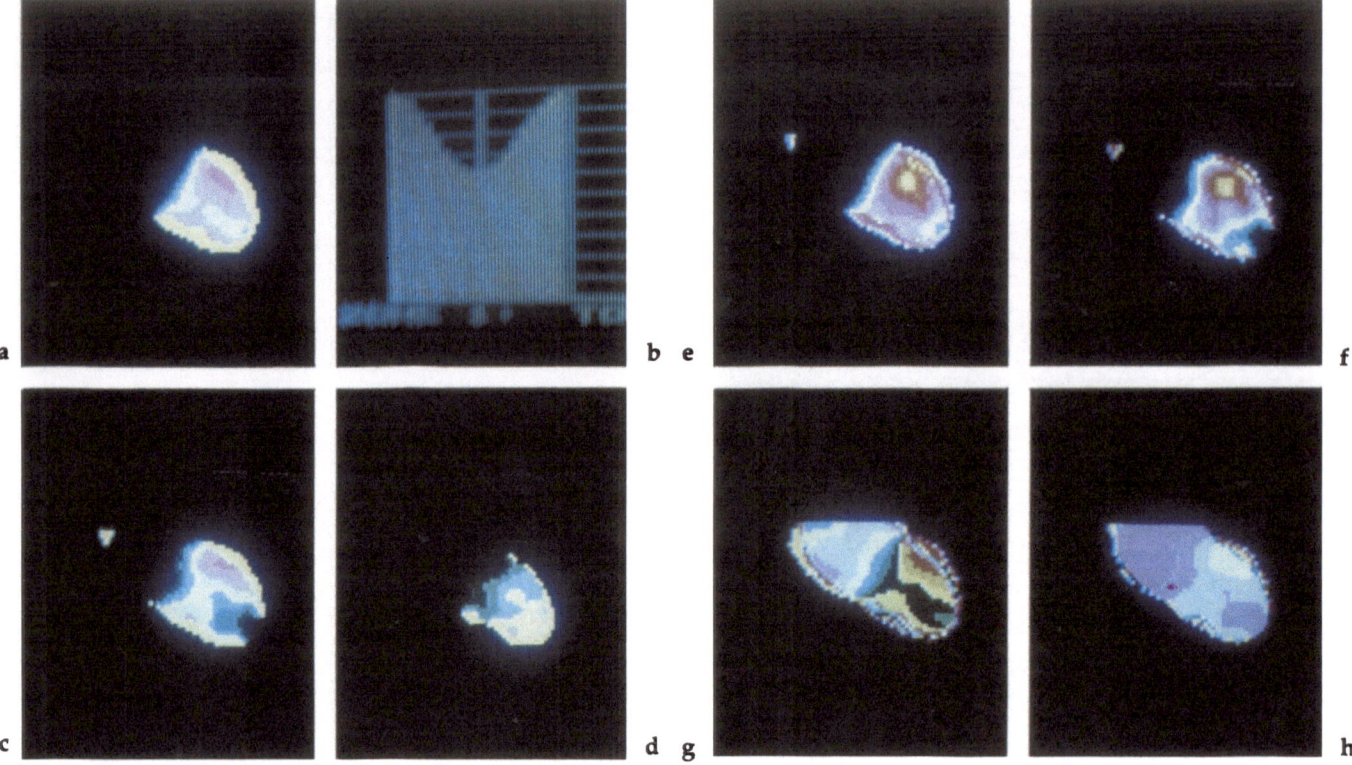

Figure 5.5 Case 3: (Rest) *LAD, circumflex and hypoplastic RCA*. 56-year-old female with recent episode of chest pain. Typical ischaemic changes extend to the apex (LAD lesion). **a**, REFI; **b**, volume curve; **c**, first half REFI; **d**, second half REFI; **e**, ejection rate; **f**, first half ER; **g**, transit; **h**, first half transit.

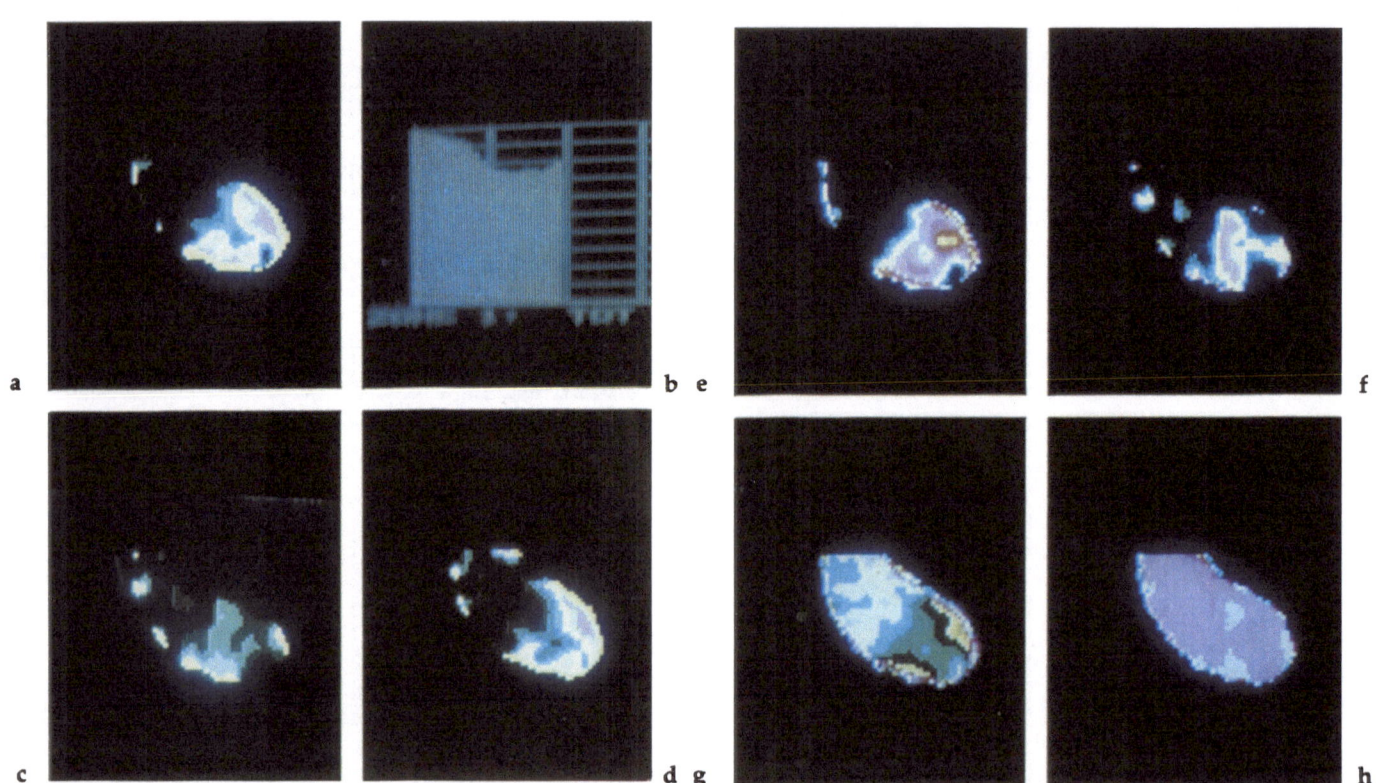

Figure 5.6 Case 4: (Rest) *Triple vessel disease*. 50-year-old male with symptoms of 'oesophagitis'. Rest study shows severe diffuse ischaemic change. **a**, REFI; **b**, volume curve; **c**, first half REFI; **d**, second half REFI; **e**, ejection rate; **f**, first half ER; **g**, transit; **h**, first half transit.

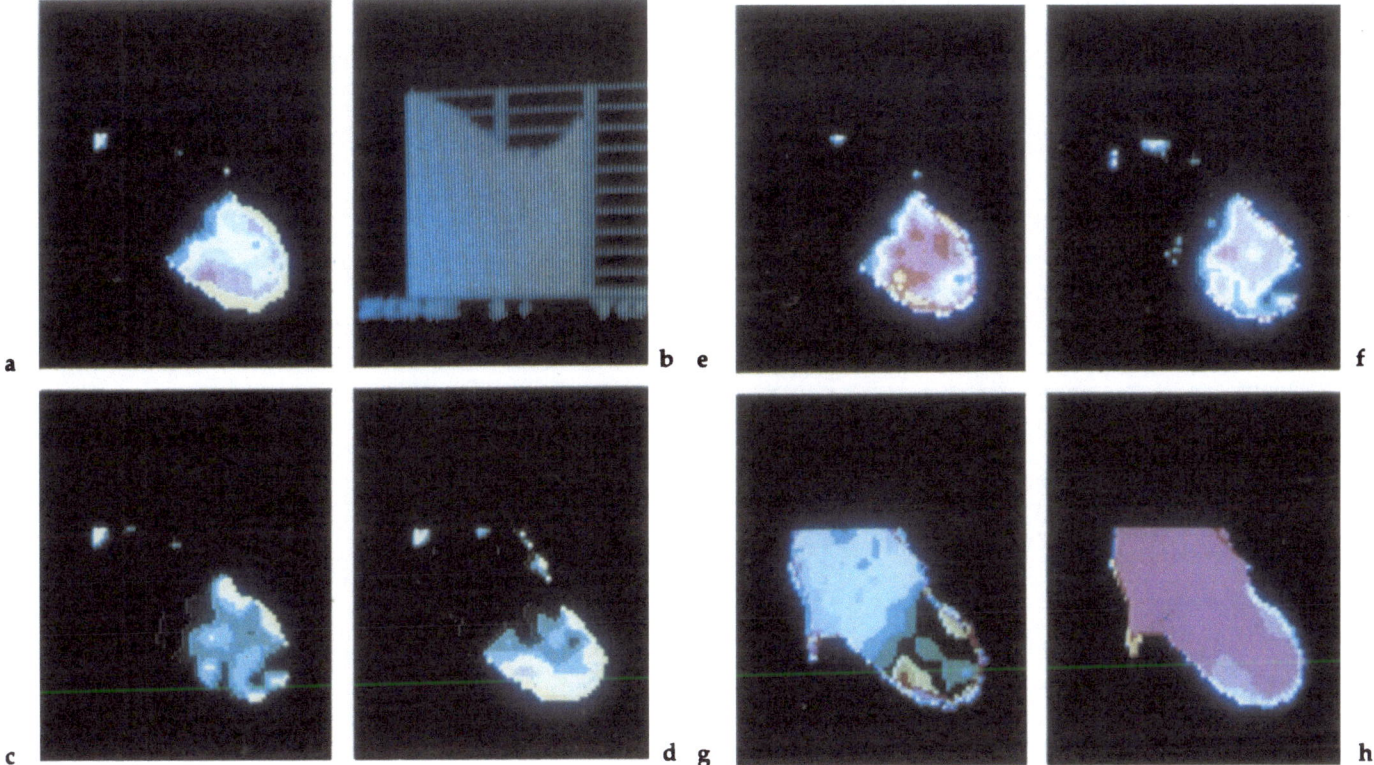

Figure 5.7 Case 5: (Exercise) *LAD and mild RCA*. 59-year-old asymptomatic male seen for 'check-up'. Typical ischaemic changes involve the anterolateral wall to apex.

a, REFI; **b**, volume curve; **c**, first half REFI; **d**, second half REFI; **e**, ejection rate; **f**, first half ER; **g**, transit; **h**, first half transit.

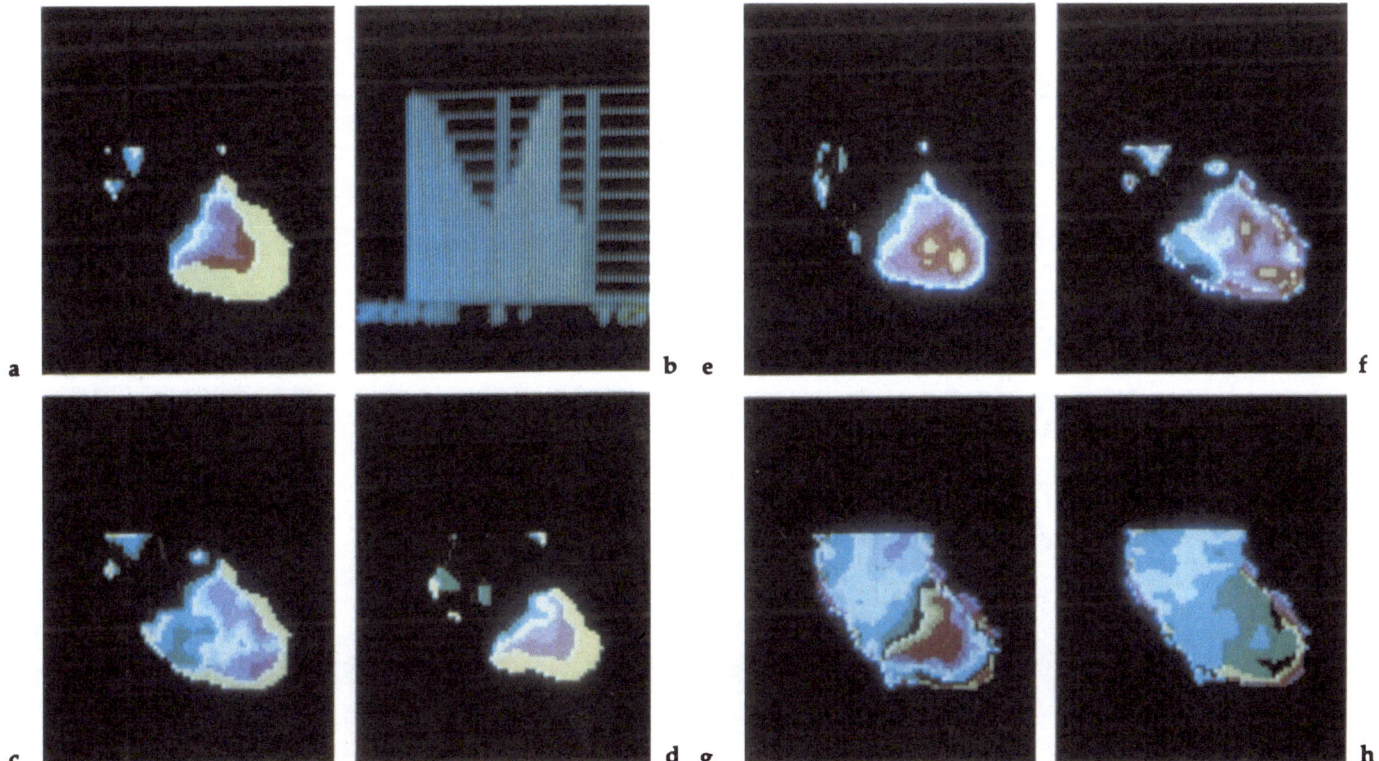

Figure 5.8 Case 6: (Exercise) *Triple Vessel Disease*. 47-year-old male asymptomatic jogger seen for executive 'check-up'. First half images typical of ischaemia, but REFI is normal. **a**, REFI; **b**, volume curve; **c**, first half REFI; **d**, second half REFI; **e**, ejection rate; **f**, first half ER; **g**, transit; **h**, first half transit.

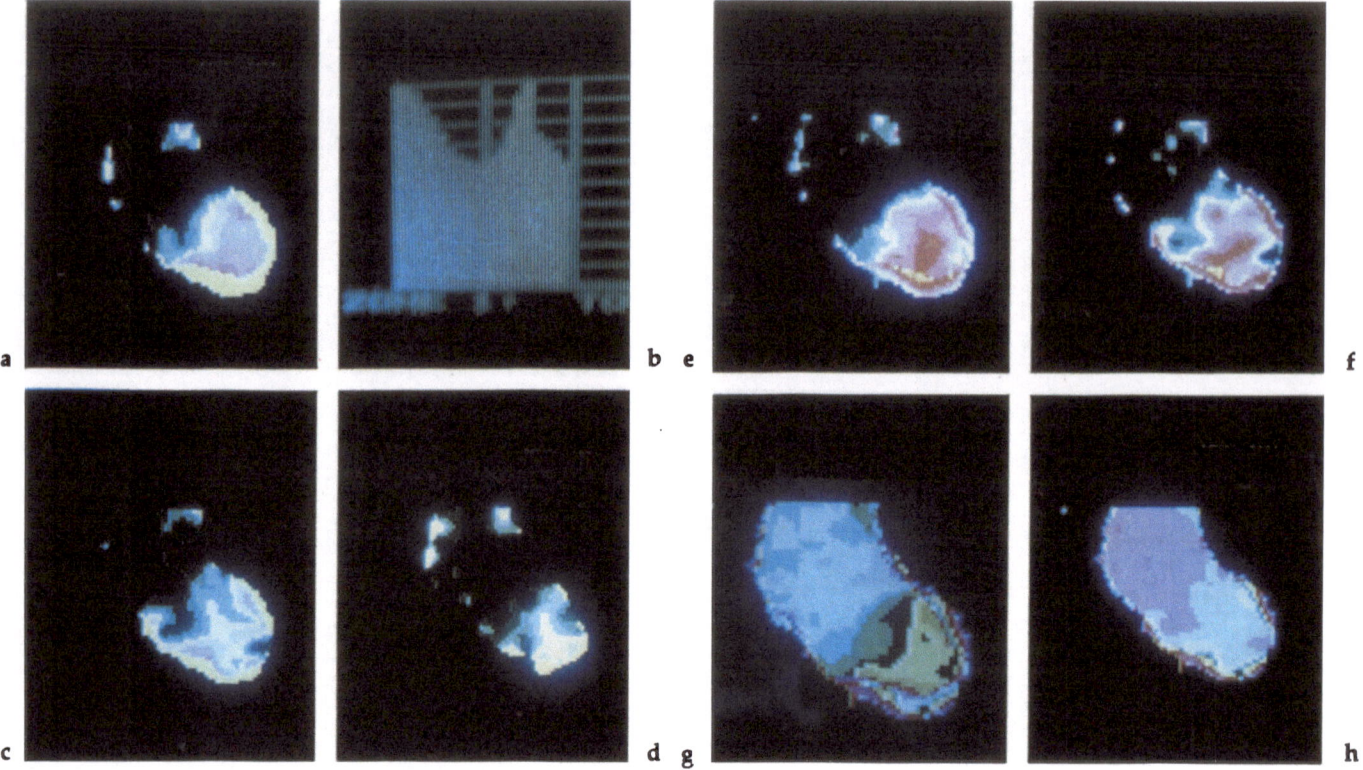

Figure 5.9 Case 7: (Exercise) *LAD and circumflex*. 36-year-old female nurse with family history of CAD. Typical ischaemic change is seen anterolaterally and inferiorally.

a, REFI; **b**, volume curve; **c**, first half REFI; **d**, second half REFI; **e**, ejection rate; **f**, first half ER; **g**, transit; **h**, first half transit.

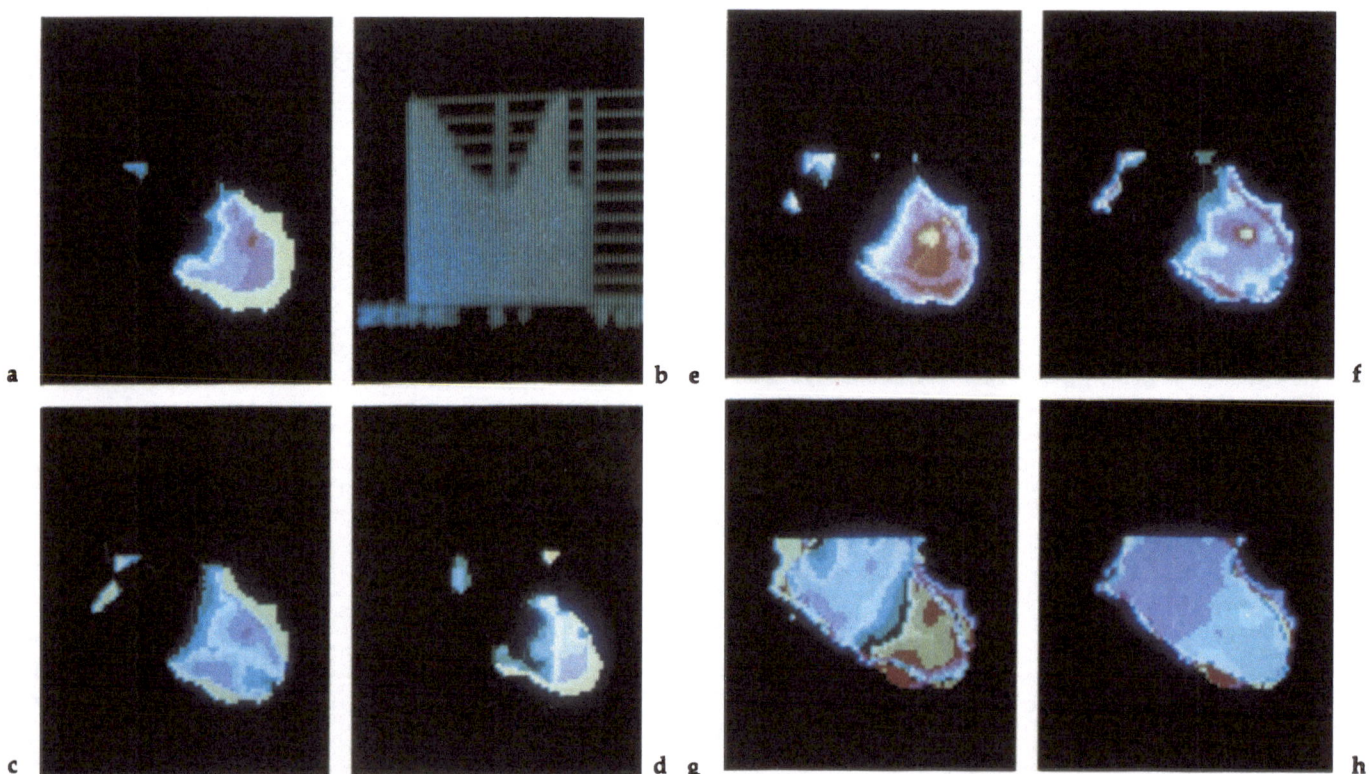

Figure 5.10 Case 8: (Exercise) *LAD*. 26-year-old male with chest pain. Early systolic wall motion abnormality extends to the apex typical of an LAD lesion. **a**, REFI; **b**,

volume curve; **c**, first half REFI; **d**, second half REFI; **e**, ejection rate; **f**, first half ER; **g**, transit; **h**, first half transit.

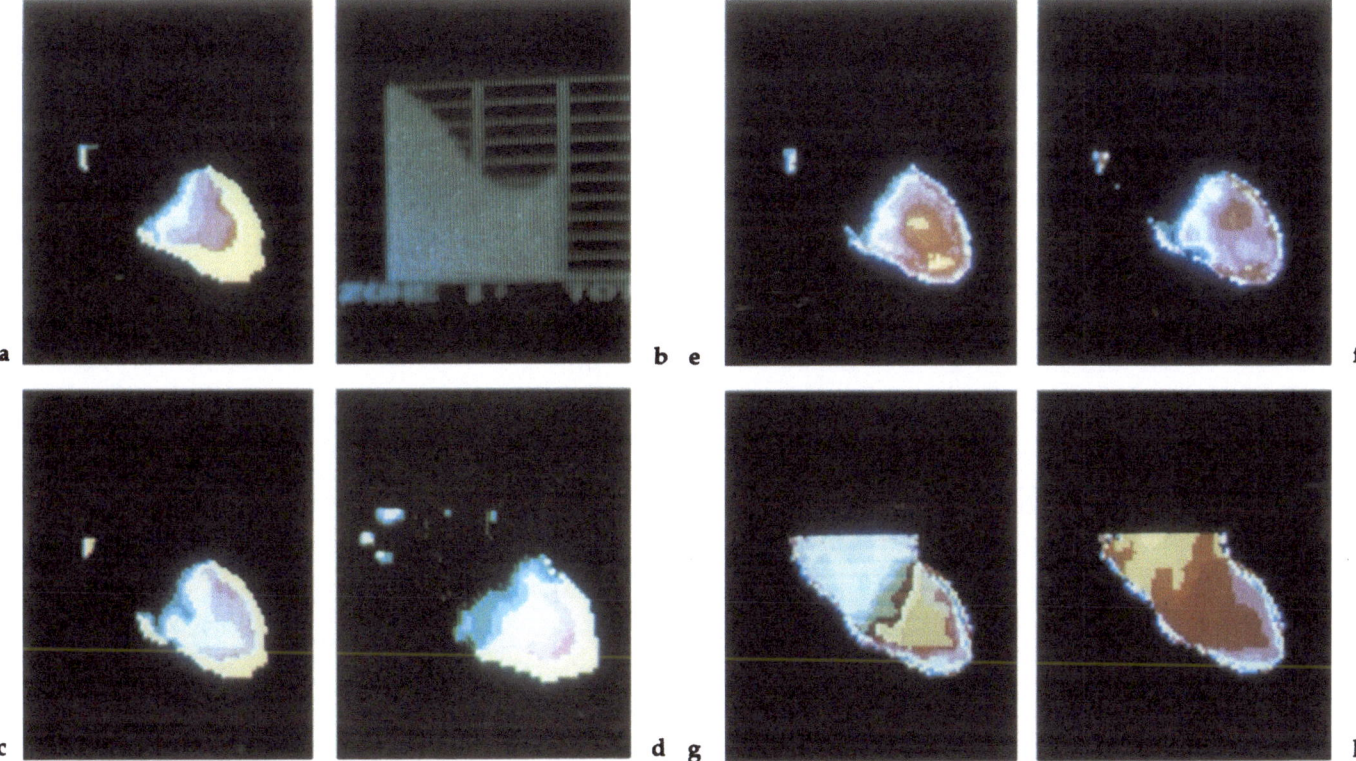

Figure 5.11 Case 9: (Exercise) *RCA and circumflex.* 50-year-old male with exertional dyspnoea. Posterior, inferior changes are seen with normal REFI and global fx

(EF=68). **a**, REFI; **b**, volume curve; **c**, first half REFI; **d**, second half REFI; **e**, ejection rate; **f**, first half ER; **g**, transit; **h**, first half transit.

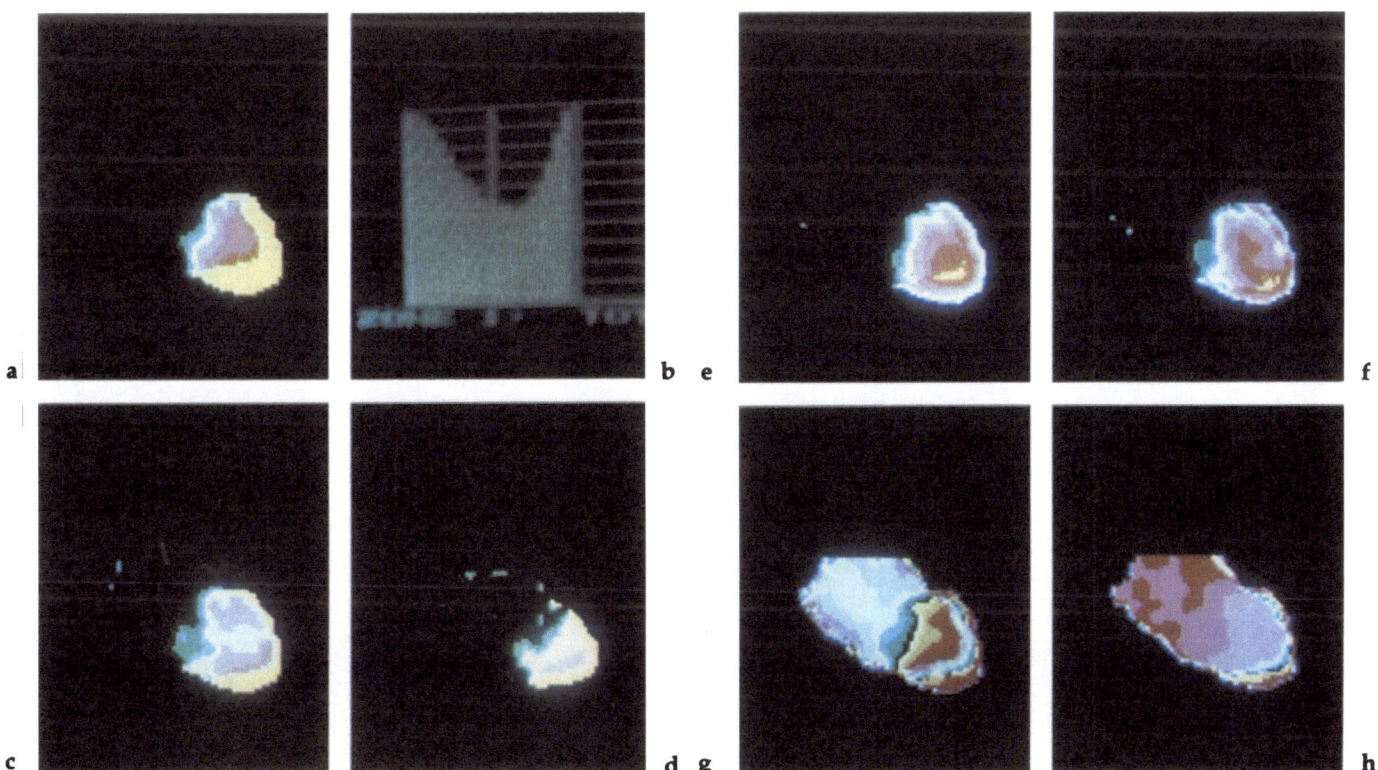

Figure 5.12 Case 10: (Exercise) *Diagonal branch of LAD.* 43-year-old male with chest pain. A focal wall motion abnormality extends to the periphery of the high lateral

wall. **a**, REFI; **b**, volume curve; **c**, first half REFI; **d**, second half REFI; **e**, ejection rate; **f**, first half ER; **g**, transit; **h**, first half transit.

6

Functional Imaging in Myocardial Infarction

N. SCHAD AND F. BRUZZONE

Prognosis in patients who had a prior documented myocardial infarct is affected by residual left ventricular function, the number of coronary narrowings and the presence of collateral flow, according to a multi-institutional study of 467 patients with an average follow-up of 50.5 months (Reale and Romeo, 1983). Invasive measurements of global ejection fractions showed no statistical difference between patients without late complications (52.86 ± 0.8 (SE) %) and with reinfarction (50.37 ± 2.3 (SE) %) respectively. However, in patients who died, the global EF was significantly lower (45.19 ± 3.2 (SE)%). Three-vessel disease was also significantly more frequent than in the other two groups together. In this study collateral flow was noted in about two thirds of the patients with or without complications or reinfarction, but in 86.8% of the patients who died during the follow-up period.

Thus, left ventricular function and coronary anatomy are the main determinants of prognosis and are of paramount importance for clinical decision making and therapy in patients with a history of myocardial infarction. Left ventricular function is mainly influenced by the extent of the infarcted zone and the degree of its malfunction, by eventual complications such as aneurysm formation, ventricular septal defect or mitral reflux, and by other coronary territories jeopardized by additional coronary narrowings. First pass radionuclide angiography can non-invasively provide information about these elements of diagnosis. Radionuclide examinations have been utilized in patients with myocardial infarction (Reduto *et al.*, 1978; Shah *et al.*, 1980). First pass studies in patients who have had myocardial infarction (Schad, 1976a,b; 1977) and functional imaging can help evaluate the following:

(1) extent and degree of malfunction in the infarcted area

(2) presence of complications such as ventricular aneurysm, ventricular septal defect, and mitral reflux

(3) degree of pulmonary congestion and involvement of right heart function

(4) response of infarcted and adjacent zones to nitrate medication, i.e. assessment of residual myocardial function.

(5) presence of other vascular territories in jeopardy.

Cine-angiographic studies have shown a constant *topographical correspondence* between the presence of Q-waves in the e.c.g. and the regional alterations of contractility. In cases of non-transmural subendocardial infarction, however, motion disorders cannot always be seen. On the other hand, in transmural infarcts, the zone of altered motion necessarily appears larger than the zone with pure scar formation, the ischaemic peri-infarction area being included in the motion disorder. Global left ventricular function at rest does not necessarily have to be depressed as long as the akinetic–hypokinetic segment is limited in size and some eventual compensatory hyperkinesia is present.

In *functional images* the infarcted zones produce the most severe dysfunction that characteristically is seen at rest (*see* Figure 4.16). In ischaemia, equivalent severe dysfunction is only produced by stressing the patient particularly in the case of severe coronary obstruction and inadequate collateral flow. Rarely, it can be observed in preinfarction angina at rest. For detailed description of the adopted functional images *see* Chapters 2 and 4.

In the infarcted segment very low *regional ejection fractions and rates* or defects are very common and usually seen during the entire systole. Defects, however, may be due to akinesia or dyskinesia, i.e. paradoxical motion. *Dyskinesia or systolic outward motion* is best seen on the so-called *regional systolic increase image* that exhibits all regions where blood increases during systole. Since due to the mathematical process only regions with a predominant increase of blood during contraction are visualized, very short-lasting paradoxical outward motion is not presented. Thus, even small zones of dyskinesia on this image are diagnostically relevant and usually point to the centre of the infarcted zone. On the other hand, with small infarcted areas some systolic tethering can still occur mimicking some wall motion (yellow band) on regional ejection fraction images. Since, however, blood is only displaced but not actively ejected the adjacent zones typically show extremely low regional ejection fractions and rates.

The most informative functional image in patients with prior myocardial infarction is the *regional mean (transit) time image* (centre of gravity) reflecting regional persistence of blood during systole (*see*

Chapter 2). Contribution from infarcted akinetic segments to outflow is minimal with the effect that regional persistence of blood from underneath the infarcted zone to the centre and outflow tract is prolonged. Thus, the longest mean times result immediately under the infarcted zone, corresponding to mean times as usually only seen in the subvalvular area or in the ascending aorta. More centrally and toward the outflow tract, other regions may also contribute to flow so that somewhat shorter but still long mean times result. In the image, 'channels' of long subvalvular mean times appear to conduct toward the peripheral infarcted segment where usually the longest times are found. Analogous images have been recently observed with nuclear magnetic resonance examinations where low flows underneath infarcts can produce intracavitary signals.

The most important *complication* particularly of anterior infarcts is the formation of a ventricular aneurysm. Functional imaging of left ventricular aneurysms is described in Chapter 7. Other complications are *mitral reflux* and *ventricular septal defects*. These can be detected on the regional systolic increase image showing systolic increase of blood or activity at the location of the mitral valve or in the pulmonary outflow tract respectively. Significantly lengthened left ventricular washout (*see below*) with normal or subnormal global ejection fraction points to an early return of blood or activity to the left ventricle due to a reflux or left-to-right shunt. The latter can also be recognized as early recirculation on the pulmonary curve and the amount of shunt can be measured with accuracy. The degree of mitral reflux can be estimated by calculation of the regurgitant fraction (*see* Chapter 13).

First pass examination has the great advantage that the passage of the gamma-emitting tracer through the central circulation and the individual heart chambers can be recorded as a curve, which originally was called a radiocardiogram and included the whole heart (Prinzmetal *et al.*, 1948). By defining discrete cardiac regions of interest and by using a gamma-camera and a projection which best separates the heart chambers from each other, it is possible to avoid obtaining composite curves due to the superimposition of heart cavities and/or large vessels. Thus, it is possible to measure *lung transit* which is prolonged with congestion and to assess right ventricular washout, a mirror of *right ventricular function*.

The injection technique should guarantee that the input into the heart, i.e. the superior vena cava, does not exceed an acceptable width since a poor injection would lengthen the entire transit to an unpredictable extent. The activity bolus injected into an antecubital vein is normally advanced to the superior vena cava by a flush of 15–20 ml saline at a flow rate of 8–10 ml/s. The bolus appears in the superior vena cava after about $0.8\,s$ $(0.74 \pm 0.3,$ $n = 109)$. The pool transit time in the superior vena cava corresponds to the width in time of the bolus input between the points of maximum inflow and outflow. It was measured in 200 injections in our laboratory and related to five heart rate groups (range 50–109). Overall pool transit time averaged $1.28\,s$

$(\pm 0.045\,s\ SE)$. Two standard deviations of the pool transit time did not exceed $2.5\,s$. The average time values did not vary significantly from one heart rate group to another, but there was a significant difference of $0.44\,s$ between the two extremes, i.e., at heart rates of 50–59 and 90–109. Thus, there is a slight tendency to a shorter pool transit time in the superior vena cava with an increase in heart rate. This observation can be explained by the normal acceleration of flow in the superior vena cava during early systole and early diastole, which occur earlier in the cardiac cycle given elevated heart rates.

Having determined the bolus-input into the superior vena cava one can measure average *peak times*, for example from the count maximum in the right ventricle to that in the left ventricle. Peak times offer a simple index of blood transit which can be obtained from ventricular histograms with little calculation. They demonstrate a consistent relation to mean transit times (Jones *et al.*, 1972), but they are heart-rate dependent. *Mean transit times* provide a very reproducible index of blood transit. They can simply be added or subtracted from each other. From the pulmonary mean transit time it is possible to derive the pulmonary blood volume and index if the cardiac output is known (pulmonary mean transit time × cardiac index = pulmonary blood volume index). Normal values, expressed as relative to superior vena cava time zero have been reported by Scholz *et al.* (1980).

Peak times and transit times become longer with decreasing heart rate because propagation of the tracer bolus is pulsatile and hence governed by ventricular function. By dividing the measured time by the medium length of one cycle during transit, one can obtain *number of transit cycles*. That is, by introducing the number of heart cycles as the time unit, one normalizes for heart-rate dependency. In fact, experiences with over 10 000 first pass radionuclide studies of the heart in our laboratory have shown a nearly constant number of transit cycles to the peak in the right and left ventricle as long as no signs of heart failure, significant lung disease, or a left ventricular ejection fraction below 40% were present (Schad and Nickel, 1981). In 200 haemodynamically normal patients peak times in seconds and number of peak cycles for the right and left ventricle have been compared for different heart rate groups and statistically validated. Only with heart rates of 50–59 beats/min slightly, but significantly, lower number of heart cycles from start of injection to peak in the right and left ventricle have been found. For all other heart rate groups no statistically significant differences could be seen.

Table 6.1 reports the average normal number of transit cycles with a superior vena cava bolus-input not exceeding $2.5\,s$ in width. Number of RV and LV washout cycles is added which reflects ventricular function, i.e. ejection fraction (Schad, 1968) provided there is no early return of activity or blood by reflux or shunt. For practical purposes one can state that a right to left ventricle transit, reflecting lung transit, of more than 9 cycles is abnormal. RV washout of more than 6 cycles and LV washout of more than 11 cycles are pathological. The computer easily counts the number of transit cycles.

Table 6.1 Average number of peak transit cycles and washout cycles in 200 haemodynamically normal subjects after compact superior vena cava input

Compartment	Average values	SE
SVC input	1.28 seconds	± 0.045
RV peak	3.97 cycles	± 0.07
washout	4.68 cycles	± 0.05
LV peak	11.17 cycles	± 0.1
washout	8.64 cycles	± 0.1
Lung transit	7.2 cycles	± 0.08

Lung transit of more than 9 cycles is abnormal. RV washout exceeding 6 cycles and LV washout exceeding 11 cycles can be considered as pathological

Thus, in patients who had a prior documented myocardial infarct lung transit is determined. If it exceeds nine cycles some *degree of congestion* can be presumed. Functional involvement of the right ventricle is indicated by prolonged RV washout, obviously, as long as concomitant severe lung disease or RV pathology can be excluded (*see* Chapter 19).

Assessment of *residual myocardial function* in infarcted and adjacent zones is of primary importance for the decision to perform bypass-grafting of the corresponding artery. Regional left ventricular function can be examined before and after nitrate administration. The regional analysis of functional images allows one to determine whether function in severely hypokinetic or akinetic regions improves after unloading the ventricle or remains unchanged thereby suggesting extensive scar formation.

When global EF, ejection velocity, and end-diastolic volumes at rest, after nitroglycerin, and postoperatively were compared (Kremers *et al.*, 1978), a significant difference was found between the resting and nitroglycerin data, but not between the nitroglycerin and postoperative data. Regional analysis on a total of 120 segments showed similar changes: no improvement of dyskinetic segments (8/120) after nitroglycerin or bypass surgery and improvement of approximately half of the hypokinetic and akinetic segments following nitroglycerin and surgery; only a small number (9/120) showed improvement after surgery that was not predicted by the results with nitroglycerin (Hellmann, 1978). The studies showed a sensitivity and a specificity of 81% in predicting potential wall-motion improvement after revascularization.

Global ejection fraction and segmental wall motion, i.e. hemiaxis shortening, have been evaluated in our laboratory in 44 patients with documented myocardial infarction (Pikal, 1980). After *nitrate administration*[*], the number of segments with normal motion (25% shortening or more) increased by 51%, the number with hypokinesia (11–25% shortening) decreased by 22% and the number with akinesia (10% shortening or less) decreased by 60%. All infarcted segments showed motion disorders: 70% of the hypokinetic and 67% of the akinetic segments improved after nitrate administration, but no response was observed in the four dyskinetic

* Isosorbide dinitrate (Ayerst).

segments. Of 59 adjacent segments, 54% showed a motion disorder: three fourths of these segments improved after nitrates. No difference was observed in the response pattern of the anterior and inferoposterior infarcts (Schad and Nickel, 1979a,b). Global EF rose after nitrate medication by an average of 6%.

With the advent of *shortlived radionuclides such as gold/Au 195m* with a half life of 30.5 s it is possible to perform repeated consecutive radionuclide injections since radiation exposure of the patient is minimal (for Au 195m, *see* Chapter 1). To assess the usefulness of a second gold 195m injection in the *LAO-view* 30 patients with prior documented myocardial infarction have been examined in the RAO and LAO projection in our laboratory. The anterior wall of the left ventricle was involved 12 times, the inferoposterior wall 24 times and strictly the apical zone only once. By the use of both oblique projections a complete correspondence with the electrocardiographic location of the infarct could be found. Similar high topographical correspondence had already previously been seen in a study of comparison between the electrocardiographic pattern after myocardial infarction and the location of severe dysfunction by the use of wall motion criteria in the RAO view (Schuberl, 1978; Schad, 1977). This preceding study has also shown that the extent of alterations in the chest leads generally underestimated the expansion of wall motion disorder. If on the admission electrocardiogram more than four leads were involved, permanent dyskinesia was found at the centre of the infarct. In the present biplane study, in 26 patients out of 30 (86.6%) diagnosis could be established by the use of the discussed signs on functional images with the RAO view alone. Four times, however, only the LAO view clearly indicated the site of the infarcted zone and its posterolateral location, in correspondence to the electrocardiographic infarct localization. Except for one strictly apical infarct the additional LAO projection provided useful information about eventual lateral or septal extension of the infarction. The second LAO view made it generally easier to determine the three-dimensional expansion of the infarcted zone. As expected, the image visualizing mean transit times were the most informative with respect to infarct location and extension in both projections, whereas the regional ejection fraction image was the less useful (Schad *et al.*, 1984b).

In conclusion, from functional imaging in myocardial infarction one gains a clinically important, accurate insight into the extent of severe dysfunction at the infarcted zone and into the actual residual left ventricular function and its response to unloading with nitrates. Additional vascular territories at risk can be discovered and from first transit curves degree of congestion and right ventricular functional involvement can be estimated. Complications such as ventricular aneurysm, mitral reflux and ventricular septal defect are non-invasively revealed on functional images and their clinical relevance can be determined on compartmental histograms.

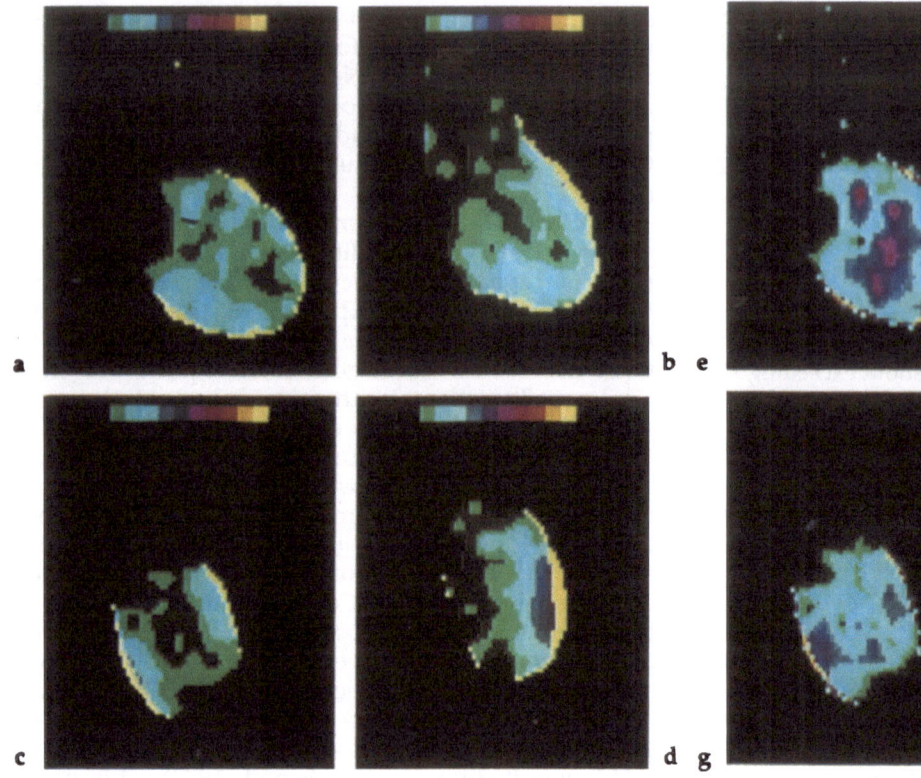

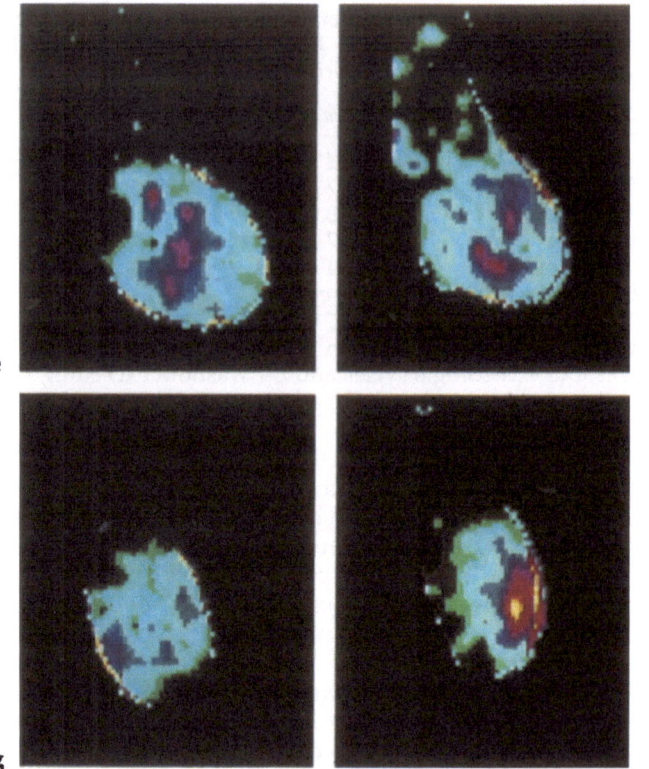

Figure 6.1 *Anterior myocardial infarction – significant LAD stenosis. Narrowing of the distal CX. Aurum 195m injection.*

a–d, REFI in two oblique projections before and after nitrate: in RAO-view significantly reduced EFs at the entire LAD-territory and posteriorly (**a**) improving anteriorly and inferiorly after nitrate* (**b**). In LAO-view defect, i.e. no EFs apical and anterolateral in correspondence to the infarcted site (**c**), after nitrates

improvement of contraction at posterolateral but some deterioration at the apical and anteroseptal side (**d**).

e–h, Regional ERs in two oblique projections before and after nitrate: in RAO-view reduced ERs along the anterior wall and posteriorly (**e**) improving in the middle and upper anterior wall after nitrates (**f**). In LAO-view defect no ERs, at apex (**g**) significantly improving laterally (**h**).

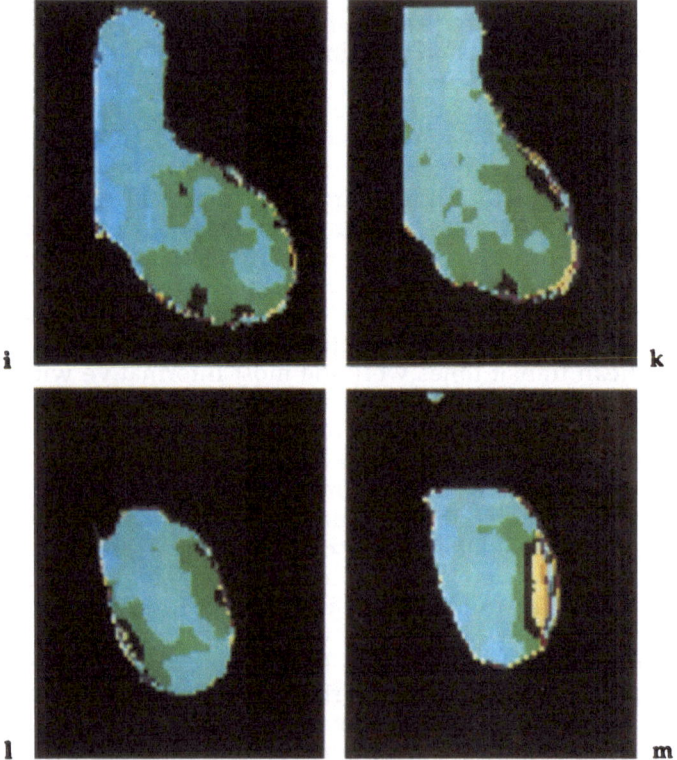

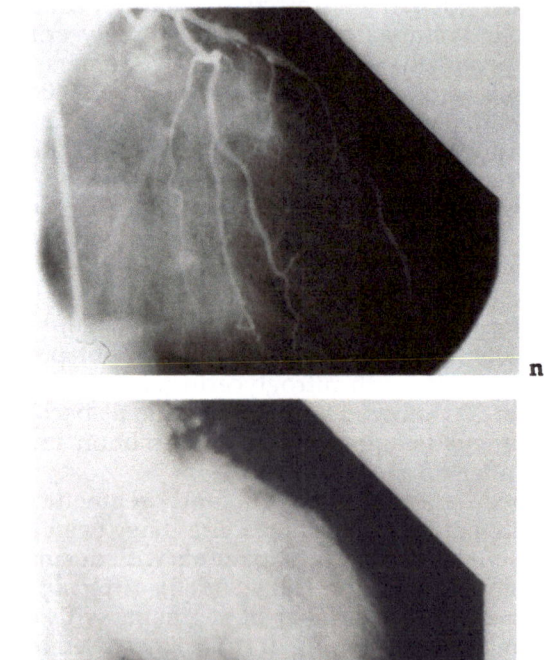

i,k,l,m, Regional MTTs in two oblique projections before and after nitrate: in RAO-view prolonged mean-times at the anterior and posterior territories with the longest times near the apex (**i**) after nitrate shortening of times at upper and the anterior wall and also at the apical region

* Isosorbide dinitrate (Ayerst)

(**k**). In the LAO-view longest mean times at the apex (**l**). Significant improvement of mean times laterally (**m**).

n,o, Coronary angiogram and levogram: significant LAD stenosis, narrowing of distal CX (**n**). At end systole severe hypokinesis of anterior apical and posterior wall (**o**).

56

Figure 6.1 *(continued)*

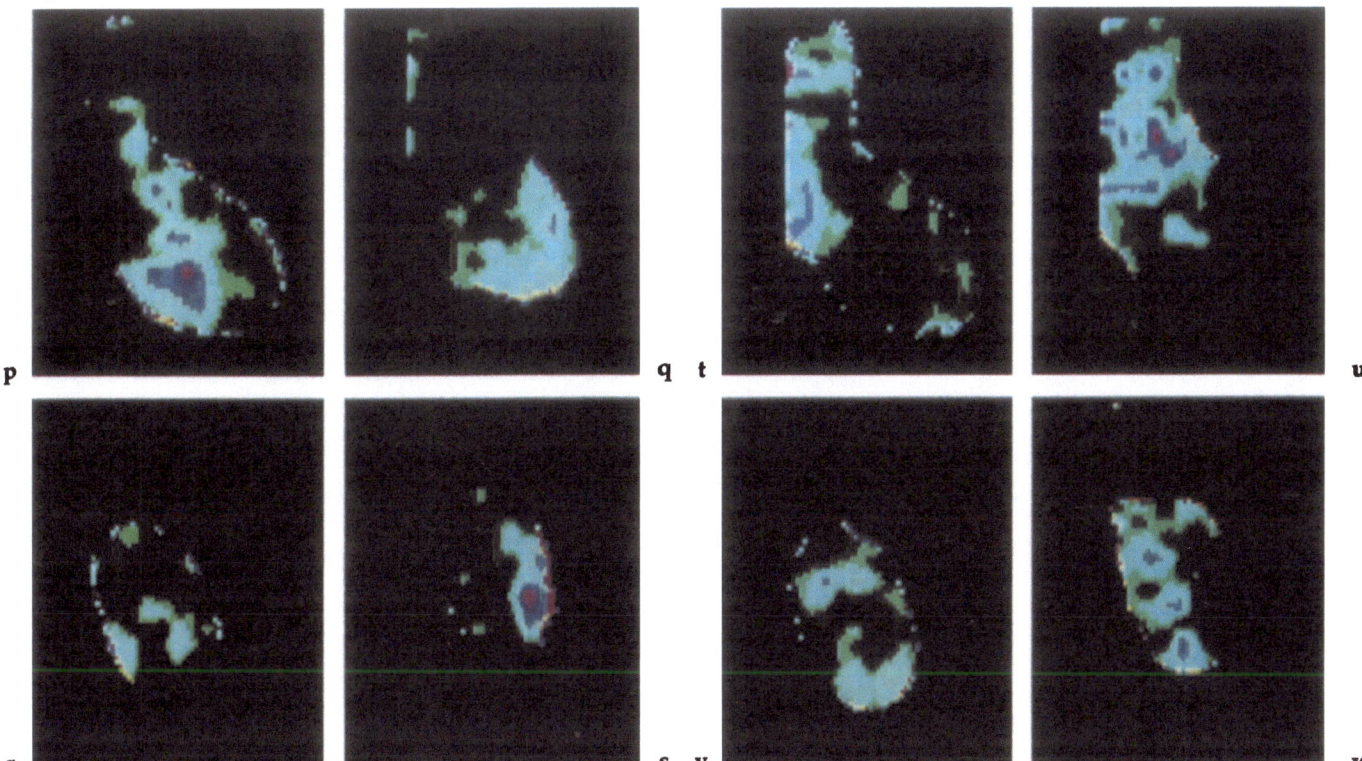

p **p–s,** Regional rapid filling rates in two oblique projections, before and after nitrates (160–175 ms): in RAO-view rapid inflow is deviated to the compliant inferior wall **(p)**, after nitrates improvement of compliance at the anterior and apical wall **(g)**. In LAO-view not initial inflow to the apex **(r)**, after nitrates inflow deviated to the lateral wall **(s)**.

t–w, Paradoxical decrease or inward motion during rapid filling in two projections before and after nitrates. In RAO-view paradoxical inward movement along the less compliant anterior wall **(t)** improving after nitrates **(u)**. In LAO-view paradoxical inward motion with inward displacement of blood at the apex and anterolaterally **(v)**, after nitrates improvement laterally **(w)**.

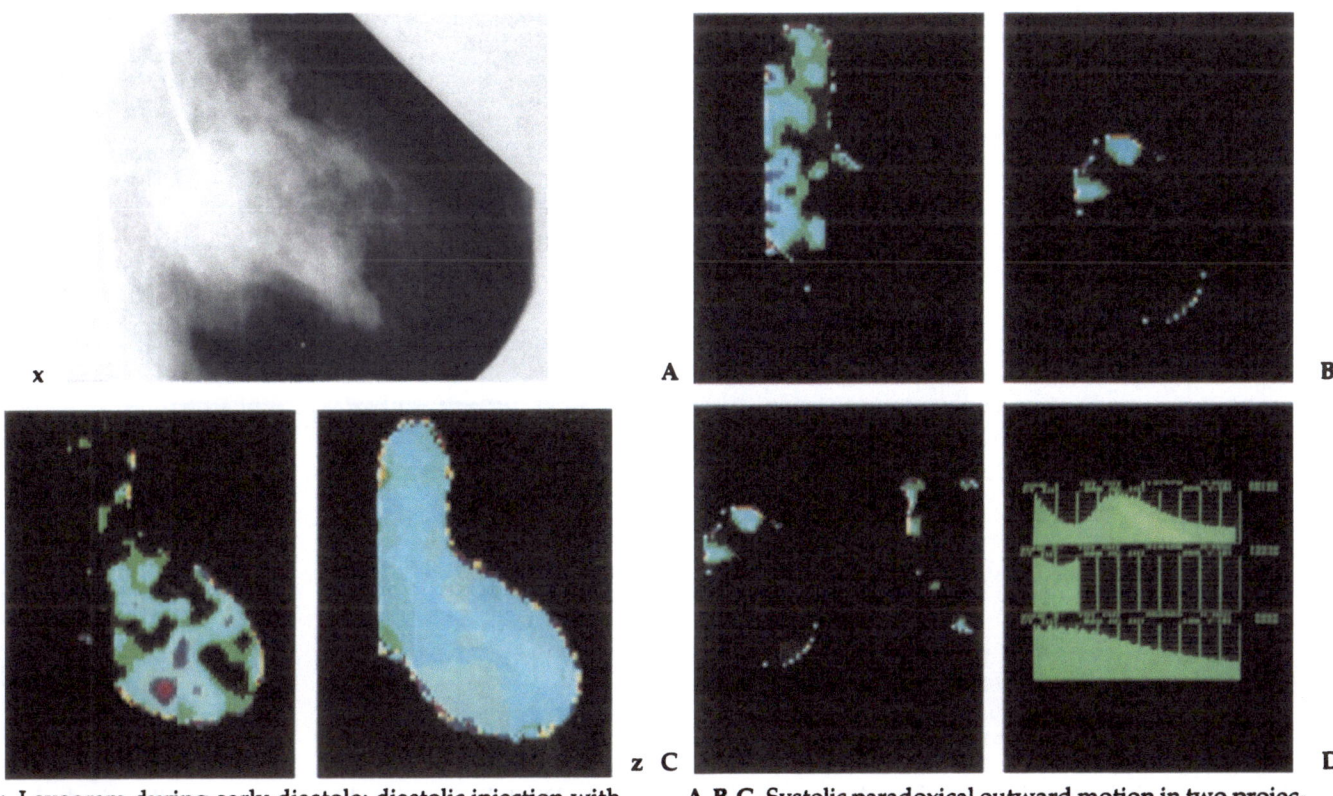

x, Levogram during early diastole: diastolic injection with distribution of contrast material mainly toward the postero-inferior wall similar to rapid filling image **(x)**.

y,z, Regional ERs during the first half-systole present a very irregular image **(y)** in comparison to the rapid filling image **(p)** lasting about the same time interval. Mean times image during rapid filling shows longest times, i.e. persistence of blood inferoposteriorly **(z)**. Compare with **(x)**.

A,B,C, Systolic paradoxical outward motion in two projections, minimal in the RAO-view **(A)** mainly in LAO-view **(B)**. LAO-view after nitrates, somewhat improving laterally **(C)**.

D, Transit curves present delayed lung transit (upper) and LV washout (lower) as well as flattened LV volume curve (middle).

57

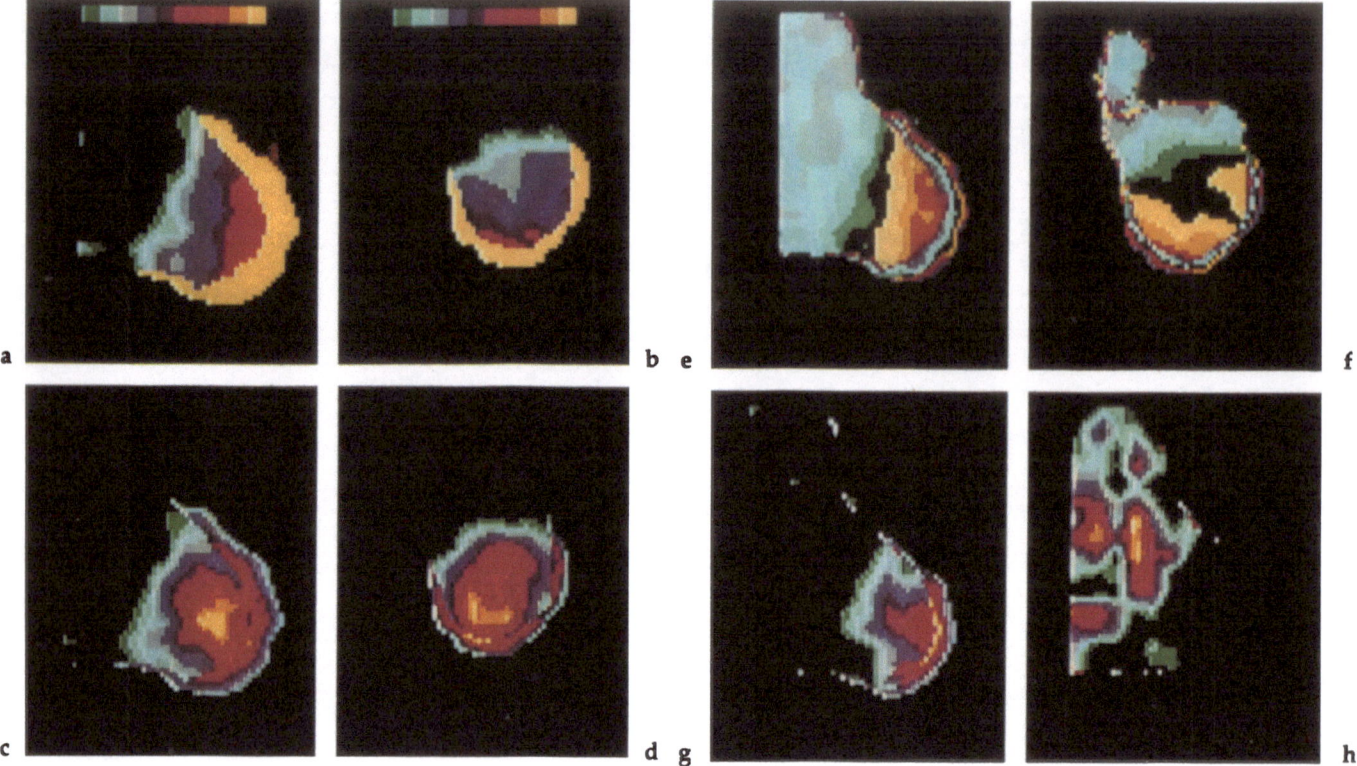

Figure 6.2 *Posterolateral myocardial infarction – Aurum 195m injection.*
a–d, In RAO-view no EFs and ERs posteriorly (defect) **(a,c)** reduced ERs at upper anterior wall. In LAO-view same loss of higher EFs posterolaterally **(b)**, significant loss of height ERs posterolaterally **(d)**.

e–h, In RAO-view a small area of prolonged mean times posteriorly **(e)**. In LAO-view long mean times (dark) advanced to the parietal posterolateral zone **(f)**. Regional rapid filling rates displays anteriorly **(g)** with defect posteriorly and paradoxical inward motion **(h)** corresponding to the circumscribed posterolateral infarcted zone.

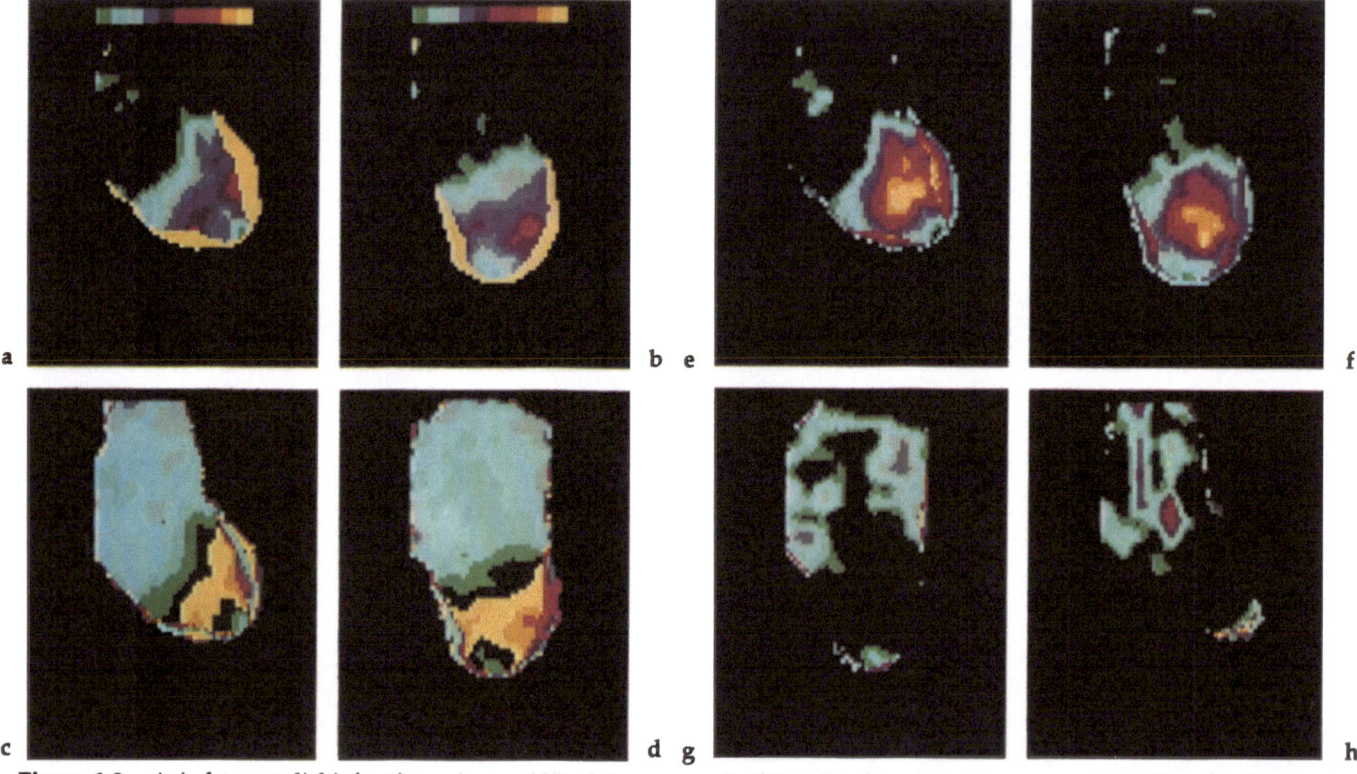

Figure 6.3 *Apical myocardial infarction – Aurum 195m injection.*
a–d, Systolic functional images: REFI in both oblique projections shows reduced EFs at the apex **(a,b)**, very long regional mean times (green) at the apex at rest pointing to the infarcted zone **(c,d)**. The two projections provide information about the three-dimensional expansion of the infarcted zone.

e–h, Diastolic functional images: rapid filling is deviated from the spared apical zone in both oblique projections **(e,f)**, paradoxical inward motion of the apex during rapid filling in both projections pointing to severe loss of compliance.

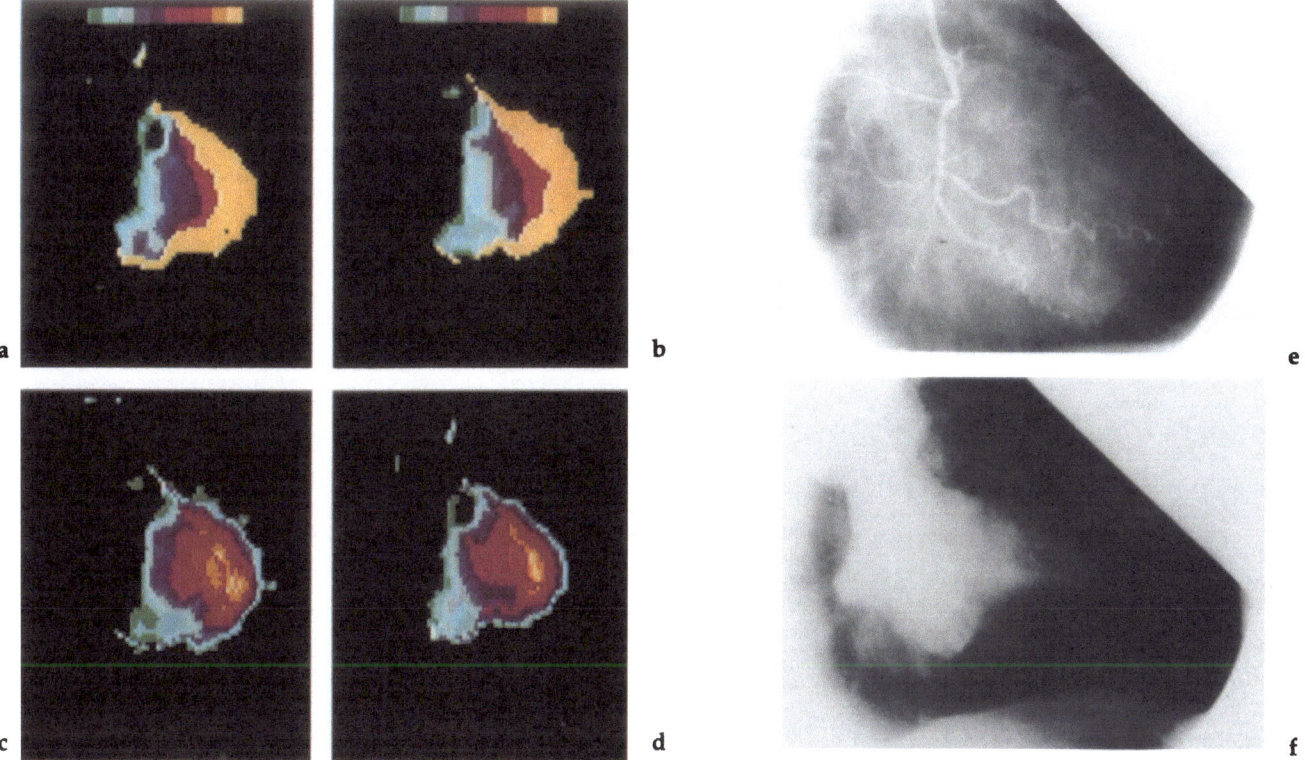

Figure 6.4 *Posterior myocardial infarction – occlusion of right coronary.*

a–d, Systolic functional images in RAO-view at rest and exercise: bulging of the posterior wall with low regional EFs and ERs at rest **(a,c)** and exercise **(b,d)**, normal contraction in the other segments.

e,f, Right coronary angiogram **(e)** shows subtotal occlusion of right coronary. End-systolic left ventricular angiogram **(f)** shows bulging of the posterior wall as already seen on the functional images.

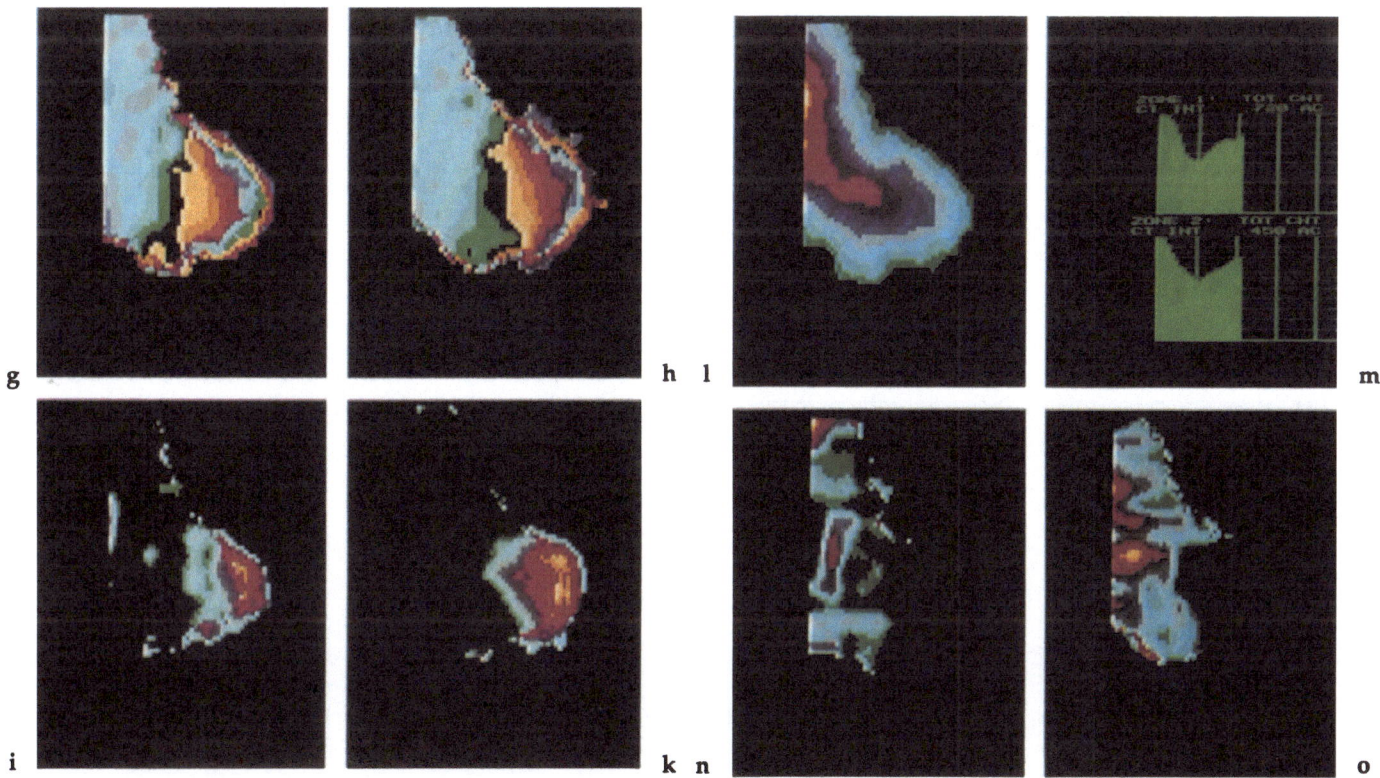

g,h,i,k, Functional images in RAO-view at rest and exercise: long mean times (dark) regionally advance into the small aneurysm **(g)**. Under stress very long mean times (green) filling into the dilated aneurysm **(h)**. Regional rapid filling rate deviated anteriorly at rest **(i)**; still some filling into the small aneurysm under stress **(k)** filling defect.

l–o, The end-systolic image of the representative cycle **(l)** corresponds to the end-systolic LV angiogram **(f)**, the volume curve **(m)** at rest is only moderately altered (upper), under stress significant flattening of global rapid filling (lower). Paradoxical inward motion during rapid filling with inward displacement of blood during rapid filling already at rest **(n)** increasing under stress **(o)**.

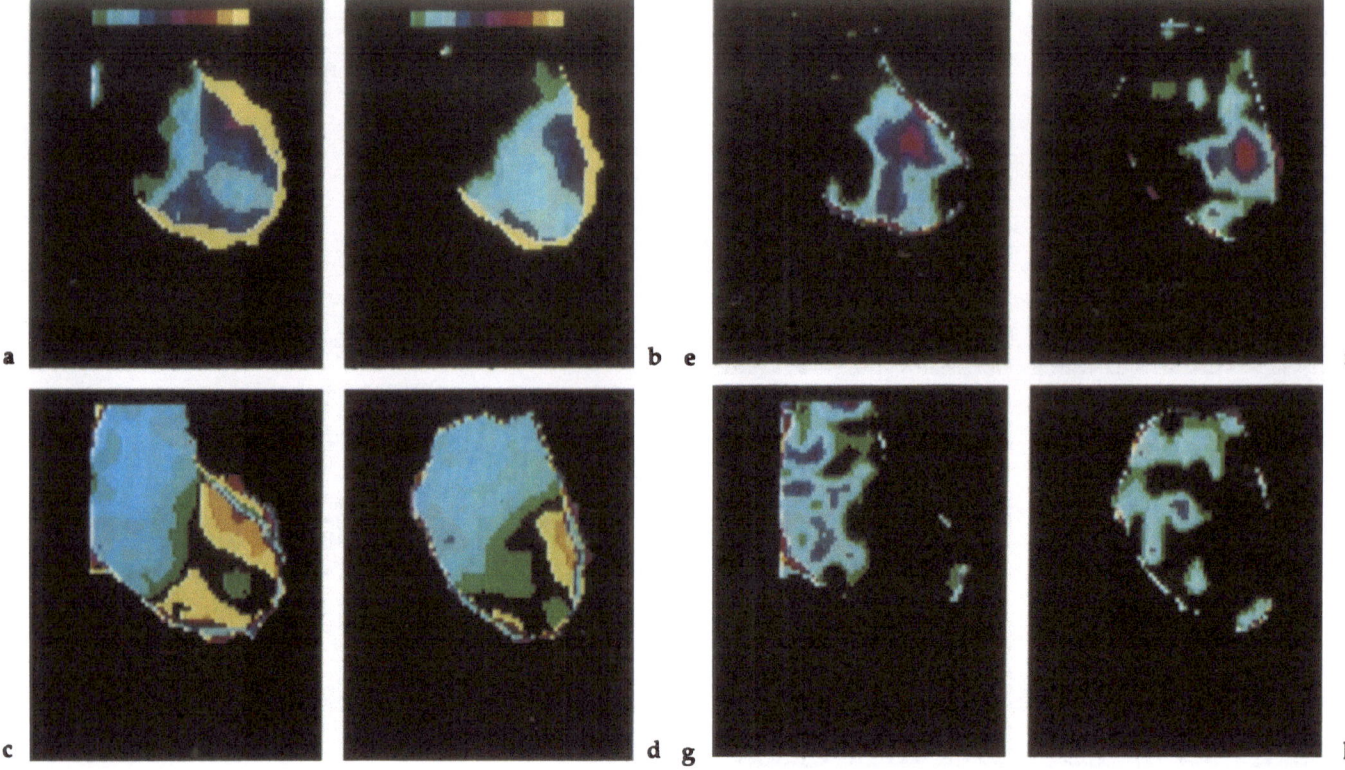

Figure 6.5 *Septal–apical myocardial infarction – Aurum 195m injection.*

a–d, Systolic functional images: loss of high EFs at the apex and septal side in both oblique projections (**a,b**) very long mean times (green) advance to the apex and septal site (**c,d**).

e–h, Diastolic functional images: rapid filling rates are deviated from the apical and septal side creating corresponding defects (**e,f**), paradoxical inward motion at apex and inferior-posterior septum pointing to zone with severe loss of compliance.

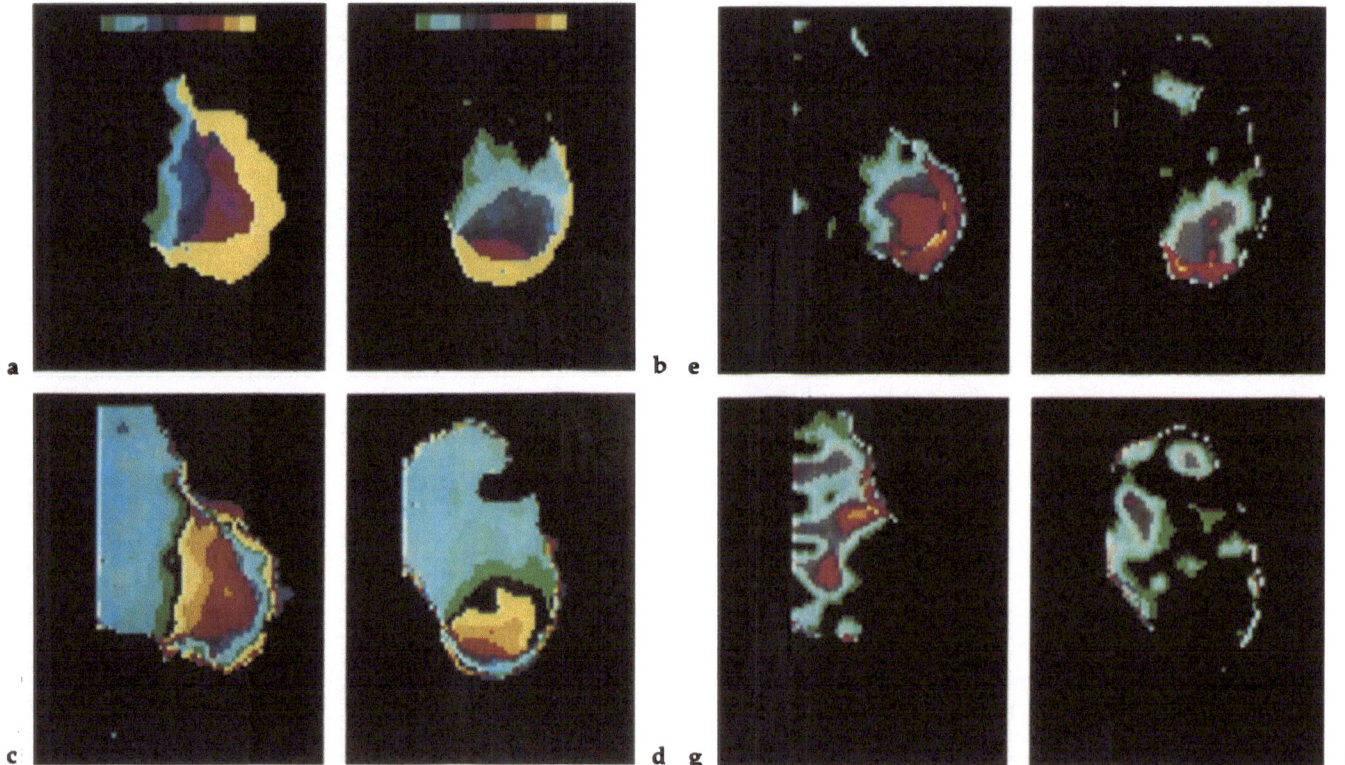

Figure 6.6 *Posterolateral myocardial infarction – Aurum 195m injection.*

a–d, Systolic functional images: loss of high EFs in a small posterior zone in RAO-view (**a**) and posterolaterally in LAO-view (**b**). Mean times in RAO-view not informative (**c**) but in LAO-view long mean times posterolaterally (**d**).

e–h, Diastolic functional images: rapid filling rates reduced in RAO-view posteriorly extending laterally (**e**) in LAO-view no rates posterolaterally (**f**). Paradoxical inward motion posteriorly in RAO-view (**g**) and posterolaterally in LAO-view (**h**).

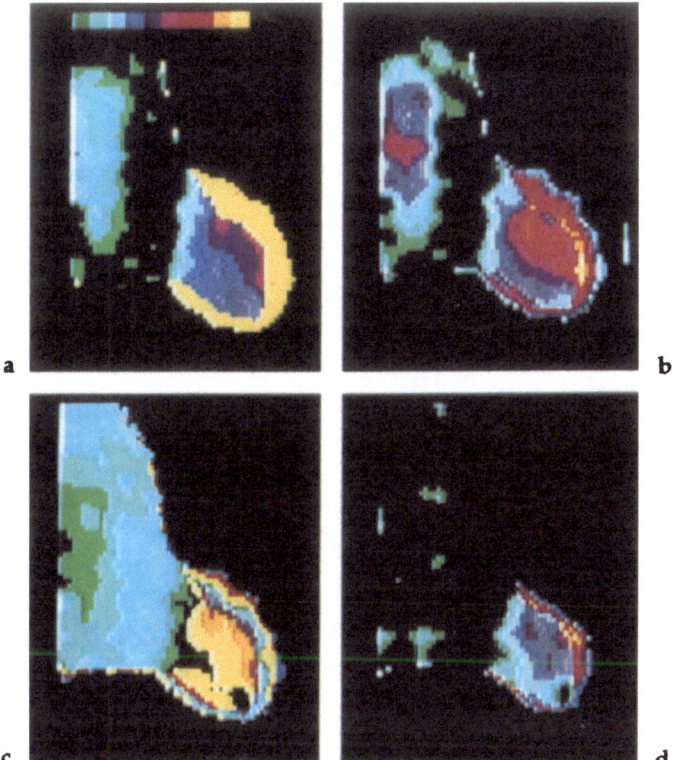

a

b

c

d

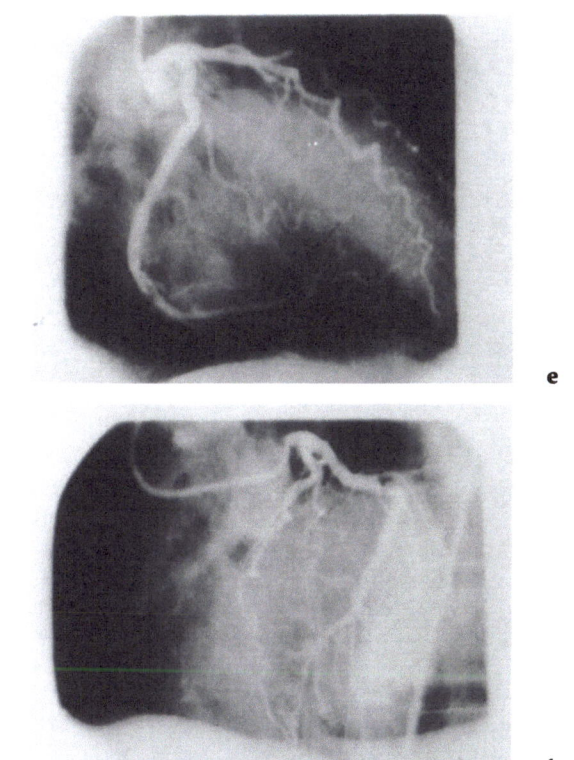

e

f

Figure 6.7 *Inferior myocardial infarction. Significant narrowing of proximal CX – peripheral narrowing of posterior-descending.*

a–d, Before nitrates: reduced EFs along the inferoposterior wall **(a)** reduced ERs at the entire inferior wall corresponding to the posterior descending territory with the retroapical minimum **(b)**. Long spherical mean times

behind the apex suggesting small aneurysm **(c)**. Anteriorly deviated rapid filling rates with retroapical spherical defect **(d)**.

e,f, Left coronary angiogram: in the RAO-view **(e)** long dominant CX with periferal narrowing of the posterior descending. In LAO-view proximal CX stenosis **(f)**.

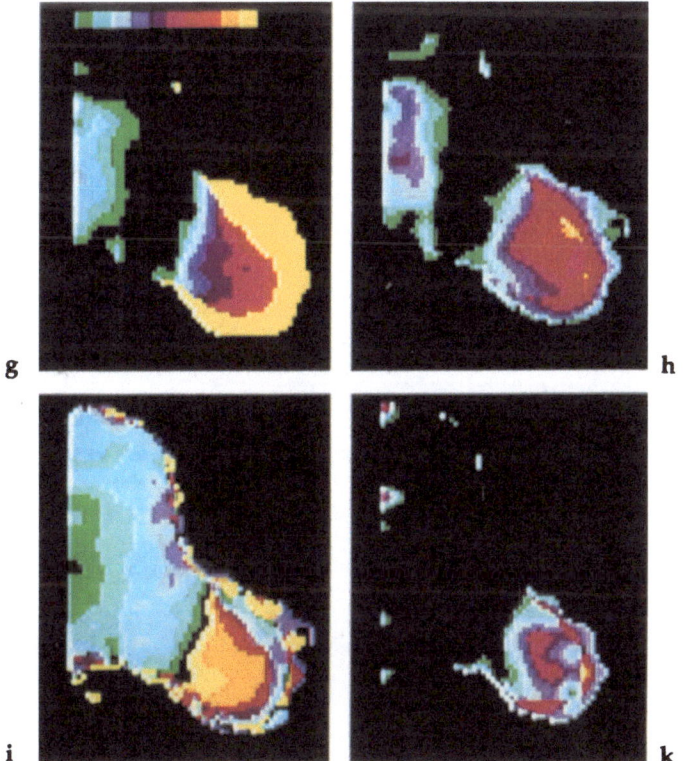

g

h

i

k

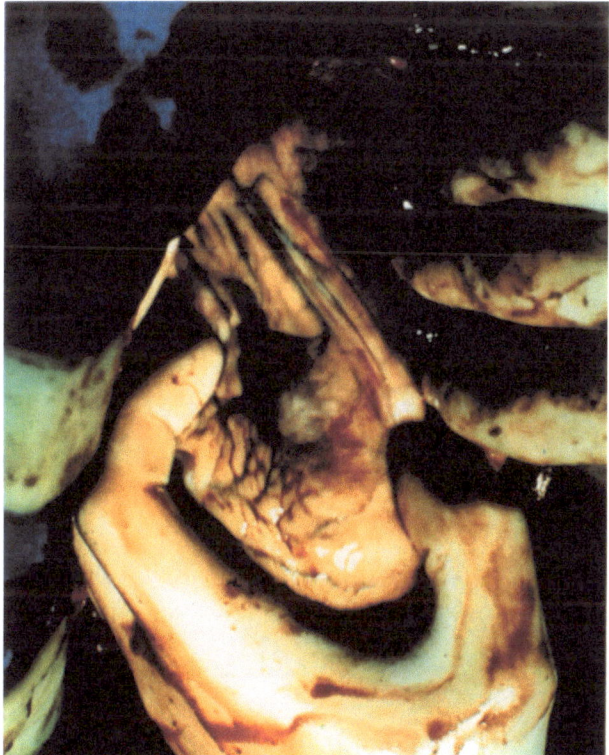

l

g,h,i,k, After nitrates: strong contraction of the anterior wall and improved EFs at the inferior wall **(g)**. Reduced zone of low ERs inferiorly **(h)**. Spherical long mean time behind the apex disappeared. Somewhat prolonged mean times at the CX territory (orange), **(i)** after nitrates some rapid filling inferiorly with displacement of spherical zone to the apex **(k)**. Nitrates improve ischaemia proximal to the small aneurysm.

l, Inferior surface of the LV at surgery shows a small aneurysm (courtesy Professor Klinner and Professor Reichart).

7

Functional Imaging in Left Ventricular Aneurysm

N. SCHAD AND F. BRUZZONE

Prognosis in patients with true left ventricular aneurysms is seriously affected by common complications such as heart failure, severe dysrhythmias, and embolization of mural thrombi. Rupture of a true postinfarction aneurysm is quite rare, because of the strength of the fibrotic aneurysmal wall and the support of the thickened pericardium. There is general agreement that a complicated left ventricular aneurysm should have surgical correction since at this stage survival rate is higher with surgery than with medical treatment. Other proposed *indicators for surgery* are an LV end diastolic pressure over 20 mmHg, an increase of mean pulmonary pressure over 40 mmHG under mild stress, an LV end diastolic volume over 200 ml/m^2 and a global ejection fraction below 30%, as well as a low rate of systolic shortening of still contractile segments. The risk of aneurysmectomy was noted to be inversely proportional to the ejection fraction of the still contractile section. Survival was reported to be 100% or 90% if this ejection fraction surpassed 45% or 39% respectively (Watson *et al.*, 1975; Kapelanski *et al.*, 1978). Surgical mortality is higher if a revascularization procedure has to be added to the aneurysmectomy (Burton *et al.*, 1979).

Thus, for rational clinical management of patients with left ventricular aneurysms one should know:

(1) the preserved function of the still contractile segments

(2) the presence of other vascular territories jeopardized by coronary narrowings

(3) the degree of LV dilatation, congestion and right heart involvement, and the global EF.

First pass functional imaging enables one to determine these diagnostic elements non-invasively.

Definition of a left ventricular aneurysm may be structural or functional. Structurally, a left ventricular aneurysm forms a localized, thin-walled, fibrotic protrusion beyond the ventricular surface involving the free wall or the septum, or both. Most postinfarction aneurysms are located at the anterior or apical left ventricle, although posterobasal and septal aneurysms may occur infrequently. Large aneurysms tend to be lined with laminated mural thrombus. The wall of the aneurysm can calcify, the parietal pericardium is often thickened and adherent to the overlying epicardium. Functionally,

the localized bulge exhibits either akinesia or dyskinesia (paradoxic pulsation) during ventricular contraction. In the latter instance, some blood enters the aneurysmal sac during systole and is stolen from forward output

Both the above structural and functional definitions present some *diagnostic limitations*. The aneurysm wall may still contain viable myocardial cells within densely fibrotic tissue as can also be seen in healed myocardial infarction. When an aneurysm exists in a ventricle that is already diffusely dilated the characteristic bulge may protrude less or even be missed and the accurate radiological diagnosis become quite difficult. Diffuse dilatation of the left ventricle is encountered in conditions with chronic heart failure as in end-stage ischaemic heart disease or idiopathic dilated cardiomyopathy. Segmental akinesia is a common sign in transmural infarction and dyskinesia can be encountered at the centre of the infarcted zone (*see* Chapter 6). Thus, some structural and functional diagnostic elements may also apply to transmural infarcts particularly if they are large.

Systolic functional images are of considerable help in the detection of left ventricular saccular aneurysms (Figures 7.1 and 7.2). The diagnostic clue is given by the spherical pattern or dysfunction with a minimum or defect at the ventricular periphery and gradually increasing functional levels or shells toward the centre of the ventricle. The aneurysmal zone is usually well-delineated by the surrounding still contractile areas presenting much higher functional levels. When in regional ejection fraction and ejection rate images the parietal zone shows systolic functional defects *dyskinesia* may be discovered in the image of regional systolic increase. Not infrequently, under the paradoxic wall motion an area is visualized where blood or activity predominantly increases during systole, particularly if the patient is somewhat stressed. (For discussion of dyskinesia, *see* under myocardial infarction, Chapter 6.) Sometimes, however, with apical aneurysm a sharply rather linearly delineated defect can be observed which can be caused by thrombus formation as seen by comparison with left ventricular angiograms. Thus, haemodynamic stasis not only favours development of mural thrombus, but by its gradual decreasing toward the ventricular cavity causes the characteristic functional pattern of gradual spherical changes seen on functional images.

Since the aneurysmal zone is usually well delineated from the remaining contractile ventricle, one can eliminate this zone from the end diastolic and stroke volume image and calculate per cent volume contained in the *contractile part of the ventricle*, estimate absolute volume and compute its ejection fraction (Figure 7.1). Additional dysfunction in these zones points to complicating coronary narrowings. A mild stress or an attempt of unloading the ventricle by administration of nitrates proved to be useful to determine the functional reserve of the remaining contractile ventricle.

The *regional mean transit time image* directly represents a rather round and compact parietal area of long mean times or persistence of blood or activity, the counterpart of severe focal, peripheral haemodynamic stasis. Indeed, by the aid of this sign it becomes possible to detect even a very small single aneurysm (*see* Figure 6.7). Multiple 'spots' of long parietal mean times, however, rather point to large infarcted areas still containing some parts with viable myocardium than to a well delineated saccular aneurysm. If regional mean time images are equivocal the gradual spherical improvement of function in regional ejection fraction and rate images from the periphery to the centre of the ventricle aid in clearing the diagnosis. Degree of concomitant congestion and, eventually, right heart functional involvement can be established from lung, ventricular histograms (*see* Chapter 6) and RV-functional imaging (*see* Chapter 19).

In conclusion, functional images can supply important information needed for rational management of patients with ventricular aneurysms, i.e. about the global LV-function, the contractility of the remaining segments, additional vascular territories at risk and the degree of congestion.

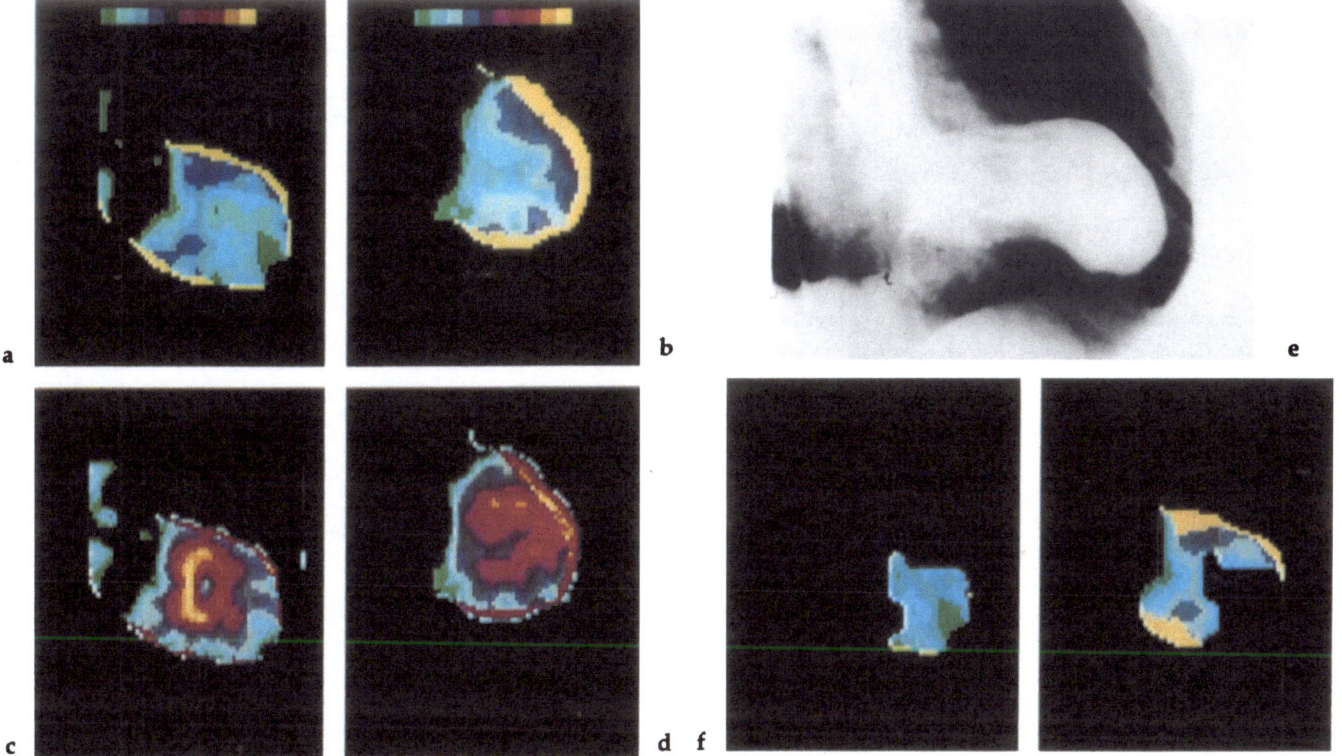

Figure 7.1 *Large anterior-apical aneurysm. Aneurysmectomy (8 × 3 cm): follow-up after 5 years.*

a–d, Systolic functional images before and after 5 years after aneurysmectomy in RAO view. Spherical zone with low EFs anteriorly and defect at the apex (**a**). After surgery (**b**) improvement of contraction of the anterior and inferior wall. Similarly improving of ERs (**c,d**).

e, End-systolic left ventricular angiogram shows the spherical aneurysmal sac and upper anterior and posterior contracting wall segment.

f,g, The zone of the aneurysmal sac (**f**) can be separated from the contractile part of the left ventricle (**g**) for which a separate EF can be computed. High regional correspondence with end-systolic levogram (**e**).

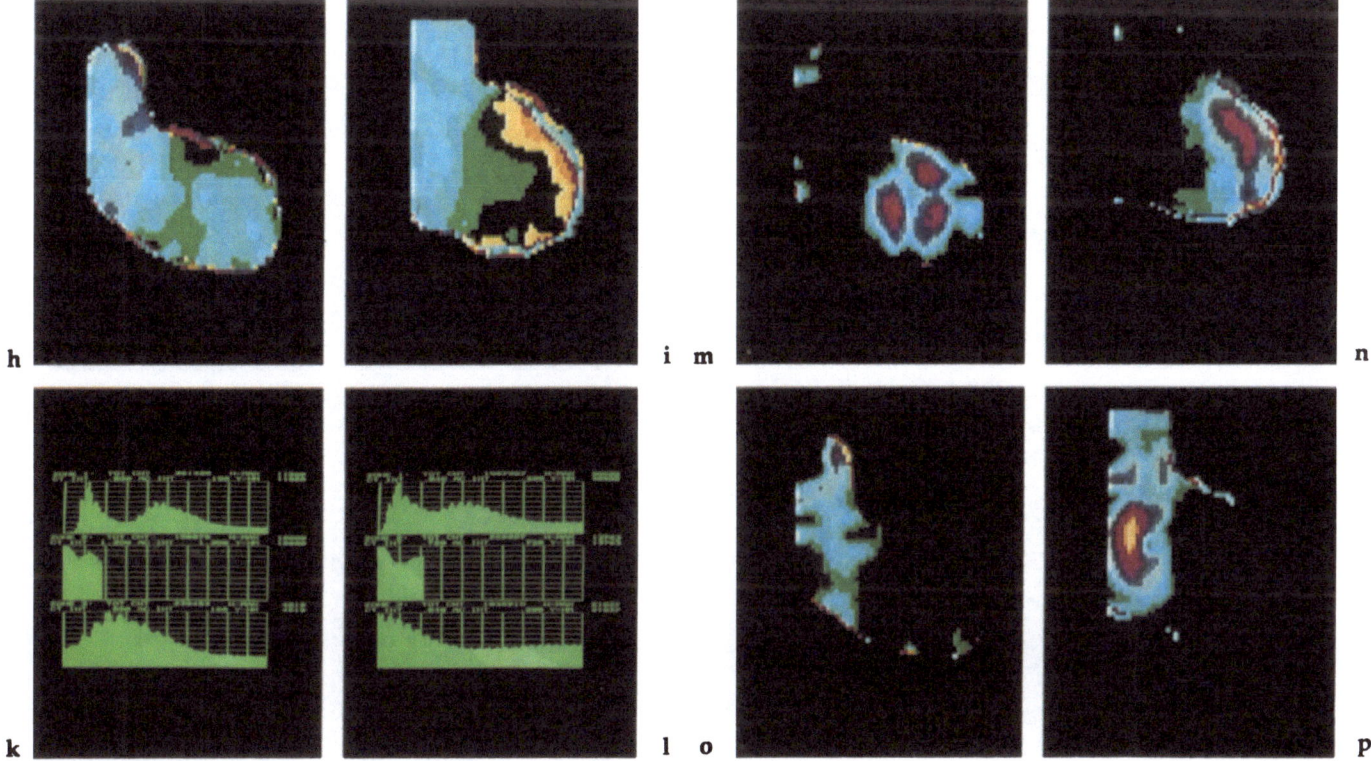

h,i,k,l, Very long spherical mean times (light green) delineate the aneurysmal sac (**h**). 5 years after aneurysmectomy significantly shortening mean times along the anterior wall (**i**). Transit curves (**k**) show somewhat delayed lung transit (ten cycles; upper), reduced global EF (middle) and delayed LV wash-out (lower). Improvement after surgery (**l**).

m–p, Diastolic functional images: rapid filling rates spare the apical, superoapical and retroapical zones corresponding to the not contracting aneurysmal segments (**m**). 5 years after surgery significant improvement along the entire anterior and apical zone (**n**). Paradoxical inward motion during rapid filling at the apical and retroapical zone (**o**) disappearing after surgery (**p**).

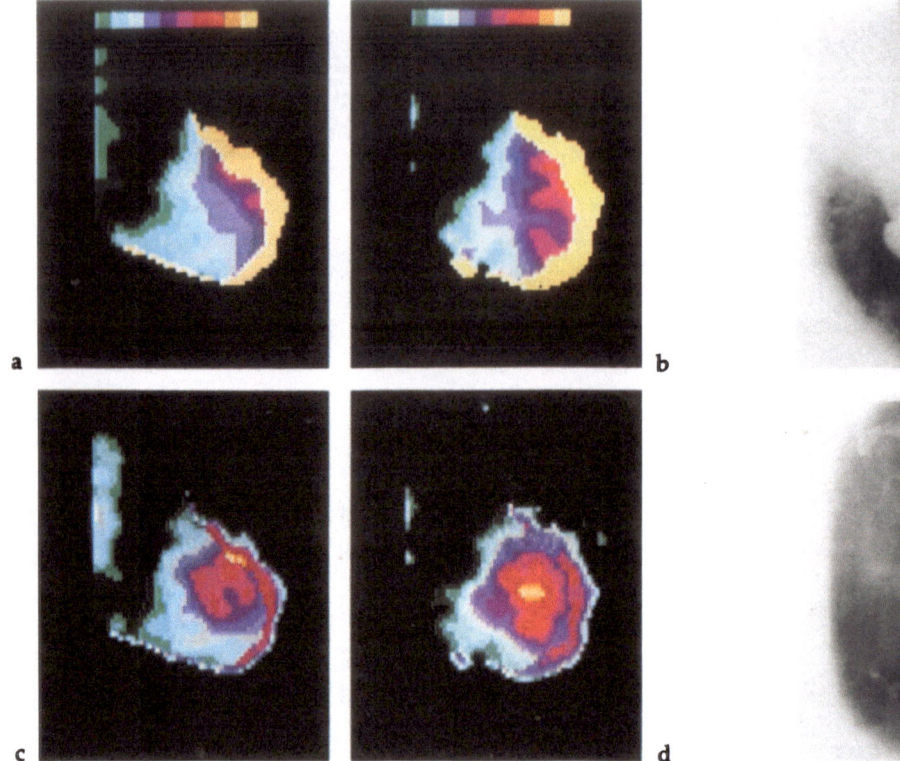

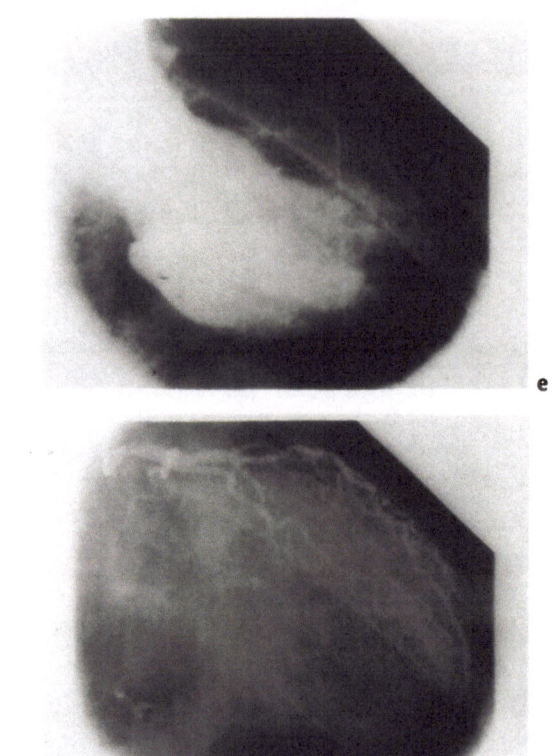

Figure 7.2 *Large inferior aneurysm – total occlusion of RC significant stenosis at the CX, LAD and diagonal (later bypass grafts).*

a–d, Systolic functional images before and after nitrates in RAO view: large inferoposterior zone extending laterally with low EFs (**a**). Significant improvement after nitrates at the anterior and probably also marginal territories (**b**).

Regional ERs also show the wall delineated inferoposterior dysfunction suggesting RC and CX involvement (**c**). Significant improvement after nitrates (**d**).

e,f, End-systolic left ventricular angiogram showing the large inferoposterior aneurysm and some hypokinesis at the anterior wall (**e**). The angiogram shows the LAD and CX stenosis (**f**).

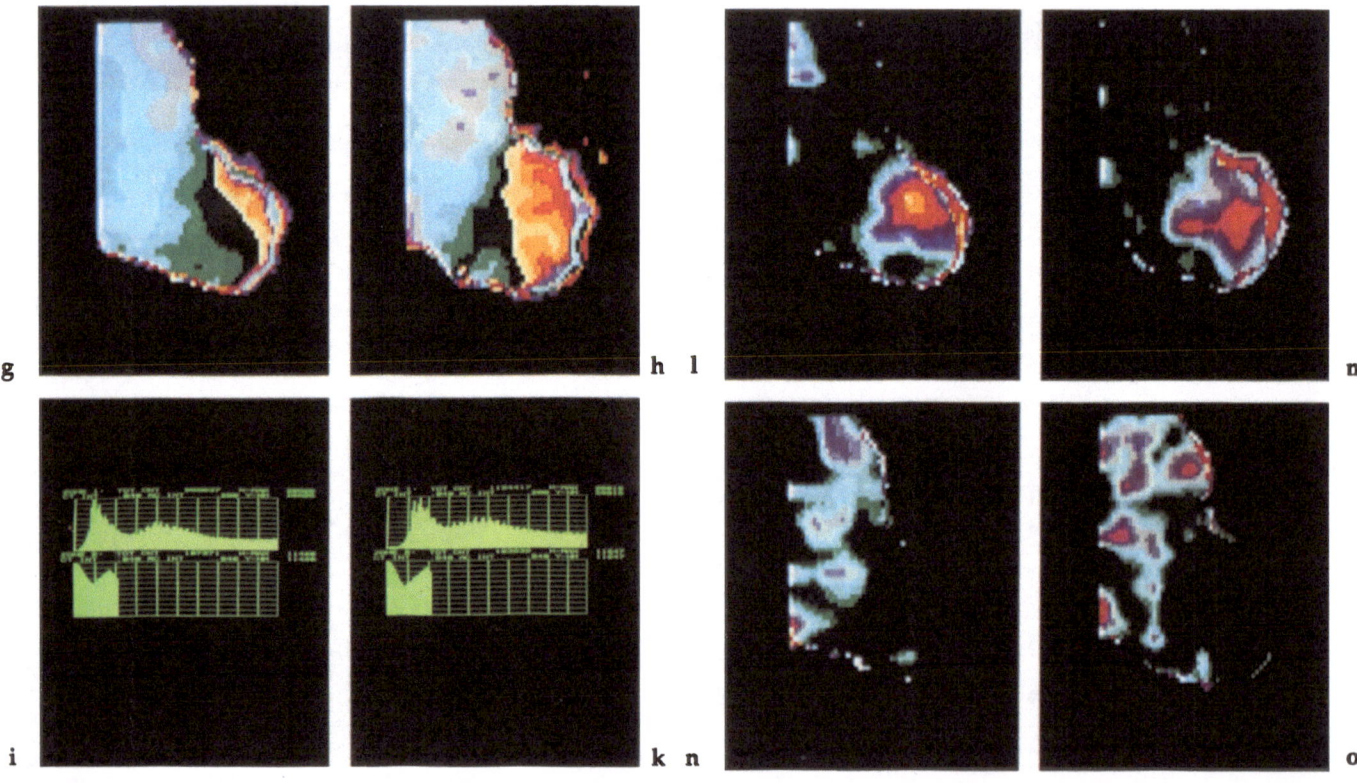

g,h,i,k, Long mean times at a large zone of the infero-posterior wall suggesting an aneurysm or a large infarct (**g**). After nitrates significant improvement of the anterior wall (**h**). Somewhat prolonged lung transit (11 cycles, upper, **i**) improving after nitrates (**k**). Increase of EFs after nitrates (middle).

l–o, Diastolic functional images before and after nitrates in RAO view. Rapid filling rates are deviated anteriorly (**l**) and deteriorated inferiorly and posteriorly after nitrates (**m**). Paradoxical inward motion with same inward displacement of blood inferiorly (**n**), increases slightly after nitrates (**o**).

66

8

Regional Left Ventricular Function after Aortocoronary Bypass Surgery

B. REICHART, N. SCHAD, R. HATZ AND M. LUTHER

In recent decades, coronary artery bypass has advanced to one of the most important routine procedures in cardiac surgery comprising more than 50% of all heart operations. The increased incidence of coronary atherosclerotic disease in the industrialized world has led to this development. The innovators of this method were not only looking for a way to alleviate angina pectoris but also actually to prevent or limit myocardial infarction and therefore to prolong life expectancy.

Clear indications for coronary bypass exist in narrowings of at least 75% of the left main coronary artery and in severe proximal three vessel disease with good distal anatomy. There is a particular indication for symptomatic patients with two vessel disease including proximal stenosis of the anterior descending coronary artery with coexistent involvement of the right coronary artery. Also, patients suffering from stable angina pectoris poorly responding to optimal medical treatment and patients with unstable angina showing signs of preinfarction status should be considered for bypass surgery.

There is no doubt that anginal pain is relieved in most patients following aortocoronary surgery. But many questions are still open as to what effect this procedure has upon the improvement of left ventricular function. It is the main objective of this chapter to take a closer look at a technique which accurately assesses regional myocardial function in patients after revascularization. This new clinical method which proved to be reliable in screening patients for coronary heart disease (*see* Chapter 4) is also a valuable tool in the postoperative follow-up of the coronary patient.

A total of *50 consecutive patients* who had undergone bypass surgery were studied by first pass radiocardiography at rest and peak exercise. Forty-eight men and two women averaged 53.9 years (range of 38–73 years). Thirty-seven patients had a previous history of myocardial infarction more than 3 months prior to surgery. The preoperative angiography showed three vessel disease in 25 patients, two vessel disease in 15 and one vessel disease in ten. Significant stenosis was defined as a narrowing of the coronary artery equal to or exceeding 75% of its diameter.

Complete revascularization was attempted whenever possible, which meant anastomosis of all vessels measuring 1 mm and more.

The assessment of global and regional left ventricular function was done 8.6 ± 1.3 months postoperatively on an average. First pass radionuclide ventriculograms with technetium pertechnetate 99 m were performed at rest and after maximum exercise as already described. All nitrate medication was discontinued 24 hours prior to the procedure.

The ventriculograms were done in the RAO projection with the patient sitting on a bicycle ergometer. After assessment of left ventricular function at rest the patients were asked to exercise at four levels. Each level was held for 2 minutes. At the final level the patients cycled as fast as possible achieving a maximum performance of $100-150$ W. The patients' heart rate increased during exercise from $85.1 \pm 16 \, \text{min}^{-1}$ to $150.5 \pm 24 \, \text{min}^{-1}$ ($p < 0.05$). The stress was interrupted if the patients had angina pectoris or significant ST-segment depression in the e.c.g.

The global ejection fraction was calculated in the usual way (stroke volume divided by end-diastolic volume) using self-developed computer programs stored in a micro-processor. But a new definition was found for the regional ejection fraction (Schad and Nickel, 1980a). The left ventricle was divided into three areas according to the preoperative coronary angiograms: the region of the left anterior descending coronary artery (LAD), of the circumflex artery (CX) and of the right coronary artery (RCA) (Figure 8.1). This delineation had to be done in every patient separately, since the distribution of the main coronary arteries varies. With the aid of a computer system the RAO radionuclide left ventriculograms were subdivided accordingly. Subdivision was performed on end-diastolic and stroke volume images. First, the percentage of end-diastolic volume (ratio or zonal counts to global counts) for each individual territory was computed. Whereas the end-diastolic volumes at rest and exercise are usually different, it was assumed that the percentage of end-diastolic volumes remains approximately the same for the same territory during exercise. Therefore, fine adjustments of the two corresponding zones of the two studies were necessary to obtain the percentage of end-diastolic volumes not varying more than 2% from each other. Then, the systolic changes and regional ejection fractions were separately calculated for the resting and exercise study.

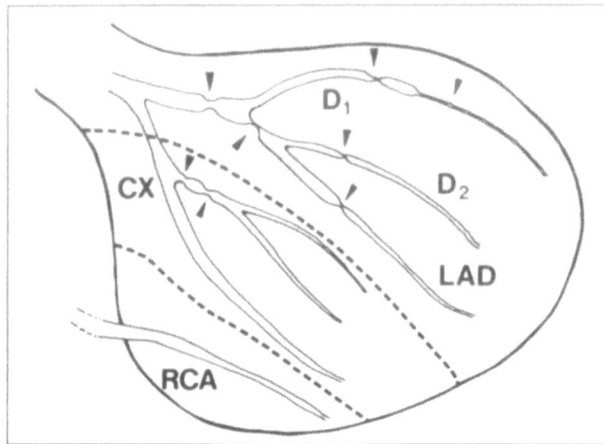

Figure 8.1 Classification of myocardial regions (RAO projection) corresponding to the vascular bed of the three major coronary arteries as determined from the preoperative angiogram (end-diastole). Schematic presentation: the arrows mark significant vessel narrowing (CX = circumflex artery; LAD = left anterior descending artery; RCA = right coronary artery; D_1, D_2 = first and second diagonal branch). The regions of the three major arteries are marked. The scintigraphic ventriculograms in end-diastole and regional stroke volume were divided into the three regions correspondingly.

In all ventriculograms the regions of the obtuse marginal branch and the septal branches of the anterior descending artery overlap as Figure 8.2 demonstrates. But the septal branch area mainly belongs to the left ventricular outflow tract where the residual volume remains at the end of systole and which shows only minimal contraction and therefore does not alter the regional ejection fraction of the obtuse marginal area considerably.

All regions were classified using preoperative coronary angiograms and operative reports. Classification depended on vascular status, degree of revascularization and diagnosis of previous myocardial infarction (history of typical chest pain, CK-enzyme level, e.c.g. pattern, coronary arteriogram, abnormal regional left ventricular motion). Finally, six groups evolved:

(1) areas of normal perfusion without stenosis

(2) completely revascularized regions without previous myocardial infarction (MI)

(3) completely revascularized regions with previous MI

(4) incompletely revascularized regions without previous MI

(5) incompletely revascularized regions with previous MI

(6) territories supplied by significantly stenosed vessels without or with previous MI, in other words, ischaemic territories, at least during exercise, without revascularization.

All bypass grafts which were closed postoperatively – the precise number is unknown – were considered 'open' in the results, since 'completeness of revascularization' only refers to the number of vessels bypassed and not to the functional result of the anastomosis.

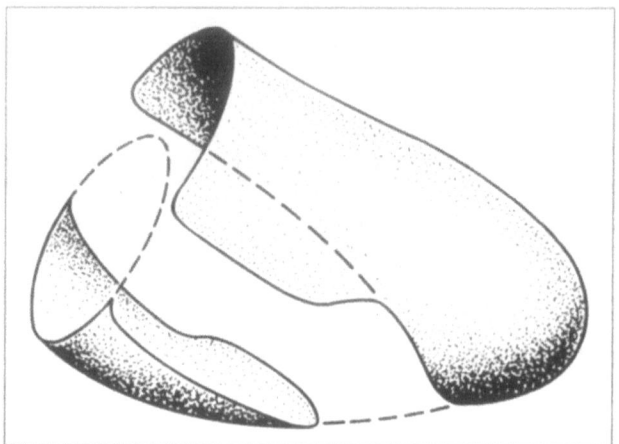

Figure 8.2 Schematic drawing of the overlap between the regions of the obtuse marginal branch of the circumflex artery and the septal branches of the left anterior descending artery. The dotted areas represent the myocardium supplied by the LAD and the RCA; the dashed ring marks the annulus of the mitral valve. (Figures 8.1 and 8.2 by permission of *Fortschritte der Medizin*, Verlagsgesellschaft mbH, 8035 Gauting, near Munich.)

The paired and unpaired Student's *t*-test was used to compare data and to obtain statistical differences. Regression curves were calculated with a Hewlett Packard Computer 67.

Altogether, the *50 patients received 161 anastomoses* (an average of 3.2 per case): two patients with one graft, four with two, 30 with three, ten with four, three with five and one with six grafts. There was one questionable postoperative myocardial infarction.

At the time of the radionuclide study 31 patients were asymptomatic, another 18 experienced intermittent mild anginal pain. In one case angina pectoris remained unchanged. Forty-three patients showed a significant increase of maximum performance during exercise on the bicycle ergometer.

In 32 patients the *global ejection fraction* increased from 52.3 ± 8 to 62.4 ± 10 percentage points during maximum exercise. In seven cases it remained unchanged, and in 11 patients it decreased from 58.9 ± 9 to 51.5 ± 8 percentage points. All changes were significant ($p < 0.05$).

Figure 8.3 summarizes the average increase or decrease of *regional ejection fractions* under stress in the six subgroups.

(1) *Group 1*: Eighteen regions were supplied by normal vessels. In 14 cases the regional ejection fraction increased after maximum exercise, remained unchanged (± 2.0 percentage points) three times and decreased once. On an average the whole group's regional ejection fraction increased by 11.6 percentage points (from 43.2 ± 13 to $54.8 \pm 12.6\%$; $p < 0.05$)

(2) *Group 2*: Altogether 55 regions were completely revascularized without previous myocardial infarction. Like most areas in Group 1 these regions usually improved after maximum exercise: REF increased in 49 cases, remained unchanged in five and decreased only once. On an average, REF improved after maximum

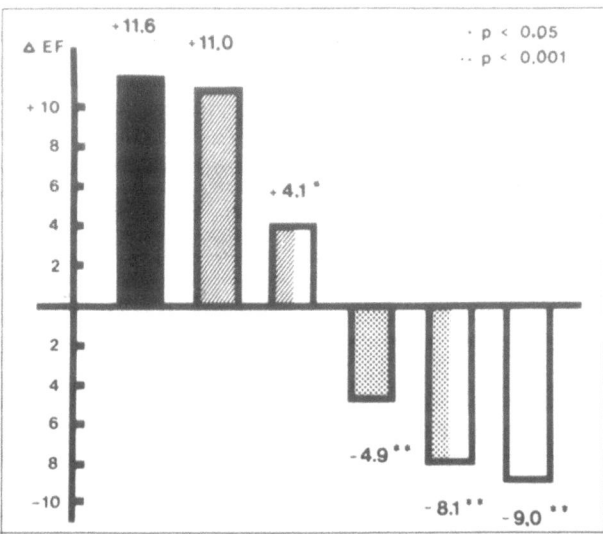

Figure 8.3 Mean values for regional ejection fraction at rest and during exercise in all six groups. Group 1, normally perfused regions: solid column; Group 2, complete revascularization, no infarct: crosshatched column; Group 3, complete revascularization, previous infarct: Group 4, incomplete revascularization, no infarct: dotted column; Group 5, incomplete revascularization, previous infarct: half-dotted column; Group 6, regions supplied by significantly stenosed non-graftable vessels, with or without infarct: open column. Δ EF is the difference between the resting and the exercise regional ejection fractions for the main vascular territories. The mean values for Groups 2–6 were compared with those of Group 1.

exercise by 11.0 percentage points (from 52.8 to 62.8%; $p < 0.05$).

In Figure 8.4 all results of a subgroup – 27 LAD regions – are put together. Almost all points – except for two – are above and to the left side of the 45° identity line. The regression line is highly significant ($r = 0.9$).

(3)   *Group 3*: Again complete revascularization was performed in the group. Yet, unlike Group 2, myocardial infarction had taken place in these regions. After exercise the REF increased in 15

Figure 8.4 Completely revascularized LAD regions ($n = 27$); regional ejection fraction (REF) at rest and during maximum exercise. The drawing includes a 45° identity line. The regression line is situated above and to the left.

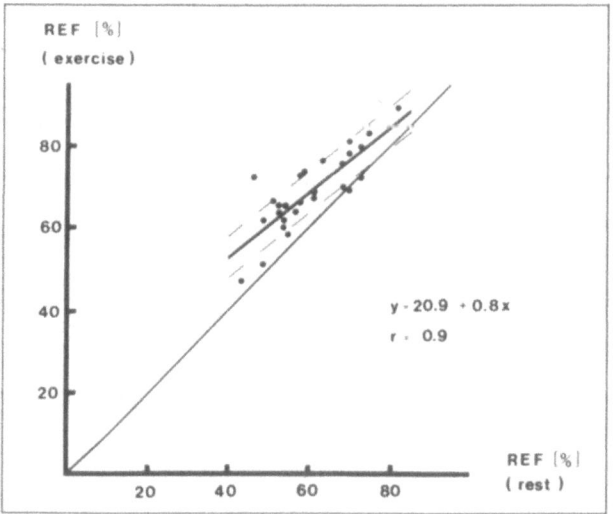

out of 25 cases, remained unchanged four times and fell in another six cases. The total group's REF, however, still increased by 4.1 percentage points (from 45.6 ± 13 to $49.7 \pm 19\%$; $p < 0.05$).

(4)   *Group 4*: All regions ($n = 19$) of this group were incompletely revascularized. No previous myocardial damage due to infarction had occurred. 'Incompletely' means that at least one vessel of an area could not be bypassed because of poor anatomy. Vessels below 1 mm in diameter were not graftable. An increase of the REF after exercise was found only in three areas. On the other hand the REF decreased in ten regions and remained unchanged in six. On average, the REF decreased by 4.9 percentage points (from 56.2 ± 14 to $51.3 \pm 10\%$; $p < 0.05$).

(5)   *Group 5*: This group ($n = 8$) consists of all regions which were incompletely revascularized and had evidence of previous myocardial infarction. After maximum exercise none of the regional ejection fractions increased. The group's total REF fell by 8.1 percentage points (from 52.0 ± 13 to $43.9 \pm 10\%$; $p < 0.05$).

(6)   *Group 6*: Finally, this group ($n = 14$) includes regions supplied by stenosed coronary arteries with or without previous myocardial infarction and no revascularization. A bypass could not be performed because of poor coronary artery quality. After exercise the REF usually fell (in 13 cases out of 14) and remained unchanged only once. The mean REF decreased by 9.0 percentage points (from 47.2 ± 13 to $38.2 \pm 13\%$; $p < 0.05$).

The comparison between regional (REF) and global (GEF) ejection fraction is illustrated by Figure 8.5. An attempt was made to correlate regional and global ejection fractions by means of a grading system. Each region received a certain amount of points. Group 1 areas (regions of normal perfusion) were given six points, Group 2 areas (regions with complete revascularization without previous MI) five and so on down to Group 6 areas which received only one point. The number of points of each region was then multiplied by the percentage of counts each territory held in regard to the entity of the whole left ventricle. The final score, an addition of three multiplications – for LAD, CX and RCA regions – was compared with Δ GEF, the difference of the global ejection fraction at rest and during exercise.

For example, patient D.G. had completely revascularized LAD and RCA areas without previous MI (areas belonging to Group 2, thus receiving 5 points each) and one highly stenotic CX region which was not revascularized (a Group 6 area, therefore only one point). The percentages of each of the three areas were: LAD 50%, CX, 44% and RCA 6%. The final score was calculated as follows: $(5 \times 0.5) + (1 \times 0.44) + (5 \times 0.06) = 3.24$. This value was then plotted against Δ GEF.

The diagram in Figure 8.5 depicts a positive correlation between Δ GEF and the calculated point grades ($r = 0.7$). The following mathematical

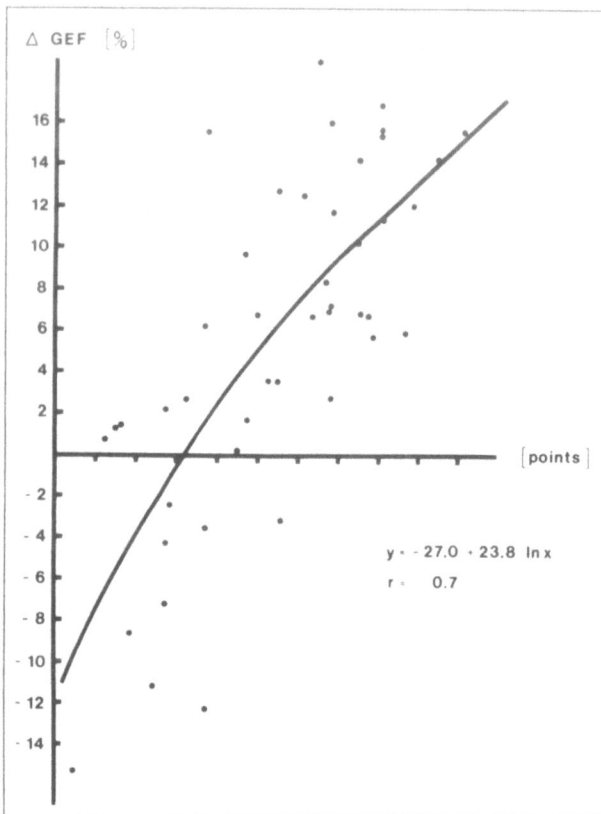

$y = -27.0 + 23.8 \ln x$

$r = 0.7$

Figure 8.5 Correlation of a score resulting from the grading of each region according to the groups 1–6, the size of the regions and the global ejection fraction (GEF); GEF is the difference in global ejection fraction at rest and during exercise. For computation of the score (points) see text. (Figures 8.3 and 8.5 by permission of the Urban & Schwarzenberg Verlag, Munich.)

equation can be used to describe this relationship: $y = -27.0 + 23.8 \times \ln x$.

Table 8.1 shows the *relationship between the global ejection fraction during maximum exercise and the extent of revascularization of the LAD region* – the largest and therefore the most important left ventricular area. The GEF of completely revascularized LAD regions without previous myocardial infarction (Group 2) improved in 24 out of 27 cases (88.9%) and in those with previous MI (Group 3) in five out of eight patients (62.5%). In incompletely revascularized LAD areas without or with previous MI (Groups 4 and 5) the GEF increased in only two cases.

Why was a new definition of the regional ejection fraction necessary?

Improvement of left ventricular function after aortocoronary bypass surgery still remains a controversial topic. The main problem is probably given by the fact that global parameters are often used to assess myocardial function, after coronary bypass. But coronary artery disease does not impair myocardial tissue and contractility in all parts of the ventricle to the same degree. Instead, this disease damages well-determined segments of the ventricular wall or septum in relation to the distribution of the main coronary arteries and its branches. Therefore, the measurement of global functional parameters does not seem to be the ideal method to prove possible improvement in left ventricular function after coronary bypass surgery.

Consequently, in the past, many investigators tried new techniques to measure regional left ventricular function. On pre- and postoperative contrast ventriculograms normokinetic and akinetic areas were grossly compared and classified (Bourassa *et al.*, 1972; Saltiel *et al.*, 1970). Changes of left ventricular hemiaxis were measured and indices calculated (Bussmann *et al.*, 1979; Leighton *et al.*, 1975; Neuhaus *et al.*, 1976; Sesto and Schwarz, 1979; Wolf *et al.*, 1978). Some authors modified the old Tenant and Wiggers technique (Tenant and Wiggers, 1935) by employing radio-opaque markers (Brower *et al.*, 1979; Hetzer *et al.*, 1976). Walton-Brodie strain gauge arches (Hairston *et al.*, 1973; Moran *et al.*, 1973) were used or, more recently, miniaturized ultrasonic dimension transducers (Hagl *et al.*, 1978; Kleinmann *et al.*, 1979). But all the above methods have one very important limitation: they are all invasive and some of them (Hagl *et al.*, 1978; Hairston *et al.*, 1973; Kleinmann *et al.*, 1979; Moran *et al.*, 1973) can only be used during surgery or shortly thereafter. Therefore, a newly defined regional ejection fraction was introduced (Schad and Nickel, 1980; Reichart *et al.*, 1982) and measured at rest and after maximum exercise during the early postoperative period.

Why was the first pass technique used in RAO projection? The first pass technique is a non-invasive method which enables the investigator to look at regional myocardial function in RAO projection. Altogether it has mainly three advantages. First, the method is not invasive, and the procedure bears practically no risk. Second, measurements are made when the radionuclide bolus travels through the left ventricle at which time the right ventricle has practically no residual radioactivity. In contrast, the pool technique – where all four chambers are simultaneously filled – would not result in a clear separation between the right and left ventricle in most views of the heart. Activities in both chambers would overlap in the RAO projection. Finally, the RAO projection with its largest extension of the left

Table 8.1 Relationship between global ejection fraction and the degree of revascularization of the region of the anterior descending artery ($n = 50$)

| Global ejection fraction | LAD normal perfusion (*n* = 1) | Complete revascularization | | Incomplete revascularization | | LAD regions with significantly stenosed coronary arteries (*n* = 0) |
		without previous myocardial infarction (*n* = 27)	*with myocardial infarction* (*n* = 8)	*without previous myocardial onfarction* (*n* = 10)	*with myocardial infarction* (*n* = 3)	
Increased	1	24	5	2	—	—
Unchanged	—	1	2	3	2	—
Deteriorated	—	2	1	5	1	—

ventricle permits maximum spatial separation of the vascular territories of the main coronary arteries. Furthermore, the entire transverse diameters of the left ventricle are viewed best in this projection.

This method has only one major drawback: approximately two thirds of the circumflex area are covered by the left ventricular septum which in the upper portion is vascularized by the left anterior descending coronary artery. However, these upper parts of the septum belong mostly to the left ventricular outflow tract that normally show minimal contraction and therefore may account for an error of just 10–20%.

The assessment of the effects of coronary artery bypass surgery was mainly based on the *dynamics of the regional ejection fraction from rest to maximum exercise.* Since the exact method of subdividing the left ventricle into three vascular territories has not been done before, no comparable data exist in the literature. Yet the three regions of the left ventricle responded to exercise like the total left ventricle is reported to do: normally the global myocardial ejection fraction significantly increases after maximum exercise. However, if diffuse severe coronary artery disease exists, maximum exercise results in myocardial ischaemia; and consequently deterioration of the global left ventricular ejection fraction is observed. Kent *et al.* (1978) and Rerych *et al.* (1978a) described a decrease of the global ejection fraction during exercise by 12–15 percentage points.

Successful aortocoronary bypass surgery may reverse the ischaemic reaction after maximum exercise: according to Kent *et al.* (1978) 17 out of 23 patients demonstrated an improvement of global ejection from 39% preoperatively to 53% postoperatively. Finally, Kamath *et al.* (1979) reported an increase of global ejection fraction by 8 percentage points.

Not all cases of complete revascularization led to an increase of the regional ejection fraction. Some causes for this might have been a decreased blood flow in the venous graft (Chesebro *et al.*, 1976), a very high regional ejection fraction already at rest – which could not increase very much during maximum exercise – or a bypass occlusion (Deeg *et al.*, 1980).

As mentioned earlier, graft occlusion was disregarded and combined with the standard deviation of the mean. In a preliminary study of 30 patients functional results of bypass grafts have been compared with postoperative coronary angiograms (Deeg *et al.*, 1980). Out of 95 vein grafts eight were found to be occluded. These involved the corresponding regions: four cases to the LAD, three to the RCA and once to the CX. In six of these cases there was a marked decrease of the regional ejection fraction during maximum exercise. In two cases there were increases of 5.1% and 4.3%. In the latter two cases the LAD was stenosed 75%, distal to one or two large diagonal branches (Figure 8.6). Functional images, however, revealed poor function at the apical LAD areas. It was concluded that coronary angiograms are only needed when radionuclide angiograms show deterioration of regional territorial function with exercise.

In what manner are the global ejection fraction and the regional ejection fraction related to one another? The global ejection fraction represents a precise balance between the regions of the three main coronary arteries and all major branches: LAD, CX and RCA. If all three regions can be completely revascularized and none of them presents a history of myocardial infarction, the GEF usually increases, as it did in seven patients. But in most cases coronary artery disease does not alter each region in the same manner. For example, a ventricle might have an LAD area which shows normal perfusion, a CX area which was completely revascularized without previous MI and an RCA region which was incompletely revascularized because of high grade and diffuse coronary artery disease. In such a case the GEF cannot accurately measure the degree of improvement of left ventricular function after bypass surgery. The separate evaluation of the function in each individual region may help the investigator to explain why the GEF during maximum exercise increases, remains unchanged or even decreases. However, the GEF – being only a ratio between stroke volume and end-diastolic volume and therefore without dimension – does not represent a simple addition of REF values, as Figure 8.5 shows. The largest revascularized territory is the LAD region which constitutes on the average 58% of left ventricular myocardium. If this area was completely revascularized without evidence of previous MI (Figure 8.4), the GEF improved in 24 out of 27 cases (88.9%). Although, in cases of incomplete revascularization the chances of improvement decreased markedly: the GEF increased only in two out of 14 patients (14.3%) (Table 8.1). These results demonstrate especially that the LAD region should be completely revascularized, and that if this region has been severely damaged by previous MI, grafting of smaller vessels of the circumflex or right coronary arteries will not improve left ventricular function significantly.

The presented findings prove that successful aortocoronary bypass surgery not only relieves anginal pain – an opinion which is widely accepted – but at the same time improves myocardial function. Yet, the revascularization must be performed as completely as possible. Best results are obtained if there is no history of a large previous myocardial infarction. These important prerequisites were proved in another study of 19 patients who had diffuse coronary artery disease and who needed 5–8 anastomoses (average 5.4). The global ejection fraction rose in 13 cases in which 84.6% of the territories were completely revascularized. On the contrary, global ejection fraction deteriorated or remained

Figure 8.6 Coronary artery anatomy in two cases of angiographically proven occluded vein grafts. Both LAD vessels had, respectively, one and two well-perfused diagonal branches.

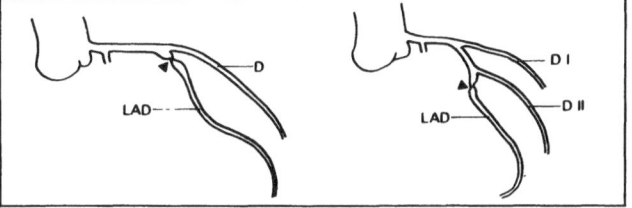

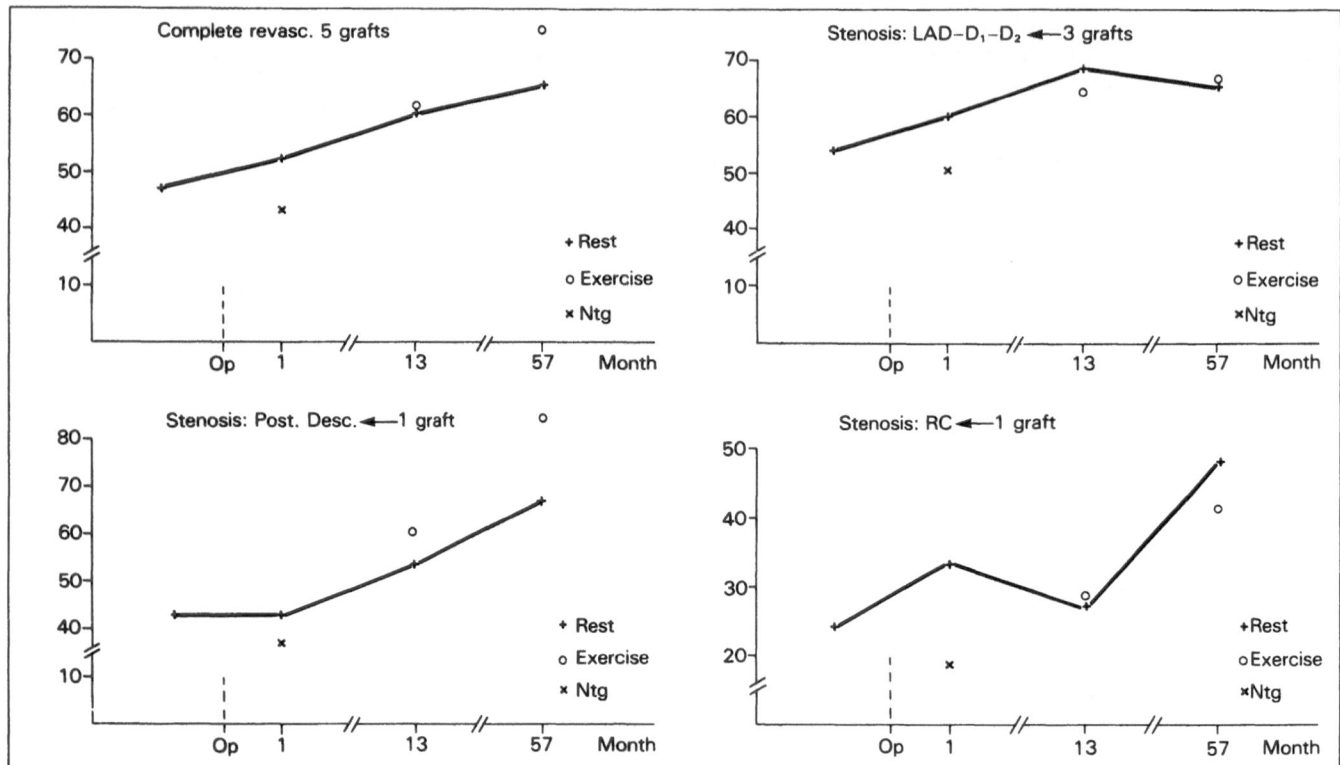

Figure 8.7 Global (left upper) and territorial ejection fractions for each coronary vascular territory (LAD: right upper, CX: left lower, RC: right lower) before and after bypass surgery during a 5-year follow-up period. Three vessel disease, complete revascularization, five grafts. Significant improvement of regional function. For functional images see Figure 8.9.

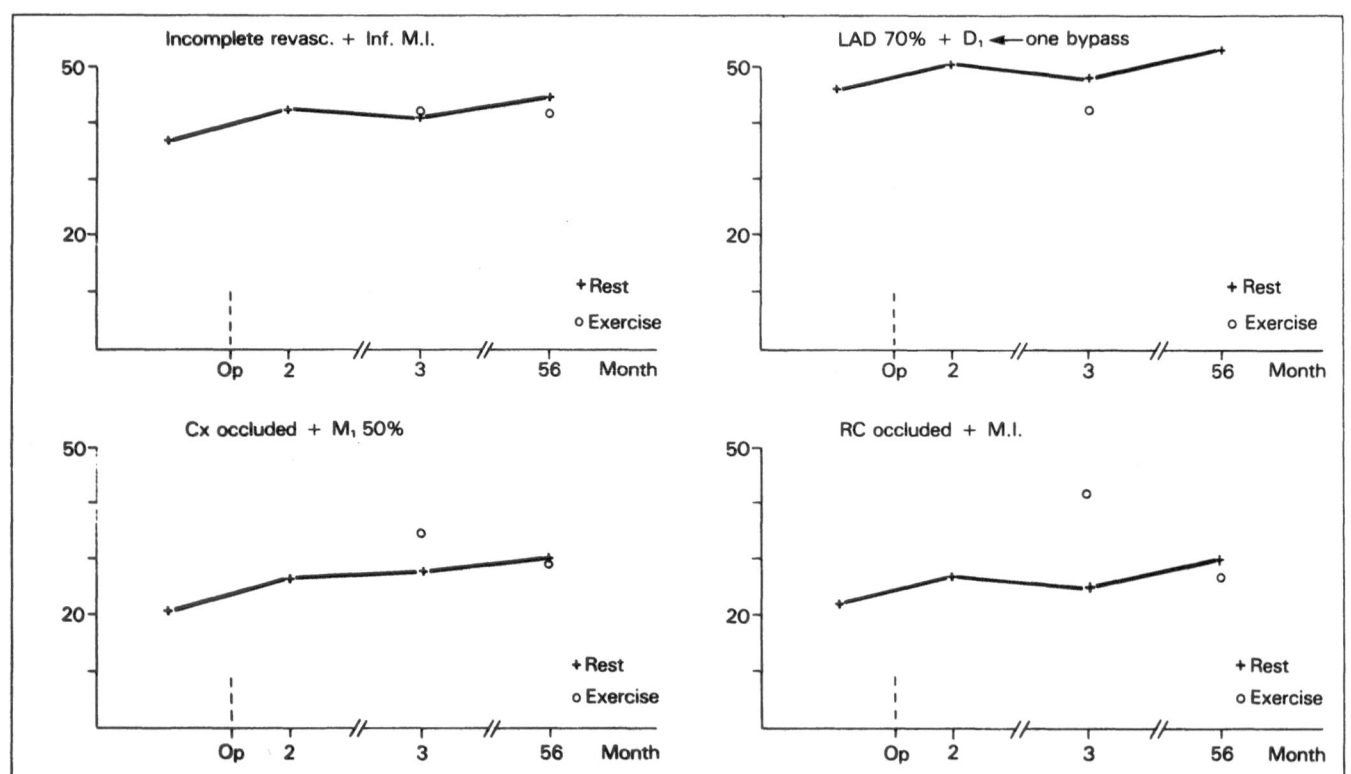

Figure 8.8 Global (left upper) and territorial ejection fractions for each coronary vascular territory (LAD: right upper, CX: left lower, RC: right lower) before and after bypass surgery during a 5-year follow-up period. Severe three vessel disease and documented prior myocardial infarction. Incomplete revascularization, one graft (LAD). Clinical improvement and 5-year survival. For functional images see Figure 8.10.

unchanged in six cases in which incomplete revascu-larization was predominant – 77% of the territories (Reichart *et al.*, 1983).

Furthermore, as presented, regional evaluation of left ventricular function performed 2–3 months postoperatively at rest and during maximum exercise allows a safe, non-invasive classification of the results of aortocoronary bypass surgery. The method may be repeated as often as necessary, an advantage which may prove very important. Long term follow-up with postoperative coronary angio-grams has revealed that brilliant early success may not last forever. Within a few years or less athero-sclerosis may progress in both the native coronary arteries and the grafts (Grondin, 1984). Repeated clinical and scintigraphic evaluations help to select the proper time for invasive investigation and possibly, eventual reoperation.

The two graphs (Figures 8.7 and 8.8) present for two patients global and territorial ejection fractions for each coronary territory before and after bypass surgery and during a 5-year follow-up period. The corresponding functional images are shown in Figures 8.9 and 8.10 respectively. For functional images of other cases and of closed bypass-grafts see Figures 8.11–8.12.

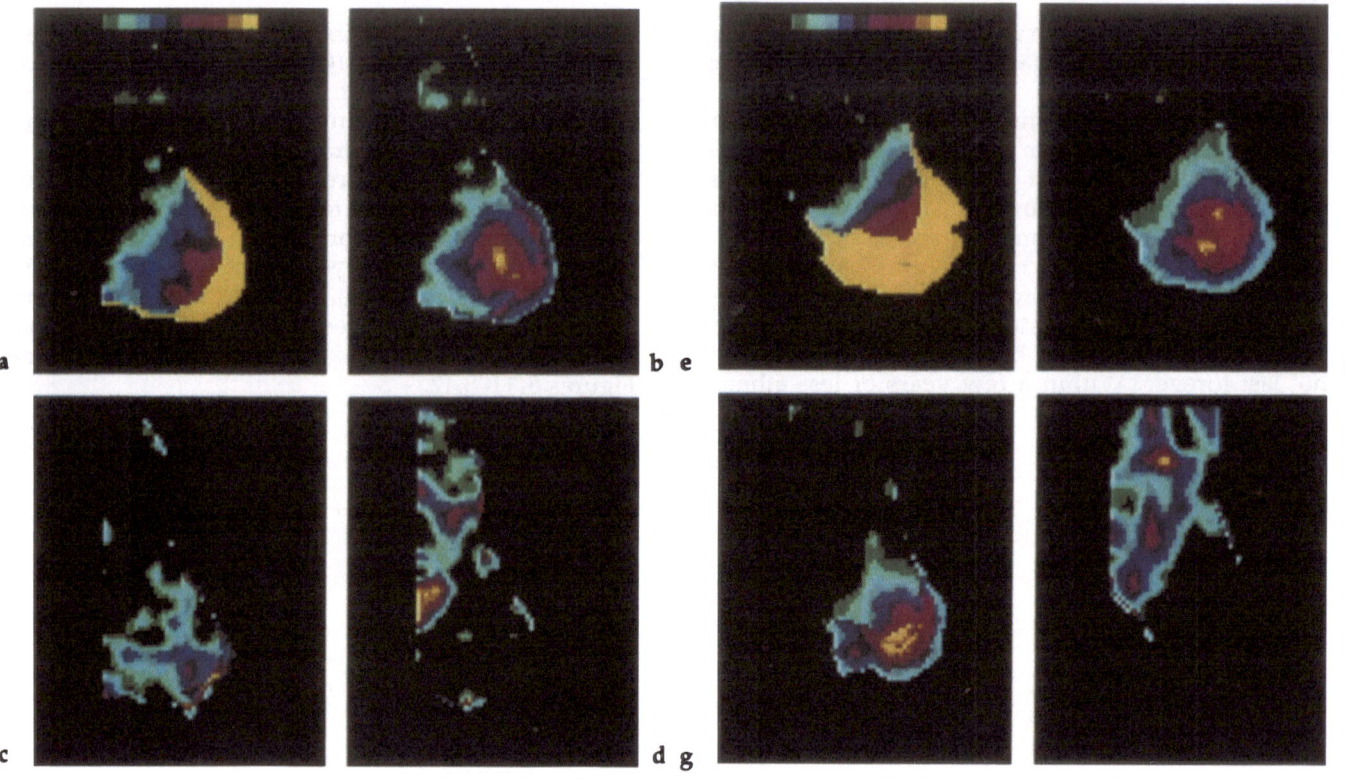

Figure 8.9 *Three vessel disease: stenosis at the LAD, D₁, D₂, CX (posterior descending), RC. 5 bypass grafts (see also Figure 8.7)*
a,b,c,d, Before surgery. Reduced EFs (**a**) and ERs (**b**) along the postero-inferior wall, low ERs at anterior wall. Rapid filling image (**c**) presents defects inferiorly, anteriorly and postero-laterally, paradoxical inward motion (**d**) during rapid filling at the corresponding areas.

e,f,g,h, 5 years after bypass surgery. Significant improvement of function in all bypass territories, EFs (**e**) and ERs (**f**). Rapid filling improved and directed as normal to the apex (**g**), paradoxical inward motion (**h**) disappeared except at upper anterior wall corresponding to the first diagonal branch. For territorial ejection fractions see Figure 8.7.

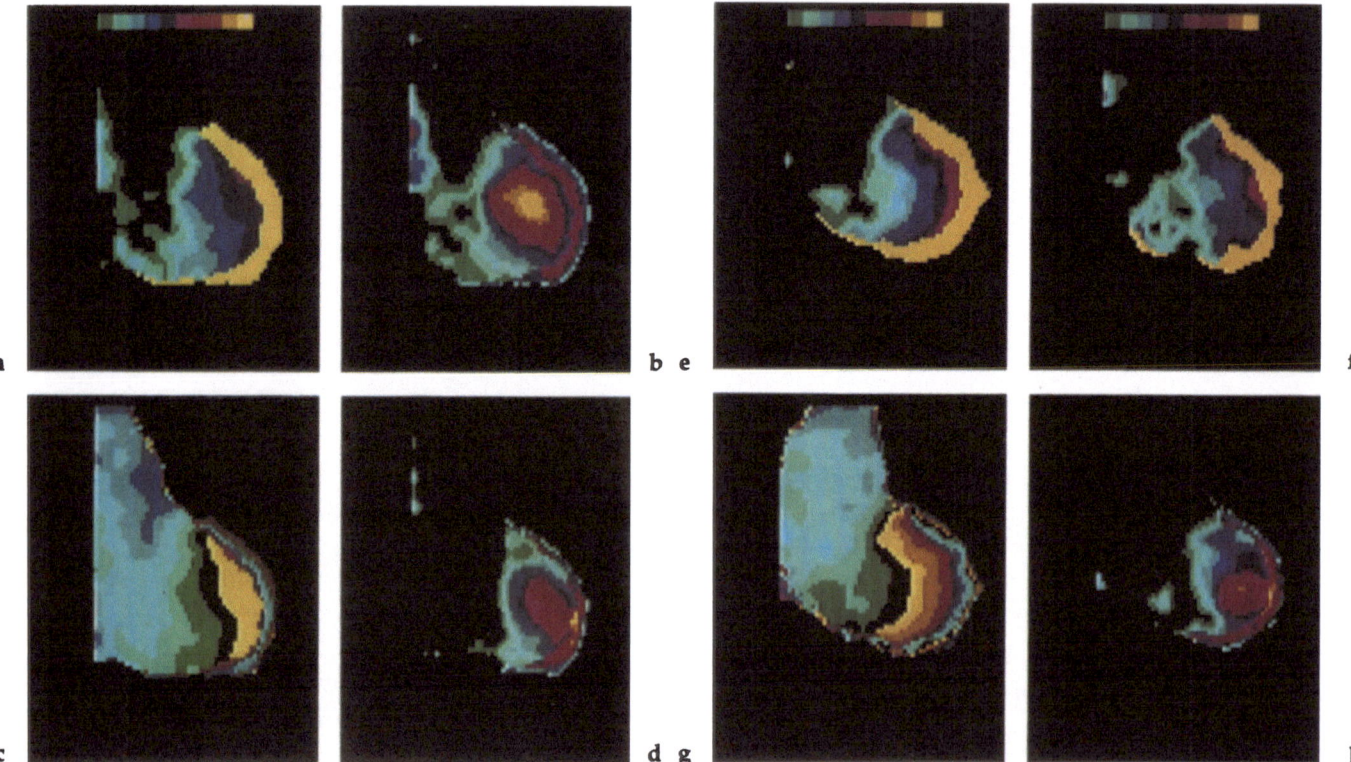

Figure 8.10 *Three vessel disease and prior inferior MI: stenosis at LAD (70%) and D₁, peripheral CX and RC occluded, M₁ stenotic (50%) 1 bypass graft to the LAD (see also Figure 8.8)*
a,b,c,d, Before surgery. Reduced EFs (**a**) and ERs (**b**) and severely prolonged MTTs (**c**) in a large infero-posterior zone extending laterally. Lowered ERs along the anterior wall. Rapid filling image (**d**) presents large defects inferiorly and postero-laterally and somewhat reduced rates at the upper anterior wall.

e,f,g,h, 5 years after incomplete revascularization of LAD: significant improvement of function at the anterior wall higher EFs (**e**), higher ERs (**f**) and lower MTTs (**g**). Rapid filling rates at the lower and middle anterior wall improved (**h**). Clinical improvement and 5 years survival. For territorial ejection fractions see Figure 8.8.

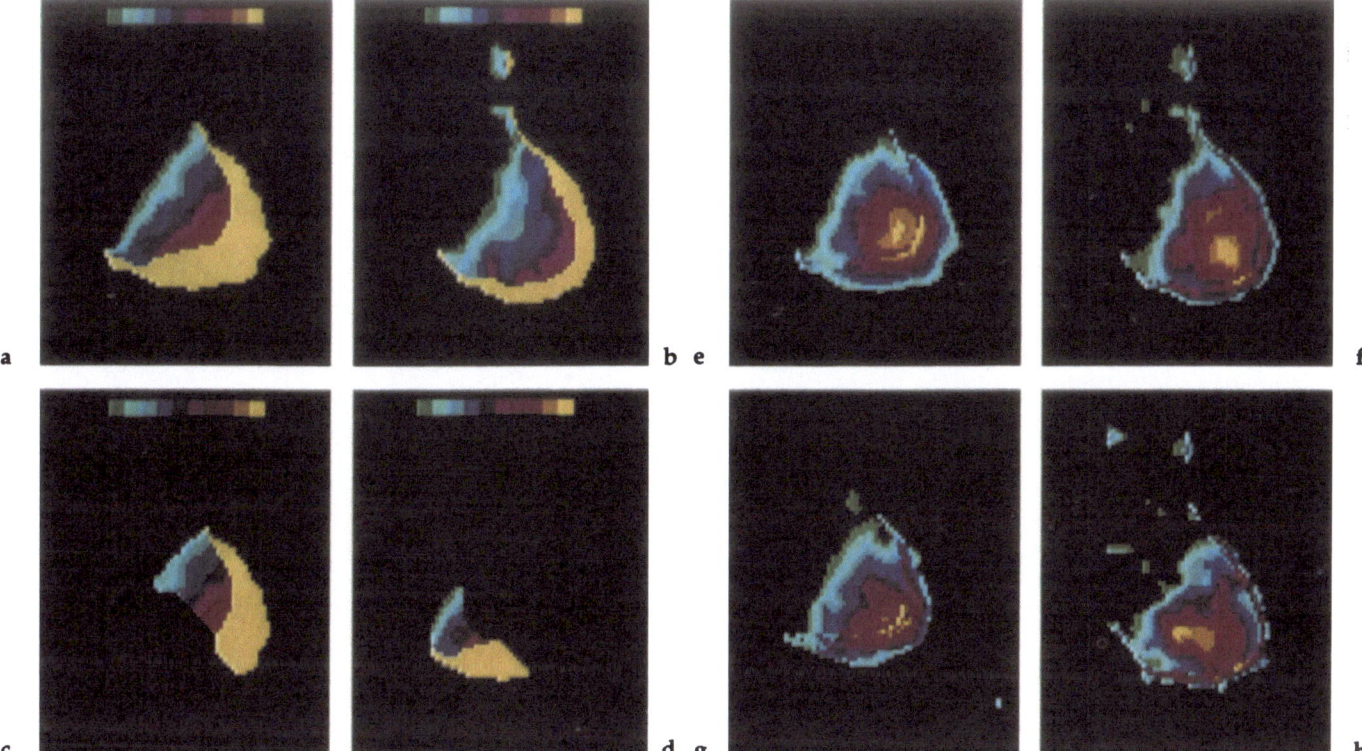

Figure 8.11 *Three vessel disease: significant stenosis at the left main, LAD, D, CX and RC. Peripheral CX occlusion. Collateral flow from RC to LAD. Bypass grafts to LAD, CX, and M. Incomplete revascularization.*

a,b,c,d, REFIs: significantly deteriorating from rest (**a**) to exercise.(**b**). LAD territory at rest (**c**), territorial EF decreasing from 63 to 53% with exercise, RC territory at rest (**d**).

Territorial EF decreasing from 60 to 42% with exercise and also CX territorial EF decreases from 62 to 37%. Global EF: at rest 63% under stress 48%.

e,f,g,h, ERs deteriorated from rest (**e**) to exercise (**f**) along the anterior wall and postero-inferiorly. Rapid filling rates deteriorated correspondingly (**g,h**).

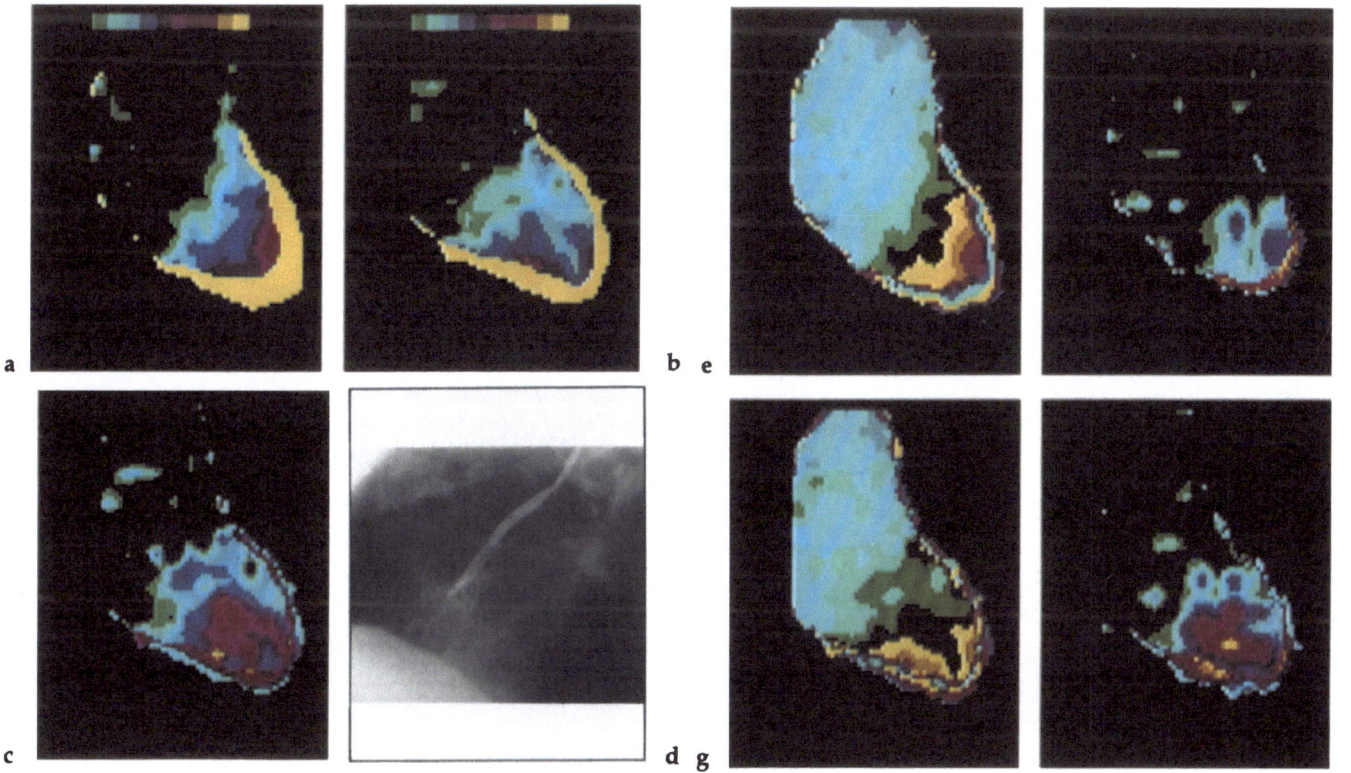

Figure 8.12 *Three vessel disease: occlusion of the LAD and proximal CX, stenosis of posterior descending and D_1. Collateral flow from RC to LAD and from D to distal LAD. 3 bypass grafts to LAD and posterior descending.*

a,b,c,d, Significant deterioration of EFs at the upper anterior wall from rest (**a**) to exercise (**b**). Severely reduced ERs at the upper anterior wall (**c**) pointing to closed LAD bypass. The graft is significantly stenosed at the point of the anastomosis, minimal anterograde flow, no retrograde flow (**d**).

e,f,g,h, Mean times already at rest prolonged at the unbypassed CX territory and also pointing to the reduced function at the upper anterior wall (**e**) with exercise severe deterioration in both territories (**f**). Rapid filling rates at rest (**g**): already defects at the upper anterior wall also seen during exercise (**h**). In these zones also paradoxical inward motion during rapid filling.

9

Coronary Angioplasty

D. PHILLIPS

Non-operative transluminal dilatation of atherosclerotic obstructions was first described by Dotter and Judkins in 1964 (Dotter and Judkins, 1964). The Dotter procedure consisted of sequential passage of rigid catheters of increasing size in relatively large, non-tortuous arteries and was not suitable for the treatment of coronary artery stenoses. In 1974 Gruntzig used a double lumen balloon tipped catheter to dilate iliac and femoral arteries and by 1977 miniaturization and cadaver experimentation permitted its use in the coronary arteries (Gruntzig, 1978). In 1979 under the support of the National Heart, Lung, and Blood Institute (NHLBI), an International Registry of Angioplasty was begun which had enrolled more than 3000 patients by 1981 (Kent et al., 1982). In 1983 more than 10 000 patients underwent transluminal coronary angioplasty.

MECHANISM

Like coronary bypass surgery, coronary angioplasty alters the abnormal coronary supply/demand ratio directly by improving available coronary blood flow to the myocardium. Inflating the fluid filled balloon tip within a stenosed arterial segment transmits lateral pressure directly to the plaque, resulting in rupture of the endothelial layer and reduction of the stenosis. The arterial wall is stretched with little, if any, compression of the atherosclerotic plaque (Hoffman et al., 1981; Block et al., 1981). Deflation of the balloon results in an immediate increase in blood flow with restoration of normal myocardial metabolism (Williams et al., 1980) and hyperaemic responses (O'Neill, et al. 1984).

The endothelial layer over the atherosclerotic plaque is denuded with splitting of the media often to the internal elastic lamina (Hoffman et al., 1981). Subsequent dilatations complete the remoulding producing a smooth appearance of the dilated segment seen on final arteriograph. Successful angioplasty can be defined in terms of percentage reduction in stenosis, pressure gradient, or normalization of ischaemic responses to exercise stress (Kent et al., 1982; Sigwart et al., 1982; O'Neill et al., 1984).

Healing may be mediated by platelet activity (Ross and Glomset, 1976). Platelet adherence and aggregation are stimulated by the denuded endothelium with exposure of medial atherosclerotic contents (Block et al., 1981). Platelet mediated thrombosis appears to be retarded by pretreatment with platelet activity suppression drugs and heparin. Continued suppression during the endothelialization period of 3–6 weeks may retard recurrence (Mehta, 1984).

In 20–30% of patients continued endothelial cell proliferation with lipid infiltration continues, producing a recurrent atherosclerotic plaque with restenosis. Pathologically, the recurrent plaque is indistinguishable from de novo proliferative plaques (Waller et al., 1983).

RESULTS

The initial NHLBI Registry described a rate of expected successful angioplasty of nearly 70%. Allowing for an initial learning curve, the primary causes for failure at angioplasty were failure to approach and cross the stenosis, while failure to dilate a crossed lesion was much less frequent (Kent et al., 1982). Because of the relatively high failure rate, optimal lesions were restricted to single, proximal, non-eccentric, non-calcified, discrete stenoses. Such selection restricted applicability to about 5% of patients who were candidates for coronary bypass surgery.

Using steerable dilating catheters with a wider selection of size and profiles of materials allowing higher internal pressurization, tortuous segments can be easily passed allowing access to distal segments of the coronary tree. Subsequent success rates of 90% or higher are achievable in selected vessels allowing a widening of the application of angioplasty. Current indications include distal, eccentric, calcified, single or multiple, discrete or complex lesions in single or multiple coronary arteries (Hartzler, 1983). Although the recurrence rate is higher, stenotic proximal or distal SVG anastomoses, midgraft lesions, and stenoses distal to SVG anastomoses often will yield to angioplasty (Block et al., 1984). Coronary angioplasty has been applied to recently occluded coronary arteries, as an intraoperative adjunct to coronary bypass surgery (Jones and King, 1984), and to symptomatic patients, who by reason of poor LV function or prior coronary bypass surgery are not felt to be adequate patients for coronary revascularization.

RECURRENCE

The interpretation of chest pain occurring during and subsequent to coronary dilatation and diagnosis of recurrence present serious difficulties in the overall evaluation of coronary angioplasty. Cardiac pain is common during the procedure and can lead to a decision to abort in favour of immediate coronary bypass surgery. Ischaemic pain arising from balloon occlusion of the coronary artery subsides promptly after balloon deflation. Longer-lasting pain may occur from subintimal dissection of the coronary artery or from occlusion of secondary branches arising from the stenosed segment.

Inapparent or trivial air embolism occurring during contrast injection may cause unexplained persisting ischaemic pain with or without e.c.g. changes. Persisting ischaemic pain may reflect coronary spasm, partial occlusion by an intimal flap or intramural hæmorrhage. If accompanied by ST segments shift, persistent pain requires repeat arteriography, further angioplasty, or urgent surgical intervention.

In the initial hours following angioplasty, chest pain of uncertain aetiology may wax and wane but if the e.c.g. remains stable only reassurance is needed. ST segment changes accompany abrupt closure of the dilated segment and more often are due to coronary spasm than thrombosis, but if not relieved by nitrates and nefedipine, urgent intervention is required to avert myocardial infarction.

Recurrent symptoms during the first 2 months of angioplasty may indicate late thrombosis or spasm in the healing dilated segment. Coronary spasm may respond poorly to nitrates and calcium-channel antagonists, and indicate a high likelihood of subsequent restenosis (Hollman et al., 1983). Symptomatic recurrence from restenosis usually appears from 6 weeks to 4 months following angioplasty; later recurrent symptoms more often indicate progression in other coronary arteries or undilated segments. Symptomatic recurrence requires repeat arteriography to identify recurrent stenosis and progression.

Recurrent stenosis not infrequently occurs without symptoms. Graded exercise testing, thallium 201 scintillography and radionuclide ventriculography were initially utilized to demonstrate effective non-operative revascularization (Sigwart et al., 1982) but later restudy identified asymptomatic recurrence by demonstrating reversion of an initial normal response to subsequent ischaemic response (Rod et al., 1984). Arteriography may demonstrate significant restenosis or progression in non-dilated segments. Repeat coronary arteriography is indicated in patients showing persisting ischaemic exercise response or reversion of normal to ischaemic response.

For the majority of patients, coronary angioplasty has been proven an effective palliative procedure for occlusive coronary atherosclerosis by repeat angiography, and a variety of non-invasive functional tests. Recurrence after 6 months' stability is uncommon and both repeat angiography and functional testing have shown stability in the dilated segment persisting for years after the angioplasty procedure (Rosing et al., 1984; Gruntzig, 1984). Rather than competing with coronary bypass surgery, coronary angioplasty widens the alternatives for palliation for patients threatened by atherosclerotic coronary heart disease.

Functional imaging offers a unique non-invasive way to evaluate patients before and after angioplasty and may prove to be helpful in long term follow-up (see Figures 9.1–9.8).

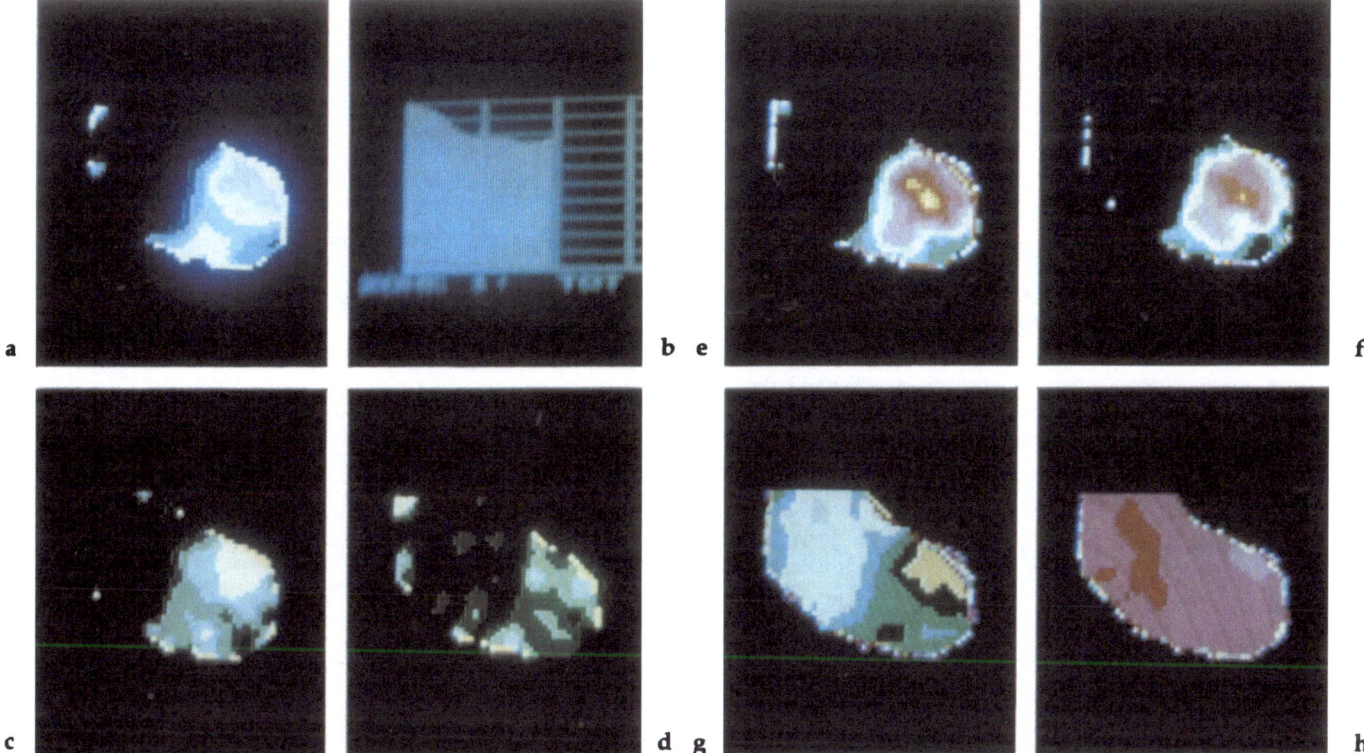

Figure 9.1 *Case 1. Preangioplasty* 85% narrowing of proximal LAD, diagonal branch totally obstructed, unchanged. Circumflex 30% narrowing. Rest anterior preangioplasty images show severe inferior and anterior lateral wall motion abnormality which extends to the left ventricular apex, most pronounced during early systole where there is reduced global function LVEF 30%. **a**, REFI; **b**, volume curve; **c**, first half REFI; **d**, second half REFI; **e**, ejection rate; **f**, first half ER; **g**, transit; **h**, first half transit.

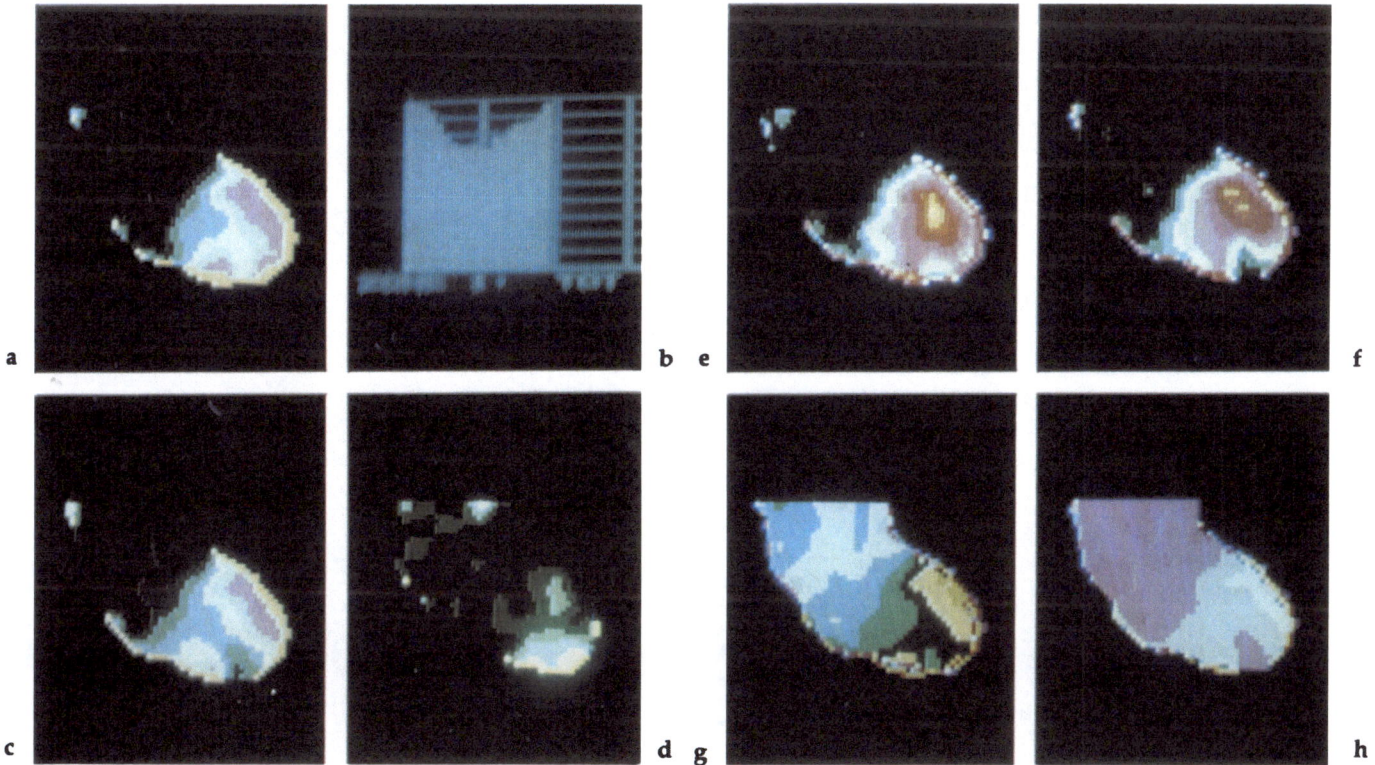

Figure 9.2 *Case 1. Postangioplasty* proximal LAD narrowing reduced to 25%. LVEF 32%, global function has improved slightly and wall motion abnormalities also appear improved following angioplasty particularly in the REFI and first half REFI images. Significant residual ischaemia is evident. **a**, REFI; **b**, volume curve; **c**, first half REFI; **d**, second half REFI; **e**, ejection rate; **f**, first half ER; **g**, transit; **h**, first half transit.

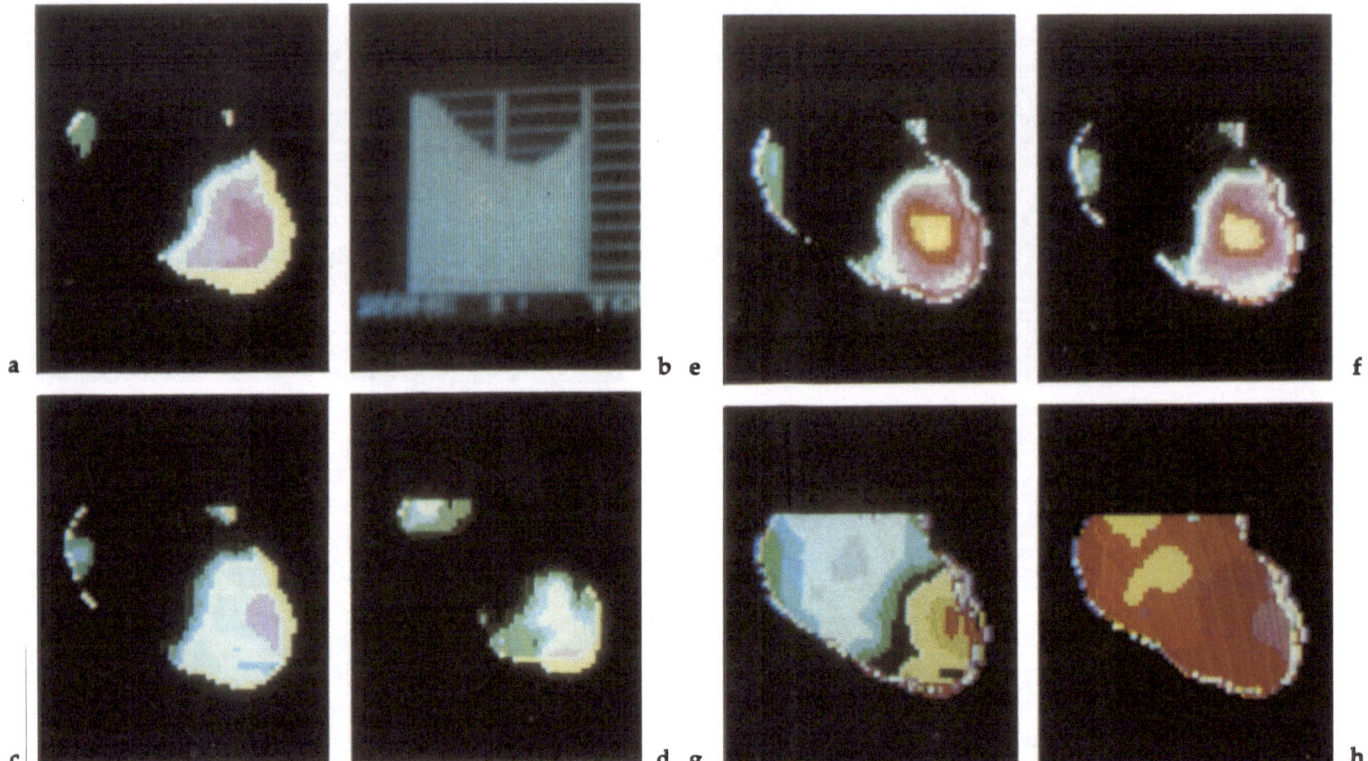

Figure 9.3 *Case 2. Preangioplasty* LAD. Total occlusion of the proximal LAD with excellent ventricular function and collateral filling through right coronary artery. LEF 51%. Rest study shows only mild apical changes which are consistent with ischaemia most pronounced during early systole in the first half REFI image and in the first half rate and mean transit images. **a**, REFI; **b**, volume curve; **c**, first half REFI; **d**, second half REFI; **e**, ejection rate; **f**, first half ER; **g**, transit; **h**, first half transit.

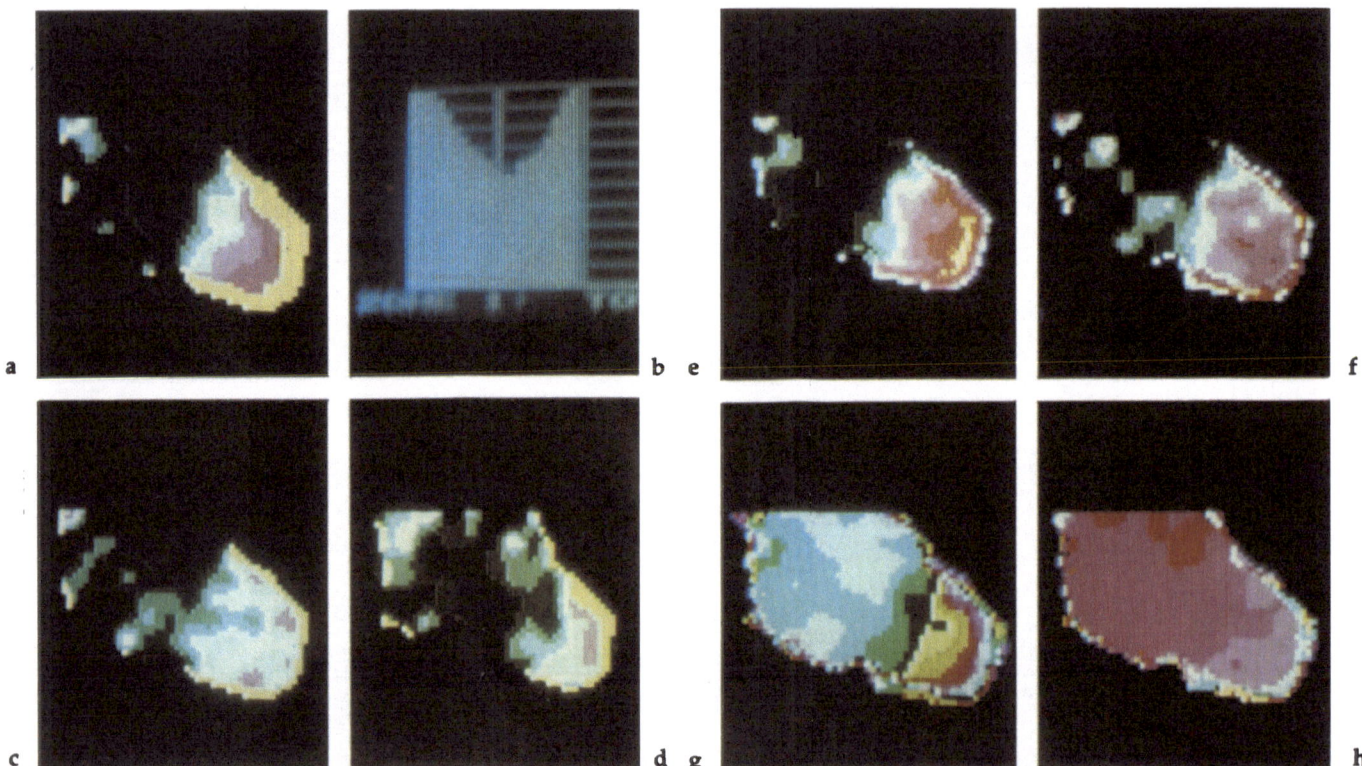

Figure 9.4 *Case 2. Postangioplasty* LVEF 51%. Global function remains good and unchanged following angioplasty. Wall motion appears slightly improved at the apex and is best appreciated in the rate and mean transit images. **a**, REFI; **b**, volume curve; **c**, first half REFI; **d**, second half REFI; **e**, ejection rate; **f**, first half ER; **g**, transit; **h**, first half transit.

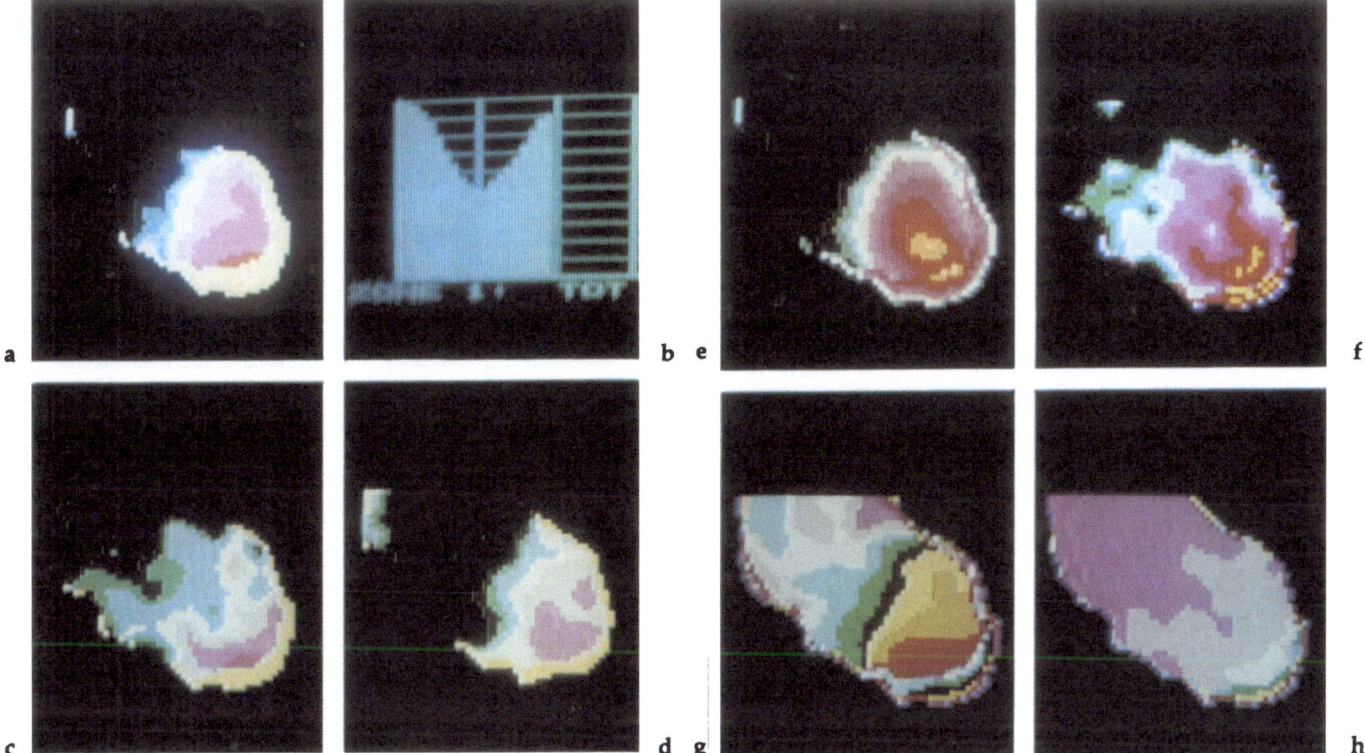

Figure 9.5 *Case 3. Preangioplasty circumflex.* Chest pain, shortness of breath, unstable angina, cardiac catheterization showed 85% stenosis of the circumflex artery and 50% narrowing of the proximal LAD artery with subtotal occlusion of the proximal diagonal branch. LVEF 45%.

RNV showed ischaemic change at rest in the region of the high lateral wall and centrally best appreciated in the first half REFI. **a,** REFI; **b,** volume curve; **c,** first half REFI; **d,** second half REFI; **e,** ejection rate; **f,** first half ER; **g,** transit; **h,** first half transit.

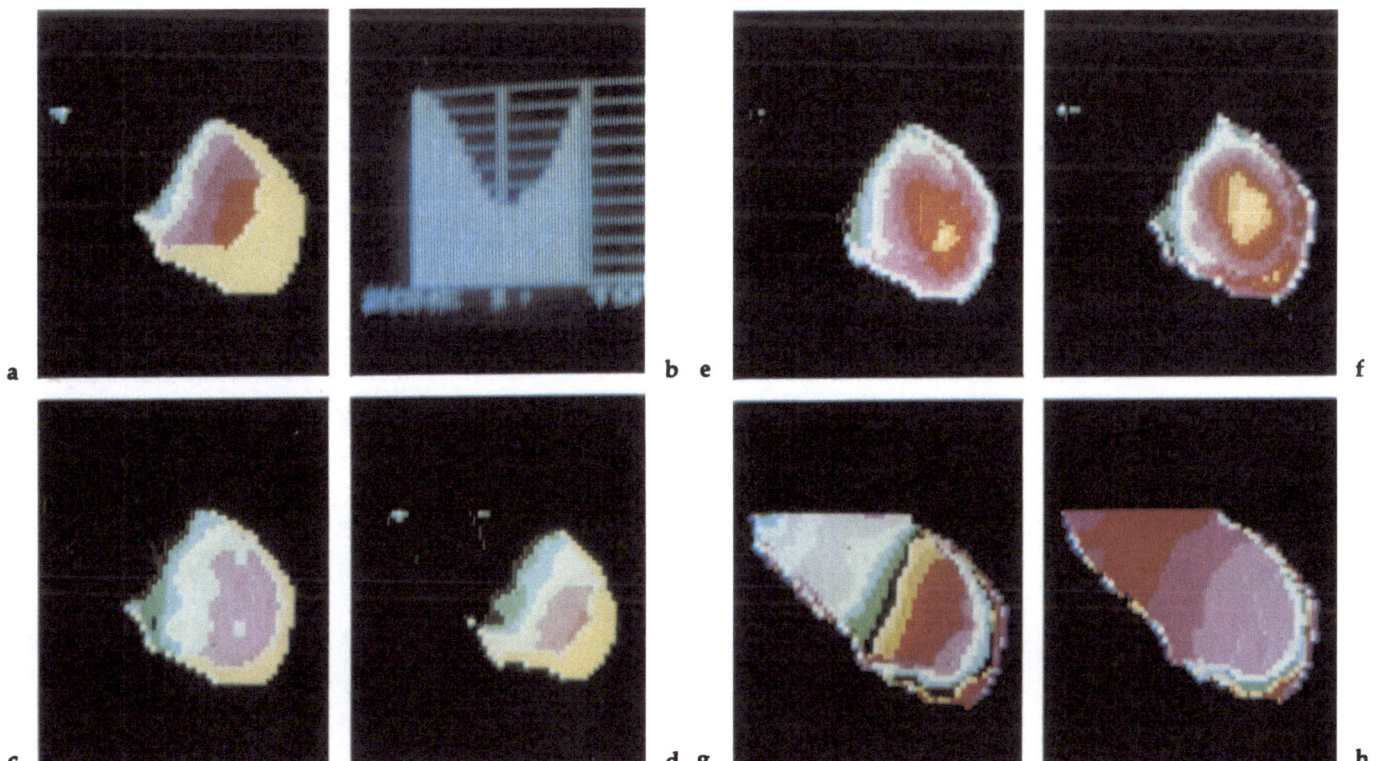

Figure 9.6 *Case 3. Postangioplasty* LVEF 62%. Global function has increased significantly following angioplasty and wall motion has also improved. The central and high lateral abnormalities previously seen are no longer

present. **a,** REFI; **b,** volume curve; **c,** first half REFI; **d,** second half REFI; **e,** ejection rate; **f,** first half ER; **g,** transit; **h,** first half transit.

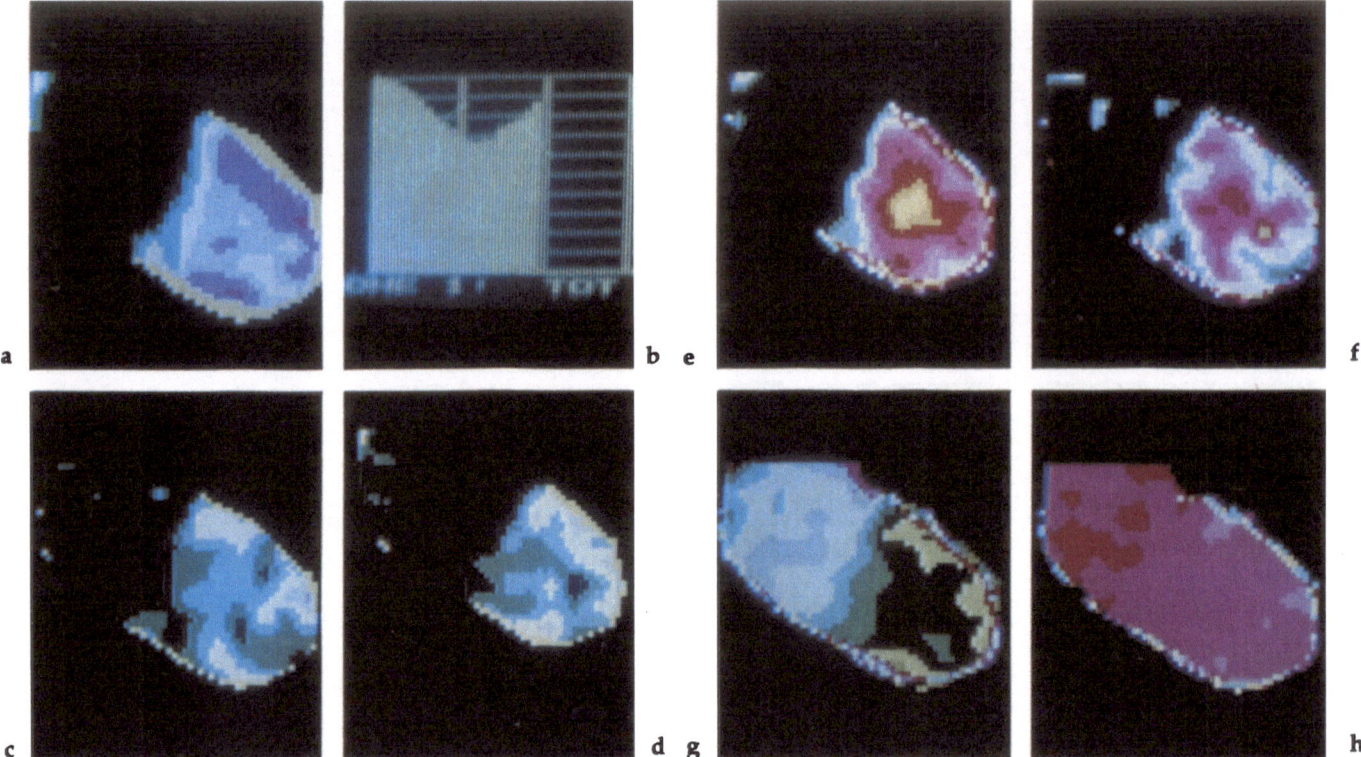

Figure 9.7 *Case 4. Preangioplasty* LAD. 45-year-old male with chest pain. 90% stenosis of the LAD coronary artery distal to the diagonal branch. LVEF 32% rest, 34% exercise. RNV images typical of ischaemia in the LAD dis-tribution. **a,** REFI; **b,** volume curve; **c,** first half REFI; **d,** second half REFI; **e,** ejection rate; **f,** first half ER; **g,** transit; **h,** first half transit.

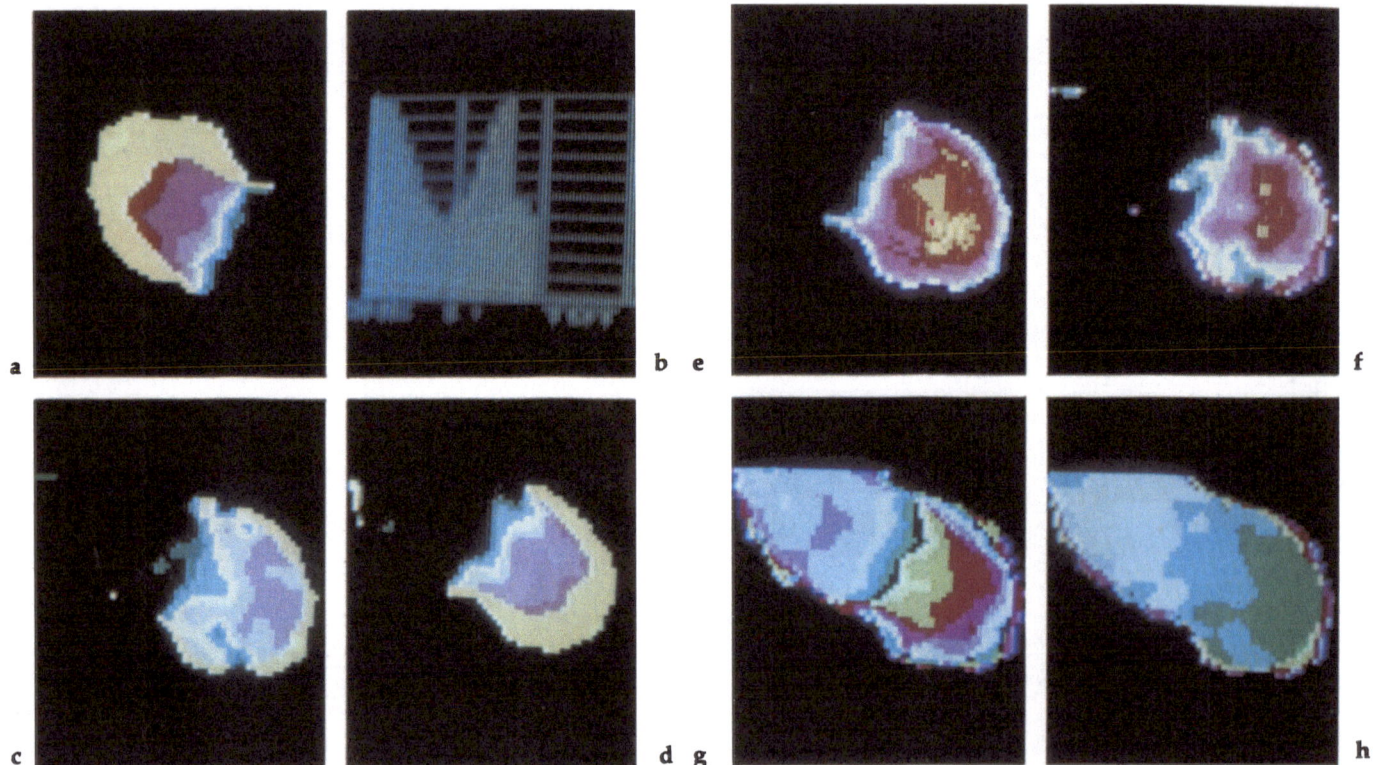

Figure 9.8 *Case 4. Postangioplasty* LAD. Global function and wall motion improve significantly following angio-plasty. LVEF 44% rest, 56% exercise. **a,** REFI; **b,** volume curve; **c,** first half REFI; **d,** second half REFI; **e,** ejection rate; **f,** first half ER; **g,** transit; **h,** first half transit.

10

Intracoronary Thrombolysis in Acute Myocardial Infarction

A. WEIKL AND N. SCHAD

Systemic as well as local thrombolytic therapy in the acute myocardial infarction aims to avoid or limit ischaemic myocardial necrosis by reopening of the occluded coronary artery. In 1974, Dotter demonstrated that one can obtain lysis of fresh intra-arterial thrombotic clot formation (Dotter et al., 1974). In 1976, Chazov reported intracoronary fibrinolysis in cases of evolving myocardial infarction, and Rentrop introduced this technique into the clinical routine in 1978 and 1980 (Chazov et al., 1976; Rentrop et al., 1978, 1980).

Schröder and colleagues reported that systemic high dose administration of fibrinolytic streptokinase (1–1.5 million units/h) resulted in lysis in about 70% of thrombotic coronary occlusions (Schröder, 1983).

Intra-arterial thrombosis develops on the basis of the following three pathophysiological factors:

(1) Haemodynamic factor: with 75% or more narrowing of the lumen of an artery blood flow is accelerated to such an extent that the Reynold's number is exceeded. Consequently, flow becomes turbulent at the stenosis and at the poststenotic segment. Turbulence, however, is one of the conditions favouring the development of intra-arterial thrombosis.

(2) Blood factors: several factors may influence coagulability, such as alterations in the lipid metabolism, postprandial hyperlipidaemia or increased production of catecholamines.

(3) Wall factor: arterial obstructions are usually arteriosclerotic with parietal deposits of lipoids and paraproteins. Secondary calcifications may develop leading to irregularities of the inner arterial surface. Then, thrombocytes may aggregate and produce vessel obstruction with peripheral stasis of blood flow that favours for extension of intravasal coagulation and thrombus formation. Atheromas are covered by a thin epithelial layer which can tear during transient blood pressure elevation so that the atheroma empties into the vessel's lumen. At these sites intravascular thrombus formation may rapidly develop.

Figure 10.1 illustrates a section of infarcted myocardium after postmortem coronarography. The open vascular territories are filled with contrast medium (white), the corresponding myocardium is well perfused (dark areas). The ischaemic zone depends on a vessel that is partially occluded by a thrombus. This thrombus is already spontaneously recanalized by three open channels. After acute myocardial infarction fresh thrombus formation causing or contributing to the infarction process could be found in up to 90% of the cases, depending on the specific anatomo-pathological technique.

Fibrinolytic therapy was performed in our clinic in 49 patients with acute myocardial infarct, in 1983 (Figure 10.2). Twelve patients underwent systemic fibrinolysis (1 million units/h). In five patients the presumably obstructed artery was later found to be open by angiography; in two the vessel was closed.

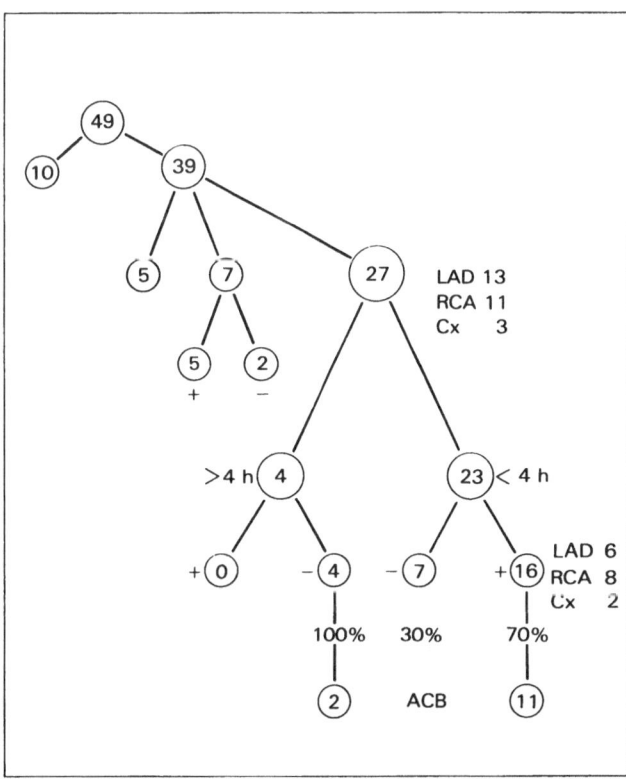

Figure 10.2 *Patients treated by fibrinolytic therapy: follow-up in 39 patients.* Of the 27 patients who underwent intracoronary fibrinolysis 23 were treated within 4 hours after the onset of pain: 70% presented a positive result. Conversely, all patients who were treated later than 4 hours from onset of pain showed a negative result.

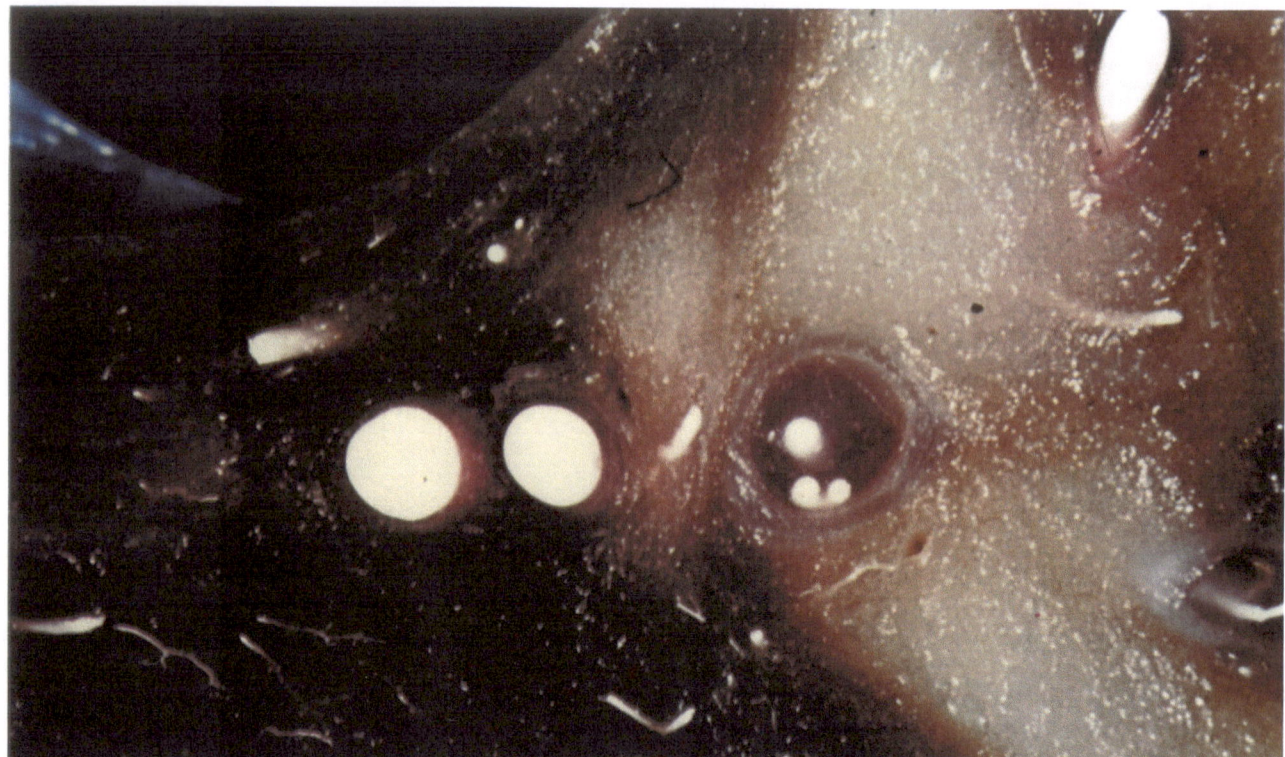

Figure 10.1 *Section of infarcted myocardium after postmorten coronary angiogram*. The open vascular territories are filled with contrast medium (white), the corresponding myocardium is well perfused (dark areas), the ischaemic zone depends on the vessel that is partially occluded by a thrombus.

In 23 of 37 patients that received intracoronary streptokinase (2–4000 units/min) the angiographic follow-up could be obtained; open arteries were found in 16 cases (69.5%). All four patients who were treated by intracoronary streptokinase more than 4 hours after onset of the myocardial infarct, had closed vessels which could not be reopened. Eleven of the successfully treated patients underwent bypass surgery.

Local application of streptokinase usually reopens the vessel within an average of 22 minutes. Precordial pain subsides, electrocardiographic ST-elevations regress, and CK-enzymes rapidly wash out. Most important, however, ventricular function significantly improves (Figure 10.3). Radionuclide angiography with functional imaging enables one to follow regional left ventricular performance non-invasively.

Precisely, the following questions which determine the prognosis and the further clinical treatment of the patient can be answered.

(1) Did function at the reopened vascular territory normalize or improve?

(2) What is the extent and degree of residual dysfunction at the treated territory?

(3) What is the functional significance of other vascular territories in jeopardy?

To answer these questions, the first pass radionuclide examination should be done at rest and exercise in the RAO view (see Chapters 4 and 8). Some examples are illustrated in Figures 10.4 and 10.5.

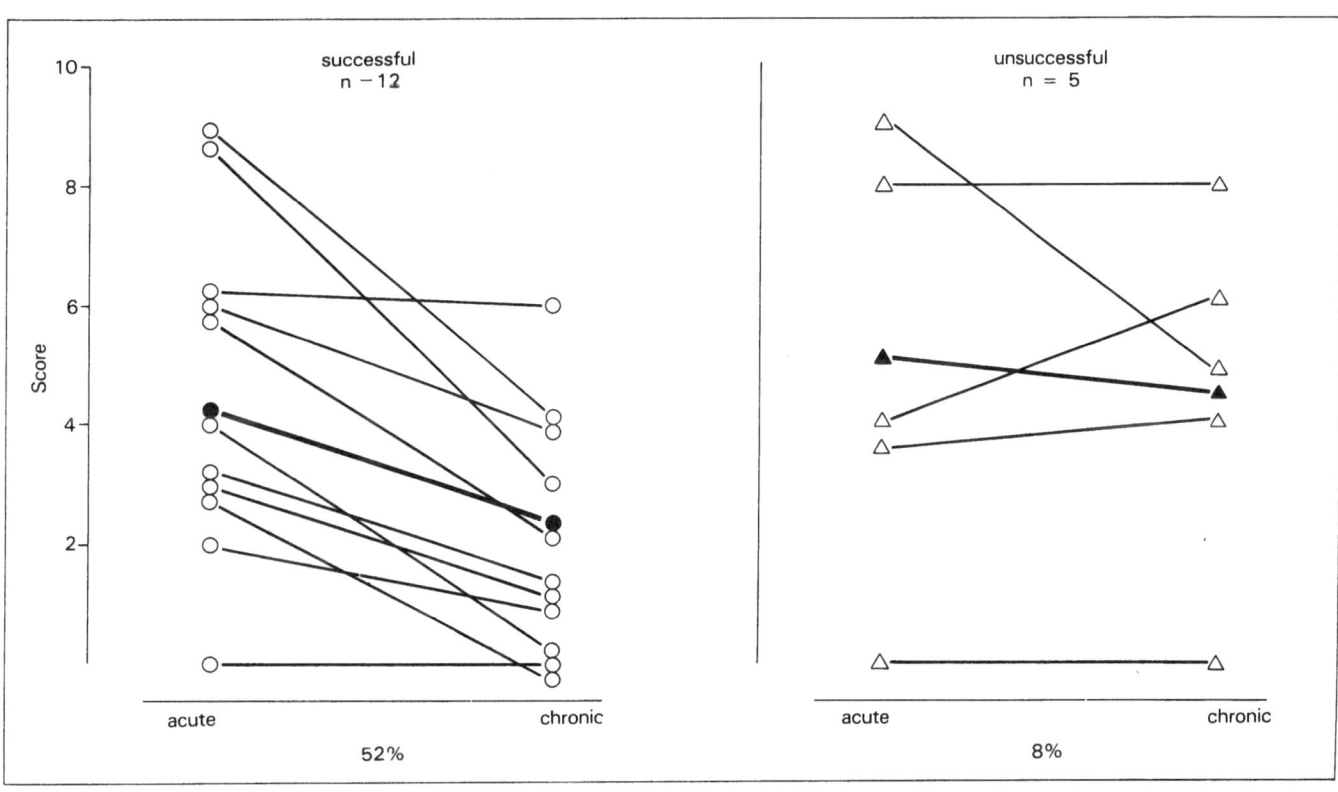

Figure 10.3 *Left ventricular function after intracoronary fibrinolysis.* Left ventricular function in both oblique projections after fibrinolysis examined with the contrast ventriculography: seven segments scored as follows:

normal = 0, hypokinesia = 1, akinesia = 2, dyskinesia = 3. Significant improvement of sequential wall motion in 12 cases.

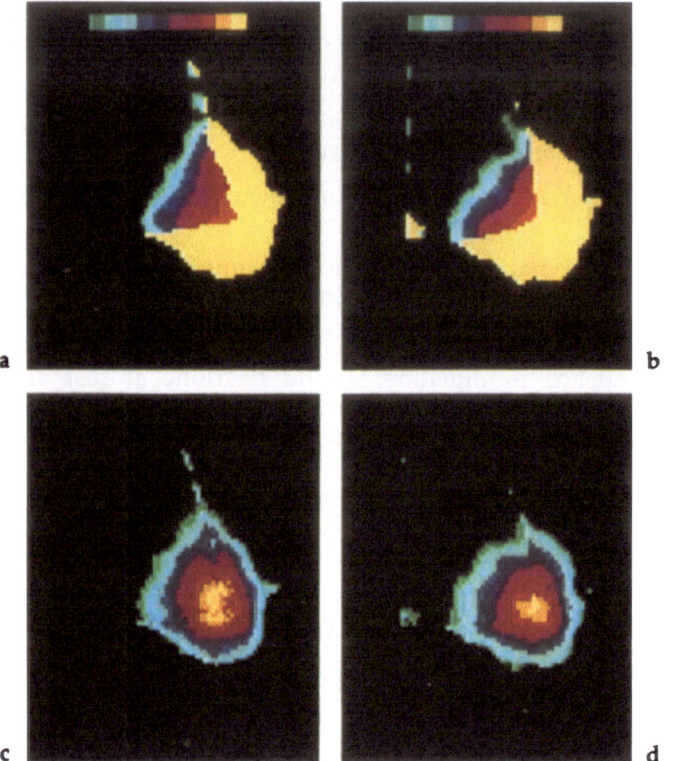

a

b

c

d

Figure 10.4 *Acute total occlusion of right coronary – lysis 1 hour after onset of chest pain. Subsequent bypass of the RC stenosis.*

a–d, Functional images at rest and exercise in RAO view: strong contraction at rest and exercise (a,b) and high parietal ERs (c,d) without any severe dysfunction in right coronary territory as usually seen in myocardial infarction.

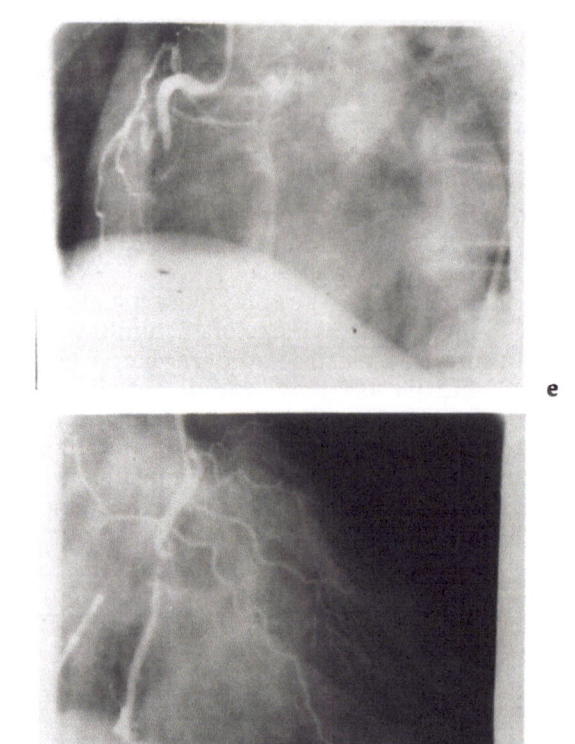

e

f

e,f, Right coronary angiogram: total occlusion of the RC (e), after lysis recanalization of the vessel (f). Lysis 1 hour after onset of chest pain.

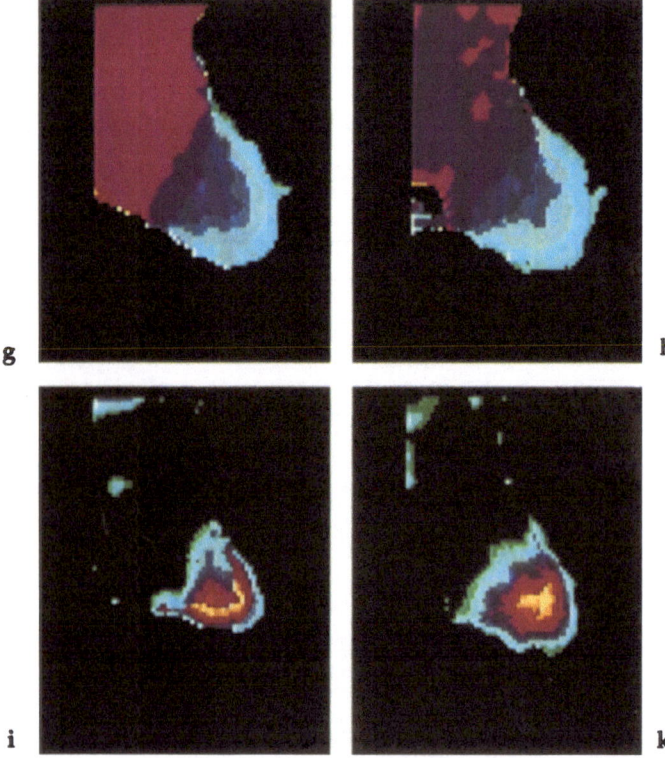

g

h

i

k

g,h,i,k, Functional images at rest and exercise in RAO view: normal mean time levels at rest and exercise; posterior mitral valve prolapse (g,h). Rapid filling at rest and exercise not deviated, i.e. directed to the apex, no defect as usually seen with infarct.

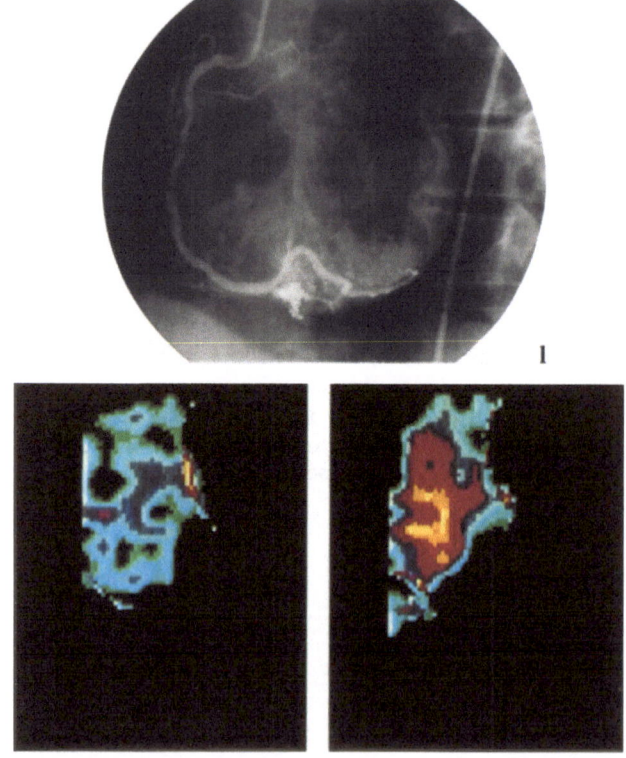

l

m

n

l, Right coronary angiogram: 8 days after lysis further regression of obstruction.

m,n, No paradoxical inward displacement of blood as regularly seen in infarcted zones.

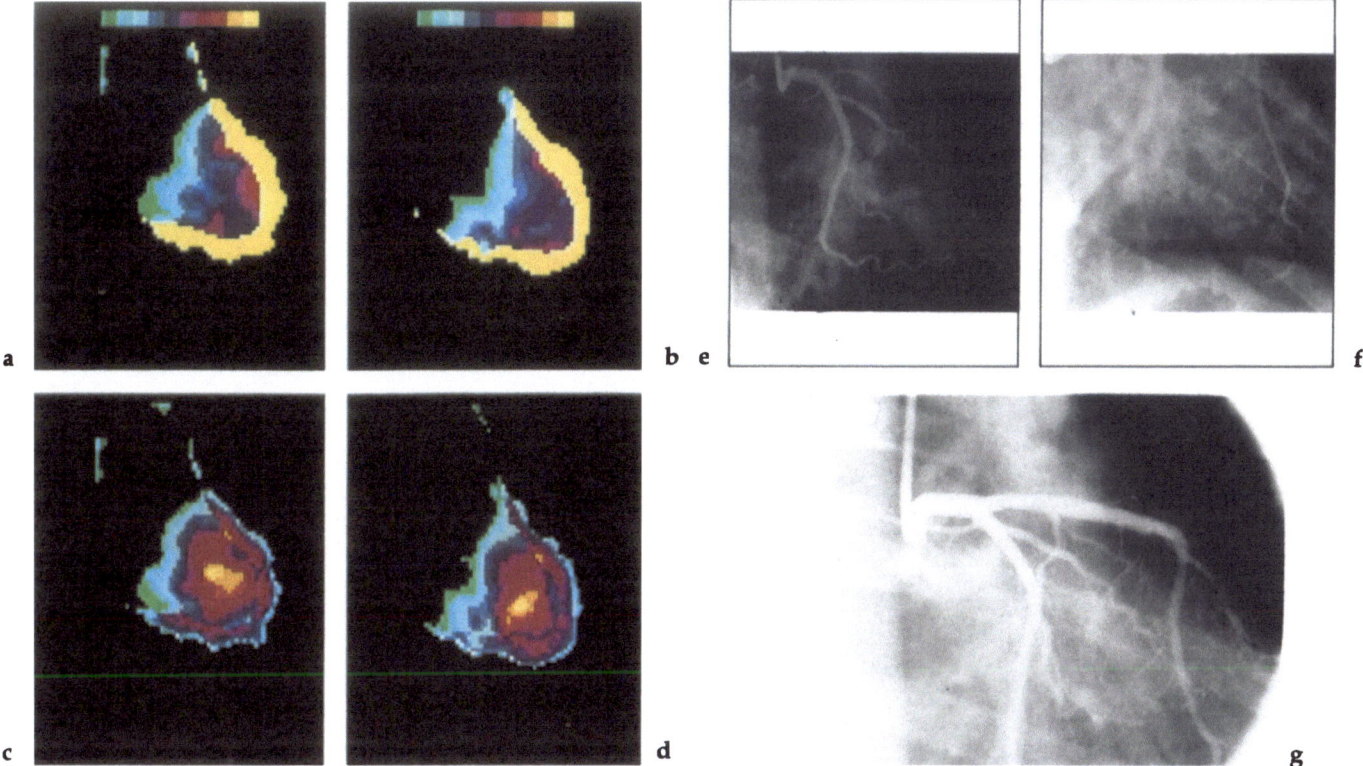

Figure 10.5 *Acute total occlusion of the LAD. Lysis 4 h after onset of chest pain. Additional peripheral occlusion.*
a–d, Functional images at rest and exercise in RAO view: under stress slight reduction of EFs at the apical and superoapical zone (**a,b**). ERs somewhat reduced along the anterior wall (**c,d**).

e–g, Left coronary angiogram shows total proximal occlusion of LAD (**e**), after lysis periferal occlusion initially persists (**f**), 10 days later the entire LAD is open (**g**).

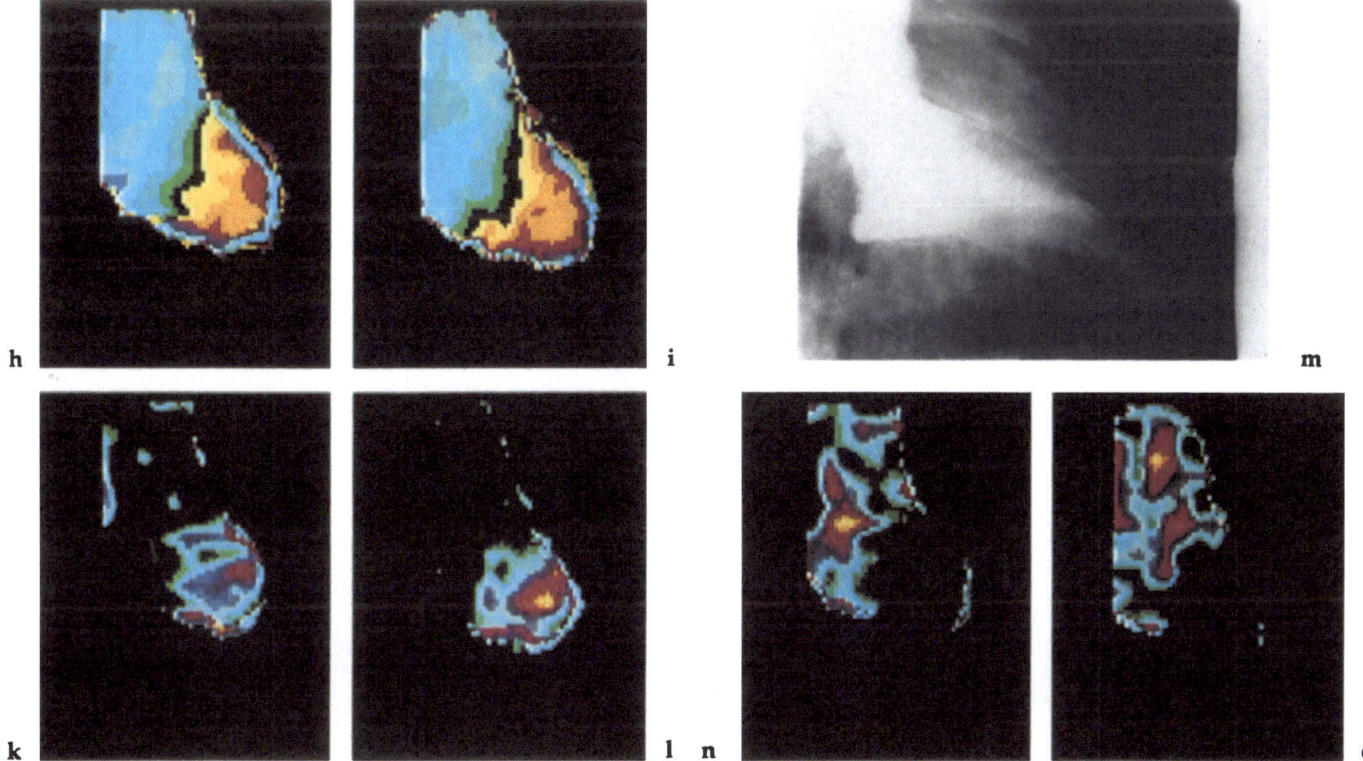

h,i,k,l, Systolic mean times at rest and exercise are only slightly prolonged (orange) anteriorly no very long times (dark, green) at the parietal zone as usually seen in myocardial infarction (**h,i**). Rapid filling rates at rest (**k**) somewhat reduced in the apical and superoapical zone improving after exercise (**l**) along the anterior wall except at a small area at the apex.

m, End-systolic left ventricular angiogram 10 days after lysis. Good contraction of the anterior wall with exception of a small apical zone.
n,o, Paradoxical inward motion during rapid filling at rest (**n**), some parietal inward motion in apical and superoapical area improving under stress (**o**).

11

Functional Imaging in Cardiomyopathy

J. W. FLEMING AND E. J. ANDREWS, JR.

Radionuclide functional imaging has added a new dimension in evaluation of patients with cardiomyopathy. Marked left ventricular (LV) dysfunction in advanced, primary, dilated cardiomyopathy may be easily recognized by clinical and other ancillary methods. However, mild to moderate, regional and global, left ventricular dysfunction is less easily recognized and occurs much more frequently than was appreciated prior to radionuclide imaging. These latter, non-specific changes may represent normal variants or residuals of myocarditis, in some instances, or developing primary cardiomyopathy in others. Thus, non-specific left ventricular dysfunction (NSLVD) with normal coronary angiograms is seen frequently in clinical practice and may mimic ischaemic heart disease in radionuclide (RN) studies (see Chapter 12). Differentiation of NSLVD and regional and global LV dysfunction associated with ischaemia remains a recurring and challenging problem.

Also RN differential diagnosis of moderately severe to severe LV dysfunction due to ischaemic versus primary idiopathic cardiomyopathy is a common problem. Findings in primary cardiomyopathy are often quite distinctive but the two conditions may be indistinguishable when ischaemia is balanced and diffuse. Although residuals of multiple infarctions may result in permanent, diffuse, LV myocardial damage, chronically ischaemic myocardial dysfunction may be reversible, in some cases. The latter is described as the 'stunned myocardium' by Braunwald (1982). Radionuclide studies before and after nitroglycerin administration sometimes can differentiate significant reversibility of LV dysfunction in ischaemic heart disease (Bodenheimer et al., 1978) (Figure 11.1). In some cases, early alcoholic cardiomyopathy and other types of cardiac myopathy also may be reversible with medical treatment. Radionuclide studies are very useful in demonstrating the relative recovery of LV function in some cases (Figure 11.2). As illustrated in Figure 11.2, improved volume changes may precede ejection fraction (EF) improvement in these cases.

Global function or EF in idiopathic dilated cardiomyopathy (IDC), depressed at rest, usually does not change very much with exercise, but according to Kirlin et al. (1984) and in our experience, in individual cases there may be moderate to marked increase or decrease in EF with exercise. In the latter instance, functional images sometimes resemble ischaemic changes.

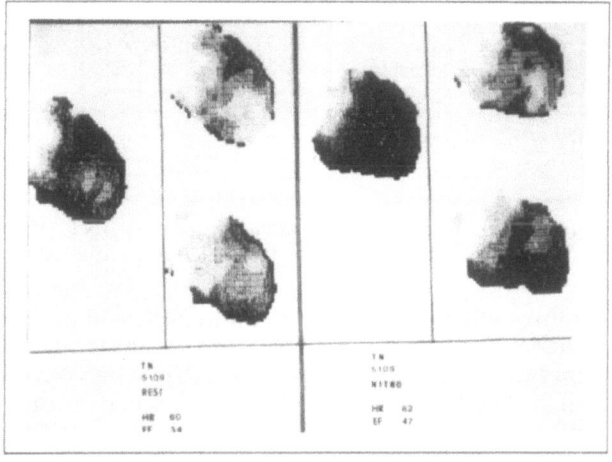

Figure 11.1 *Rest and postnitroglycerin studies in patient with ischaemic cardiomyopathy.* ANT *Left:* images show ischaemic change extending to the cardiac apex most pronounced during early systole. LVEF 34%. *Right:* apical wall motion does improve following administration of nitroglycerin. LVEF 47%. (REFI and half/half REFI).

Patients with cardiomyopathy may be seen in transitional states from early, slight cardiac involvement to advanced myocardial dysfunction. For instance, there is a wide spectrum of heart muscle abnormalities related to alcoholism (Ahmed et al., 1980). Ahmed and co-workers studied, with cardiac catheterization, a group of 54 patients with a history of heavy ethanol consumption and cardiovascular signs or symptoms. Most of these patients had more advanced LV dilatation and decreased myocardial function; however, 12 patients had normal heart size and normal or diminished LV volumes. All of these patients, including the 12 with normal LV volumes, had an increase in end-diastolic pressure or diminished LV compliance. Thus, images of diastolic filling (see Chapter 4) may show abnormalities in some patients with alcoholism and normal heart size; other similar patients may have early, transitional, global and/or regional wall motion changes at rest or only after exercise. The latter may account for some cases of NSLVD and may mimic ischaemic heart disease.

Patients with hypertrophic cardiomyopathy (HCM) or left ventricular hypertrophy (LVH) usually have hyperdynamic left ventricles and normal wall motion. However, some of these patients with HCM and some with LVH due to hypertension or aortic valvular disease may have

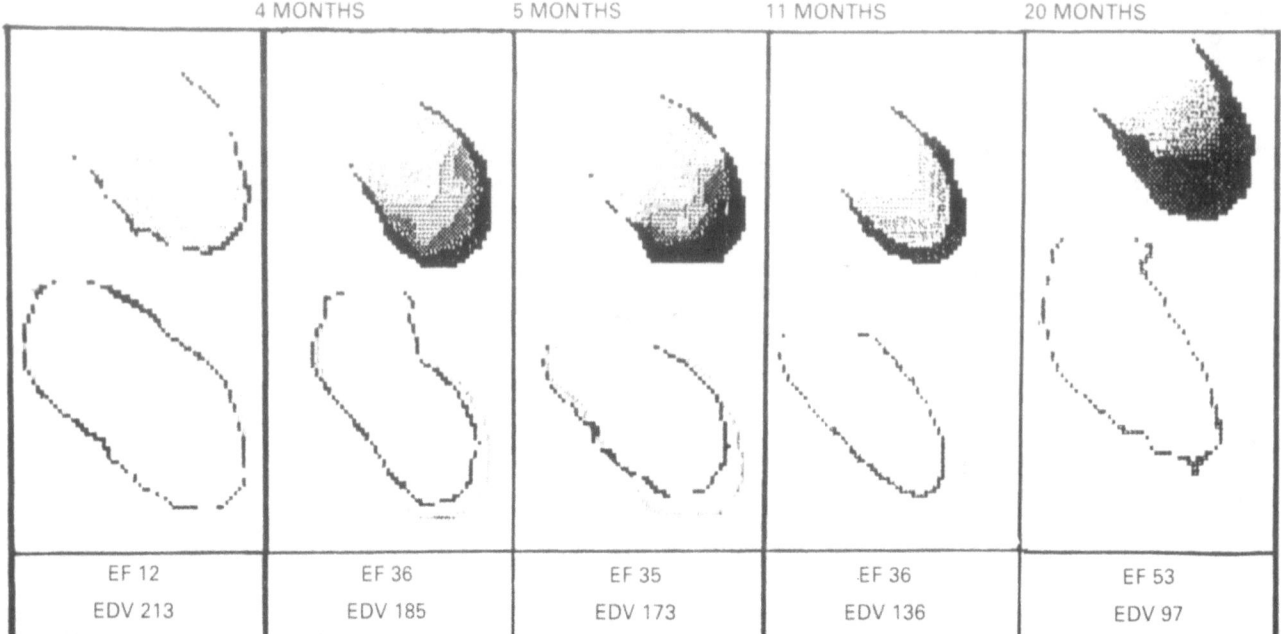

4 MONTHS	5 MONTHS	11 MONTHS	20 MONTHS
EF 12	EF 36	EF 35	EF 36	EF 53
EDV 213	EDV 185	EDV 173	EDV 136	EDV 97

Figure 11.2 *Alcoholic cardiomyopathy.* Rest, ANT, REFI. Serial studies after abstinence from alcohol. Note that the end-diastolic volume (EDV) improves earlier than the ejection fraction (EF).

findings which are very difficult to differentiate from ischaemic heart disease. Myocardial injury or degenerative changes may occur in LVH when oxygen demands of hypertrophied muscle exceed coronary blood supply (Rembert *et al.*, 1978; Bache and Vrobel, 1979; Kuhajda *et al.*, 1981; Moore *et al.*, 1980). Irreversible myocardial degenerative changes also may occur in patients with LVH with the absence of symptoms, according to Boucher *et al.* (1983a).

Examples of the more frequently encountered patterns of wall motion abnormality (WMA) as seen in association with these various forms of cardiac myopathy are presented below.

CASE EXAMPLES

Case 1: Figures 11.3 and 11.4 (alcoholic cardiomyopathy)

This patient with a history of alcoholism presented with dyspnoea on exertion. Extremely poor ventricular function was seen at rest in the radionuclide ventriculogram (RNV) with some improvement in function with exercise (Figure 11.3). The abnormal systolic images could be confused with ischaemia, particularly in the anterolateral wall, but the mean (transit) time image shows a rather diffuse homogeneous pattern, especially in the pink scale with even the first half transit image appearing homogeneous. The exercise RNV transit image remains homogeneous and symmetry is restored. This pattern is commonly seen with cardiomyopathy in contrast to ischaemia where usually there is deterioration with exercise and the transit image rarely is homogeneous.

Case 2: Figure 11.5 (alcoholic cardiomyopathy)

This 38-year-old male is an example of advanced alcoholic cardiomyopathy with a history of severe ventricular rhythm disturbances and failure. There was an EF of only 12% (Figures 11.2 and 11.5). The transit images were diffusely abnormal and quite homogeneous and little wall motion was evident. After quitting alcohol his clinical findings and RNV studies showed remarkable improvement over a year's time. The radionuclide images were used to reinforce therapy. The patient's clinical findings and images remained normal after several years of abstinence from alcohol.

Case 3: Figure 11.6 (alcoholic cardiomyopathy)

This patient has severe cardiomyopathy with cardiac failure (Figure 11.6). Global function is similar to Case 2 with an EF of 12% but wall motion pattern is distinctly different with multiple 'holes' in the functional images and the transit image shows irregularity especially during the first half of systole. These areas of decreased counts result in a 'Swiss cheese'* appearance commonly seen with nonischaemic cardiomyopathy. Exercise LVEF later was 23%.

Case 4: Figures 11.7 and 11.8 (idiopathic cardiomyopathy)

This patient has idiopathic cardiomyopathy and normal coronary angiograms (Figures 11.7 and 11.8). Ejection fraction increases with exercise; there is a wall motion abnormality (WMA) which is easily confused with ischaemia. However, the transit image remains relatively homogeneous. In addition, the first half REFI and the first half transit image do not match and are inconsistent. The latter findings favour the diagnosis of cardiomyopathy.

Case 5: Figures 11.9 and 11.10 (hypertrophic cardiomyopathy)

This patient with idiopathic hypertrophic cardiomyopathy and normal coronary angiograms was evaluated because of chest pain (Figures 11.9 and 11.10). Ejection fraction is normal but, in this case, there is a WMA at the apex, as commonly seen in patients with LV pressure overload such as aortic valve disease and hypertension. In this study, the transit time image shows a conical configuration pointing towards the apex. The maximum velocity (yellow) in the rate image remains central in the left ventricle. Ischaemia usually produces fragmentation and shift of the yellow crescent away from the ischaemic area.

Case 6: Figure 11.11 (hypertensive cardiomyopathy)

In contrast to the above case, this male with hypertension and normal coronary arteries shows a pattern seen with severe hypertensive cardiomyopathy when there is a significant decrease in global LV function (Figure 11.11). Changes at the apex could be confused with ischaemia although the transit image remains homogeneous. However, in the first half transit image, there is an island of abnormality (decreased wall motion) near the apex that does not extend to the outer perimeter of the LV image.

Case 7: Figure 11.12 (idiopathic cardiomyopathy)

This case of idiopathic cardiomyopathy in a 59-year-old female with chest pain and normal coronary arteries shows a diffuse abnormality which could be easily confused with ischaemia (Figure 11.12). However, the first half transit image remains relatively homogeneous and the crescent in the rate image remains central, although oriented closer to the apex. In contrast, with ischaemia, the crescent may be fragmented or shifted away from the ischaemic wall.

Case 8: Figure 11.13 (postpartum cardiomyopathy)

This patient had cardiac rhythm disturbances and congestive heart failure following pregnancy and term delivery (Figure 11.13). Patchy and diffuse wall motion abnormalities are noted.

SUMMARY

Experience in a limited number of patients with cardiomyopathy and normal coronary angiograms suggests that, in the majority of the cases, differentiation can be made between advanced cardiomyopathy and ischaemia. However, there is a group of cardiomyopathy patients, approximately 10% in our series, in which there are global and regional wall motion abnormalities indistinguishable from ischaemia. The distinctive patterns, commonly seen in association with advanced cardiomyopathy, have been illustrated in this chapter. The findings of some types of mild to moderate non-specific left ventricular dysfunction (NSLVD) are described in the following chapter (Chapter 12) on mitral valve prolapse and NSLVD.

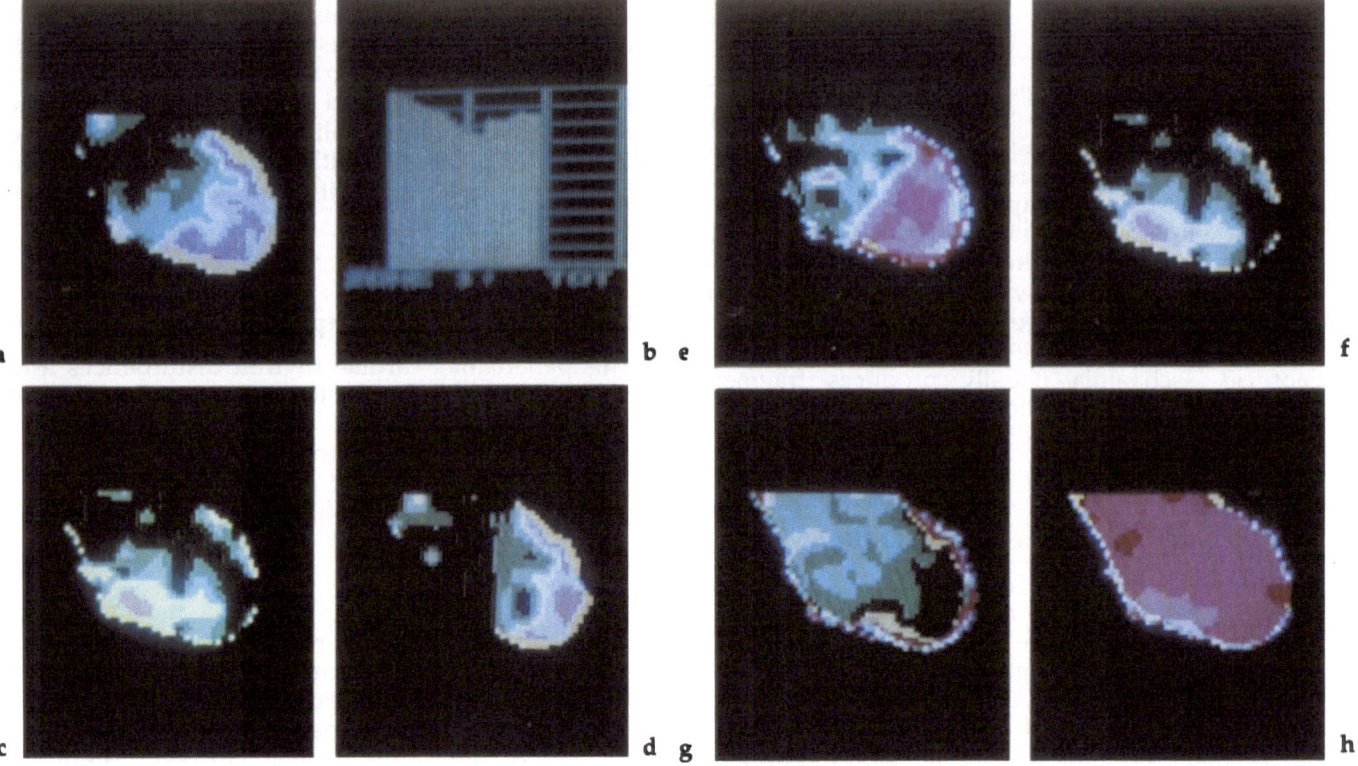

Figure 11.3 *Case 1, Alcoholic cardiomyopathy*. Symptoms of congestive heart failure with history of alcoholism. Cardiac catheterization showed severe LV dysfunction and normal coronary arteries. Rest, ANT. Parts **a** and **b**, REFI and volume curve show decreased global function and diffuse wall motion abnormality. Parts **c** and **d**, first half REFI and second half REFI show wall motion abnormality occurring both early and late in systole. Parts **e** and **f**, ejection rate and first half ejection rate images also show diffuse wall motion abnormality. Parts **g** and **h**, transit and first half transit images show a more homogeneous abnormality than is normally seen with ischaemia.

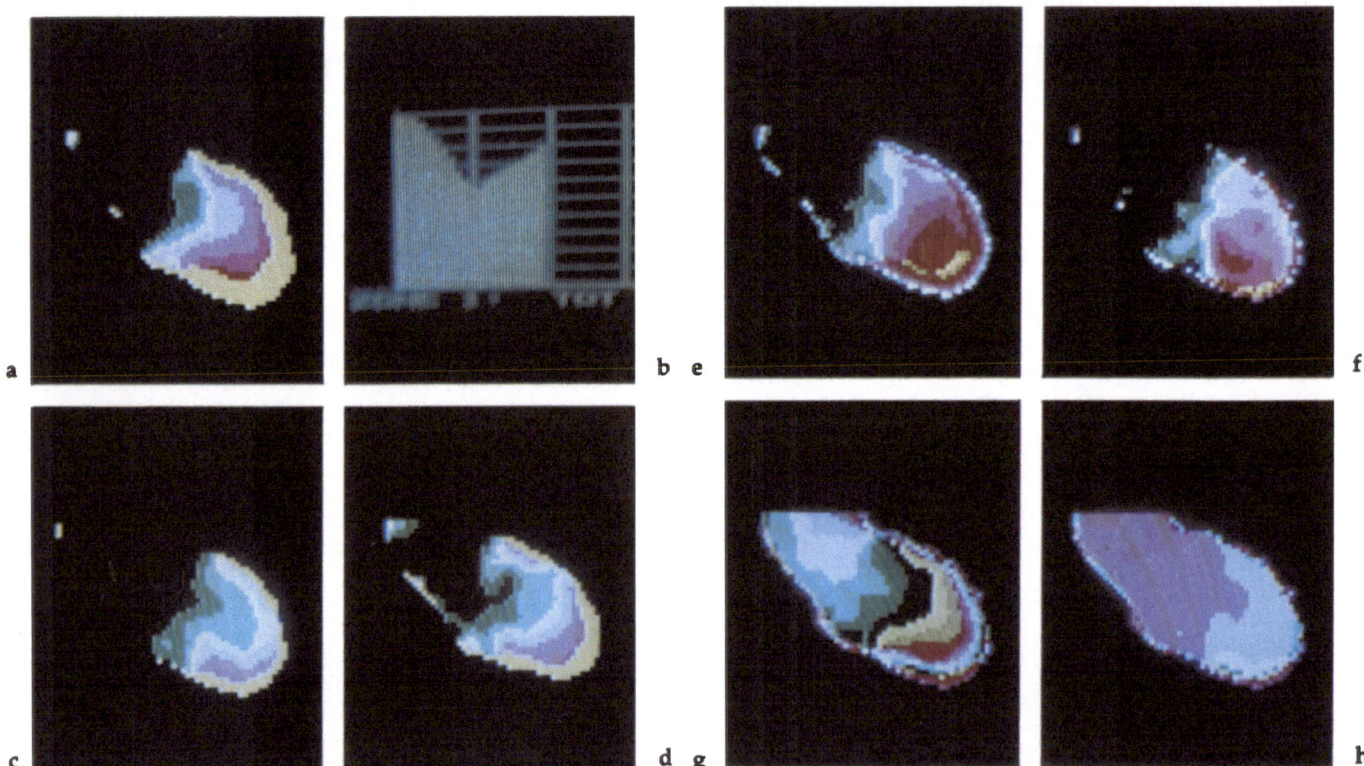

Figure 11.4 *Case 1, Alcoholic cardiomyopathy*. Exercise. Parts **a** and **b**, REFI and volume curve showed improved global function and wall motion with exercise. Parts **c** and **d**, first half REFI and second half REFI also show improvement in wall motion both early and late in systole. Parts **e** and **f**, ejection rate and first half ejection rate also show improved function remaining homogeneous. **g, h**, transit and first half transit images.

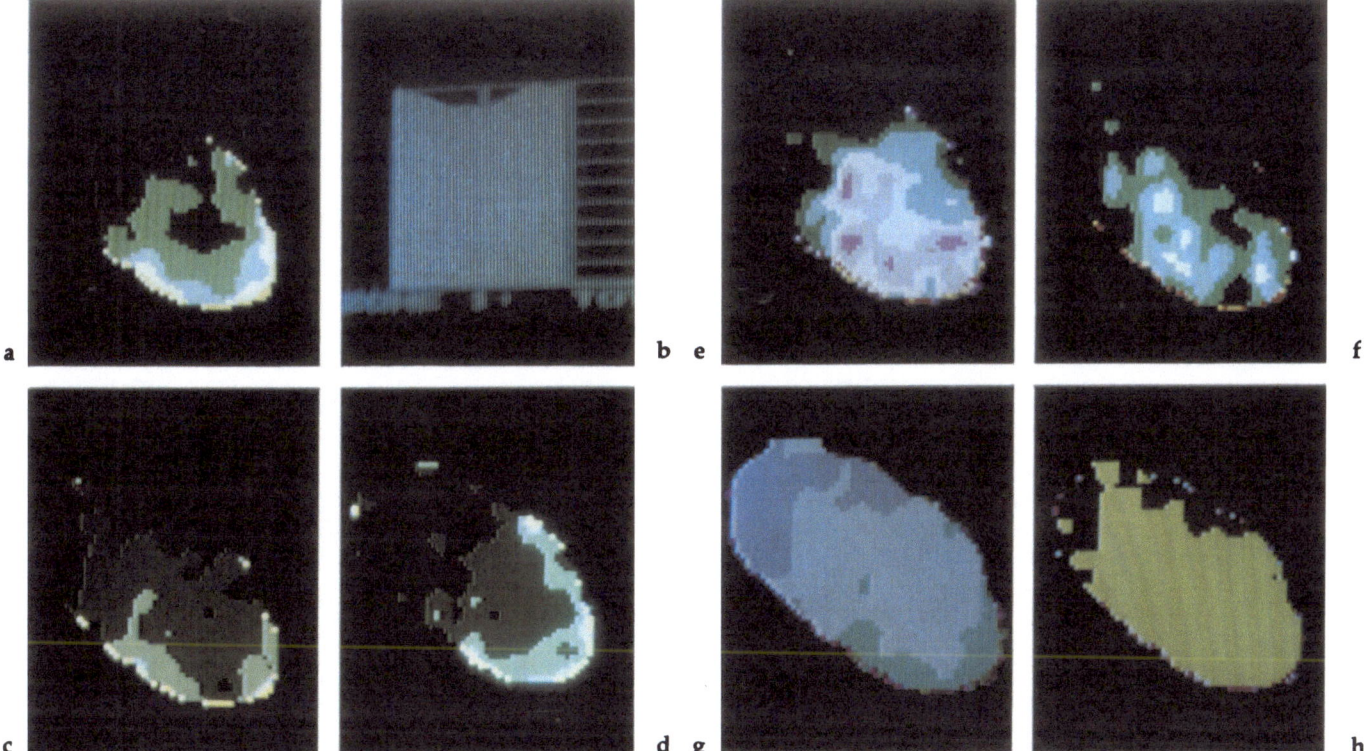

Figure 11.5 *Case 2, Alcoholic cardiomyopathy*, symptoms of congestive heart failure and rhythm disturbances. Rest ANT LVEF 12%. All images show diffuse decreased LV function with a relatively homogeneous pattern. **a**, REFI; **b**, volume curve; **c**, first half REFI; **d**, second half REFI; **e**, ejection rate; **f**, first half ejection rate; **g**, transit; **h**, first half transit.

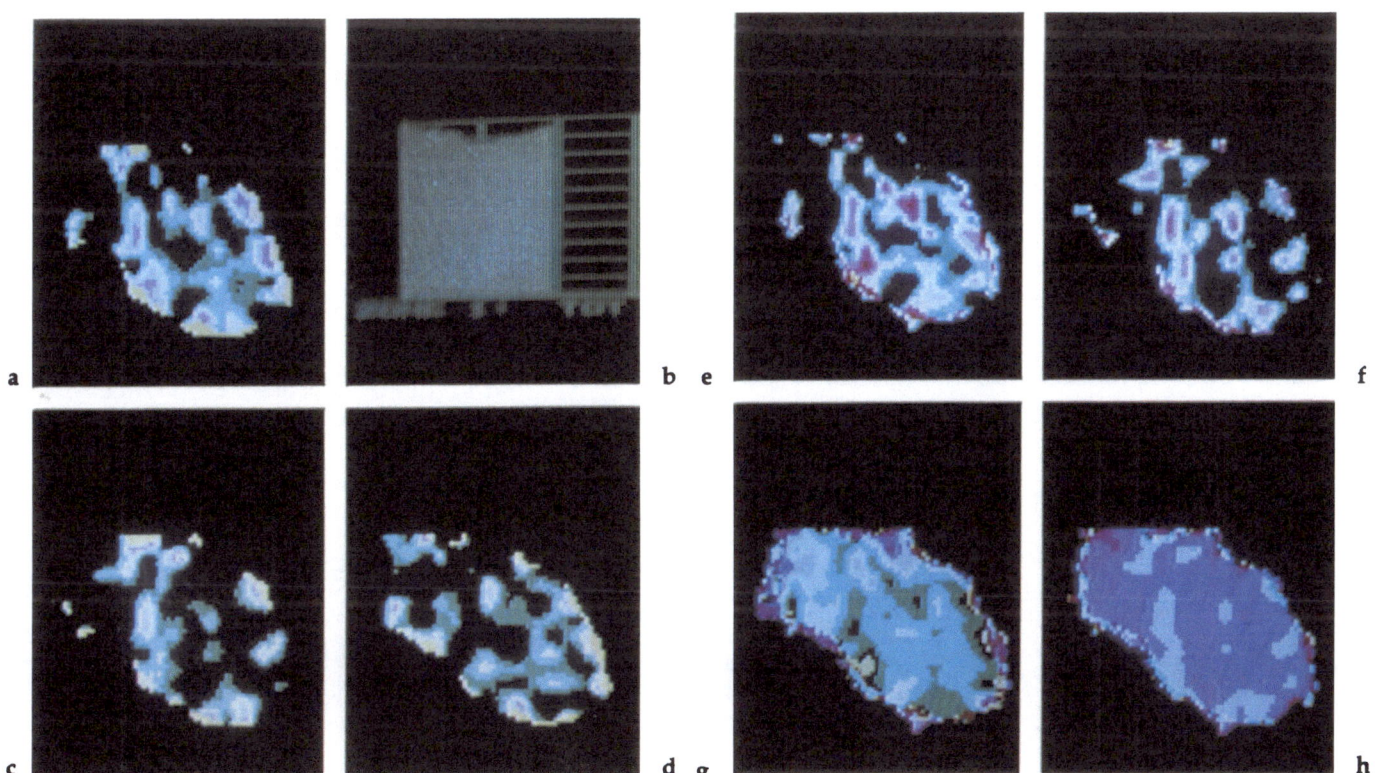

Figure 11.6 *Case 3, Alcoholic cardiomyopathy*. Rest, ANT, LVEF 12%. Symptoms of dyspnoea on exertion with no significant coronary disease found at cardiac catheterization. In contrast to the previous case, wall motion has a more patchy appearance with all images having a 'Swiss cheese' appearance. This pattern is also a common one in patients with cardiomyopathy not related to ischaemia. **a**, REFI; **b**, volume curve; **c**, first half REFI; **d**, second half REFI; **e**, ejection rate; **f**, first half ER; **g**, transit; **h**, first half transit.

93

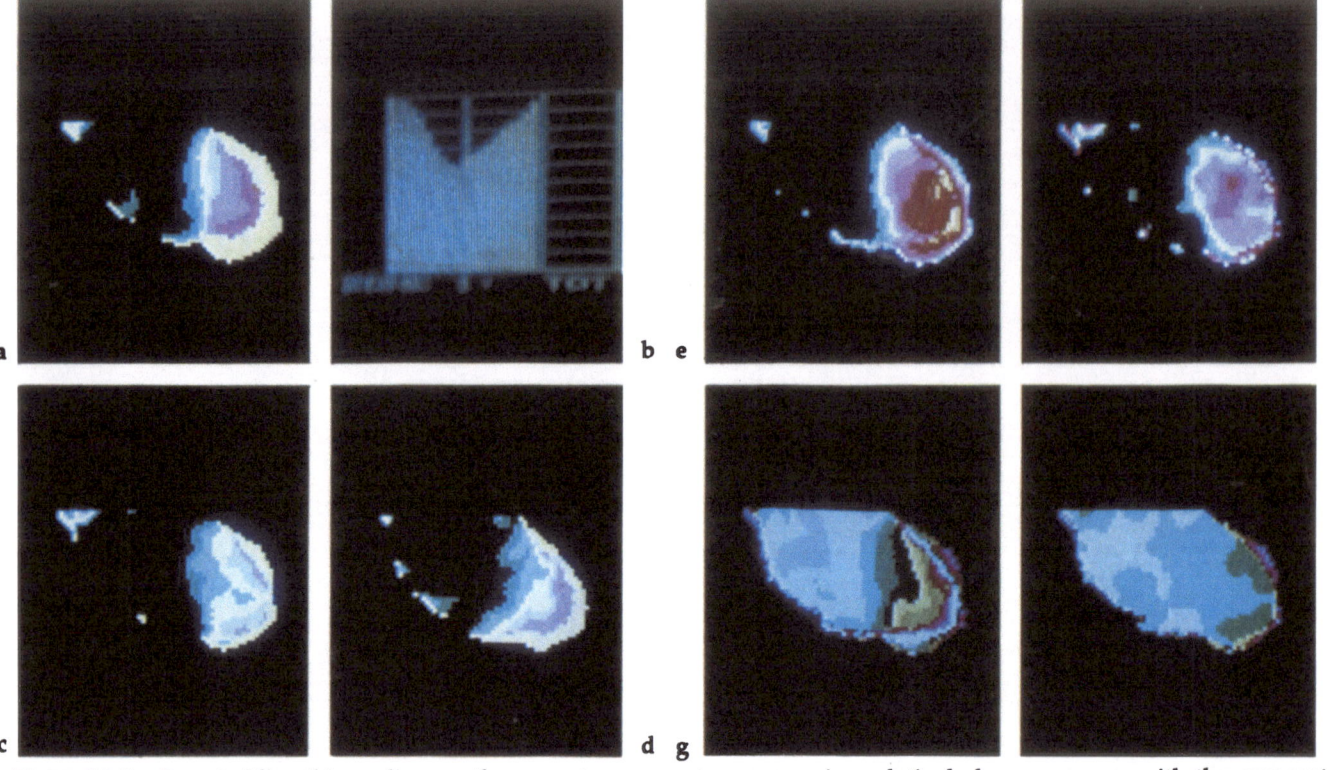

Figure 11.7 *Case 4, Idiopathic cardiomyopathy*, symptoms of chest pain. LV dyskinesia and normal coronary arteries at cardiac catheterization. Rest, ANT, LVEF 32%. All images show diffuse wall motion abnormality but the rate image remains relatively homogeneous with the crescent remaining central but near the periphery. **a**, REFI; **b**, volume curve; **c**, first half REFI; **d**, second half REFI; **e**, ejection rate; **f**, first half ER; **g**, transit; **h**, first half transit.

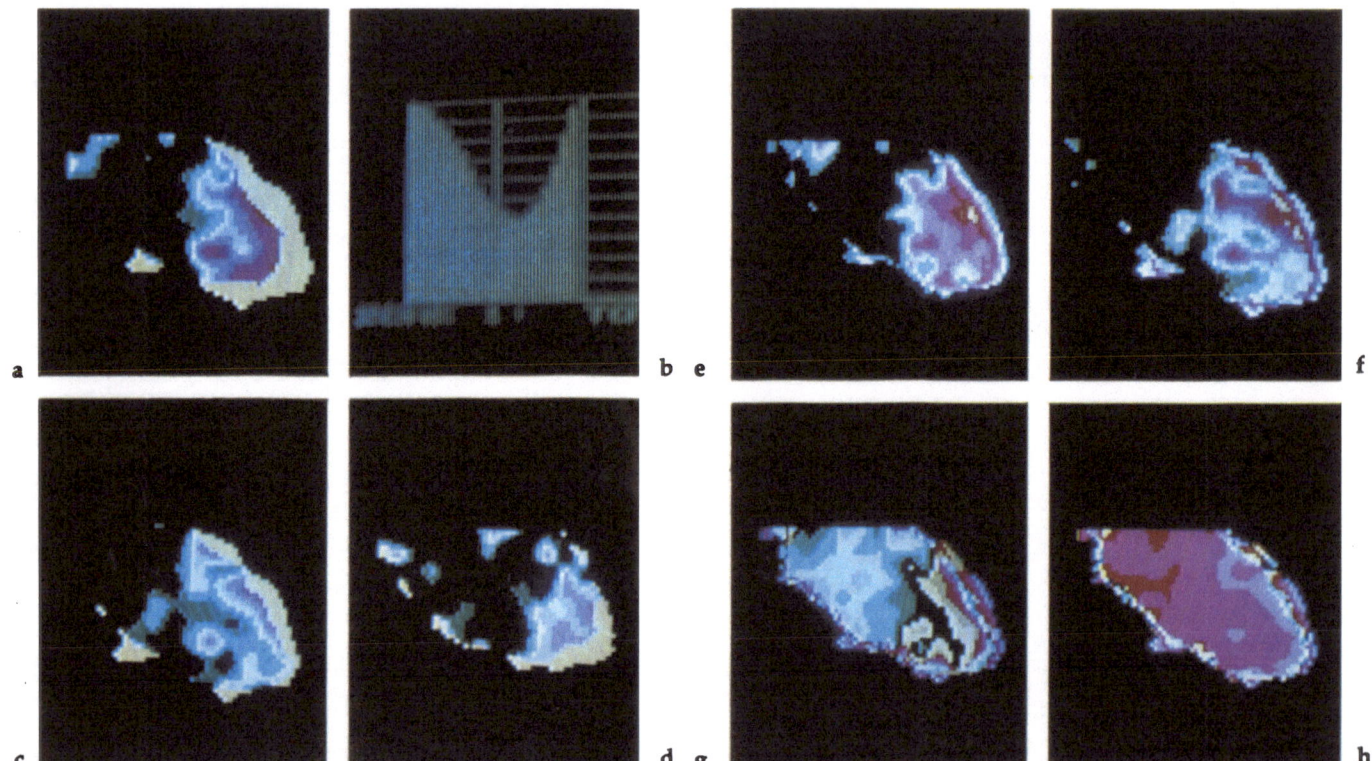

Figure 11.8 *Case 4, Idiopathic cardiomyopathy*. Exercise, ANT, LVEF 36%. Although global function improved slightly with exercise, wall motion remains abnormal becoming more pronounced serially during early systole in the first half REFI, first half rate, and first half transit time images. This pattern could easily be confused with ischaemia. **a**, REFI; **b**, volume curve; **c**, first half REFI; **d**, second half REFI; **e**, ejection rate; **f**, first half ER; **g**, transit; **h**, first half transit.

94

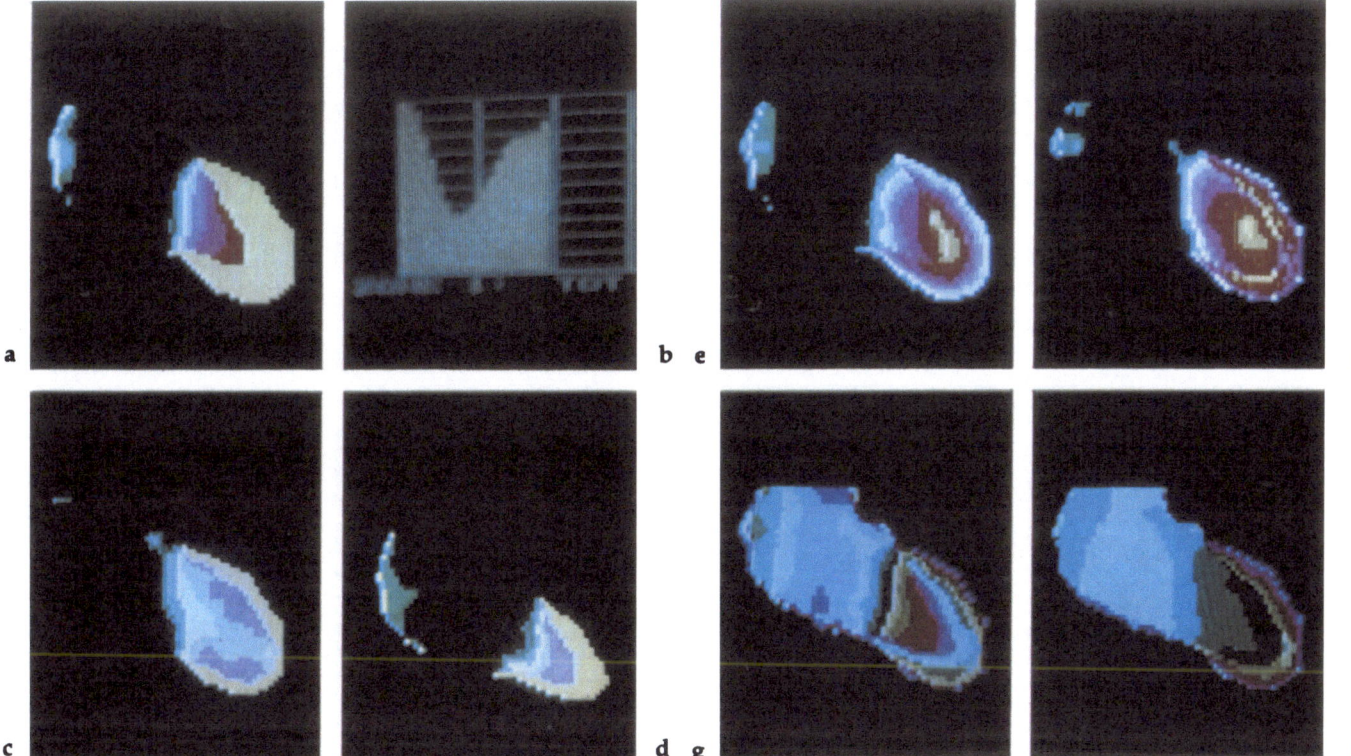

Figure 11.9 *Case 5, Hypertrophic cardiomyopathy*, chest pain. Rest, ANT, LVEF 65%. Cardiac catheterization showed normal coronary arteries and a lag in long axis shortening with elongation of the left ventricle. Images show slight decrease in apical motion during early systole with the other images remaining normal. **a**, REFI; **b**, volume curve; **c**, first half REFI; **d**, second half REFI; **e**, ejection rate; **f**, first half ER; **g**, transit; **h**, first half transit.

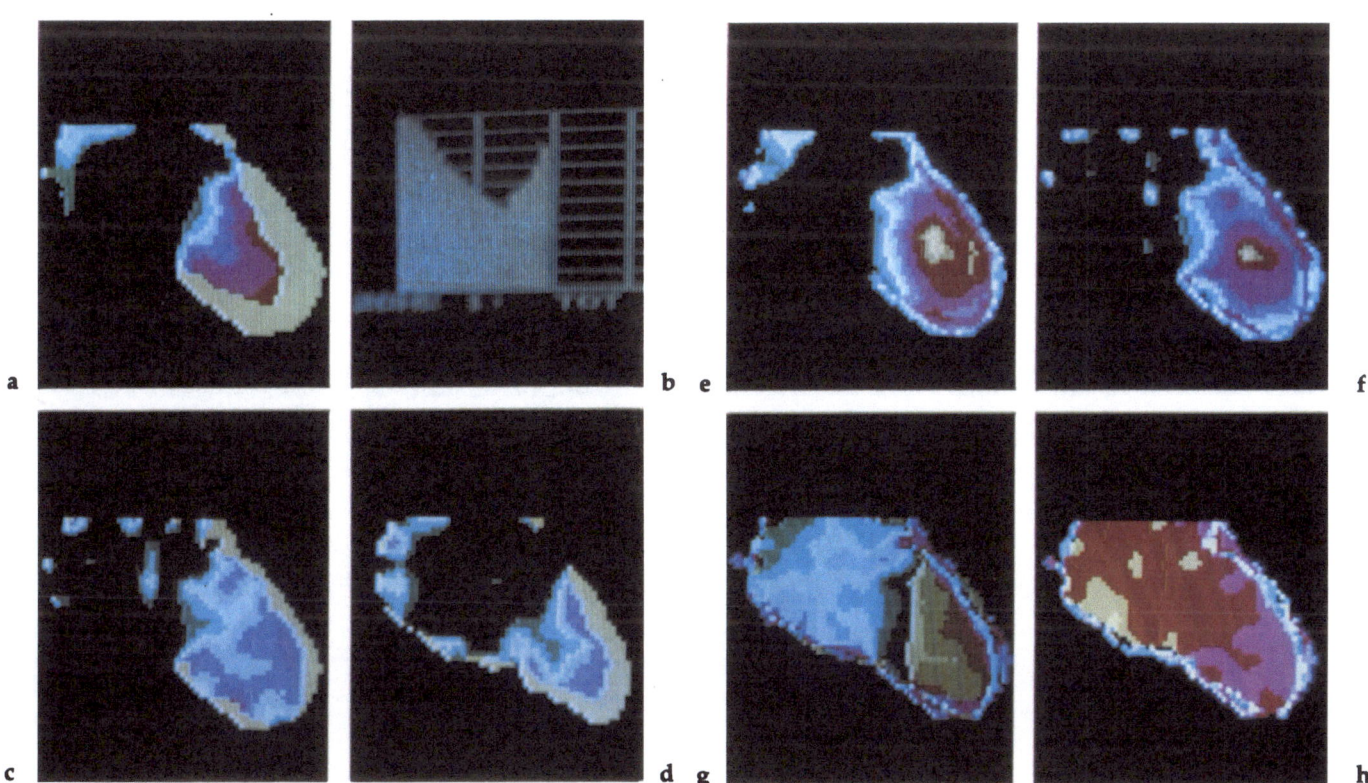

Figure 11.10 *Case 5, Hypertrophic cardiomyopathy*. Exercise, ANT, LVEF 58%. LVEF decreases slightly with exercise and apical wall motion abnormality becomes more pronounced with mean transit time and first half rate and mean transit time images becoming abnormal with decreased long axis shortening. This pattern is commonly seen with concentric LV hypertrophy, pressure overload, as well as with ischaemia. **a**, REFI; **b**, volume curve; **c**, first half REFI; **d**, second half REFI; **e**, ejection rate; **f**, first half ER; **g**, transit; **h**, first half transit.

95

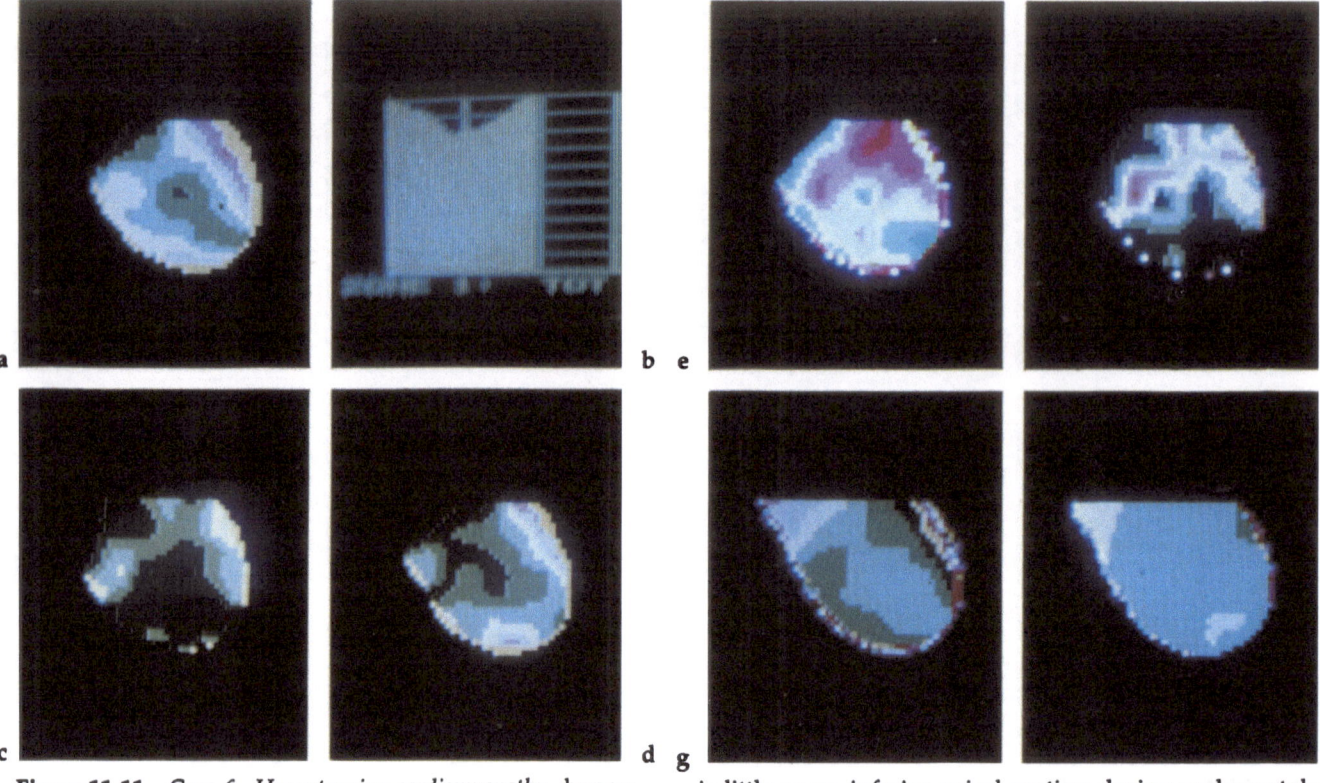

Figure 11.11 *Case 6, Hypertensive cardiomyopathy*, hypertension and dyspnoea on exertion. Normal coronary arteries at cardiac catheterization with diffuse LV dysfunction. REST, ANT, LVEF 24% EDV 252 ml. Images show diffuse abnormality which is more central and apical in orientation which could be confused with ischaemia. This is particularly true on the first half REFI image where there

is little or no inferior apical motion during early systole. This pattern is often indistinguishable from ischaemia (*see* Chapter 13, on valve disease). **a**, REFI; **b**, volume curve; **c**, first half REFI; **d**, second half REFI; **e**, ejection rate; **f**, first half ER; **g**, transit; **h**, first half transit.

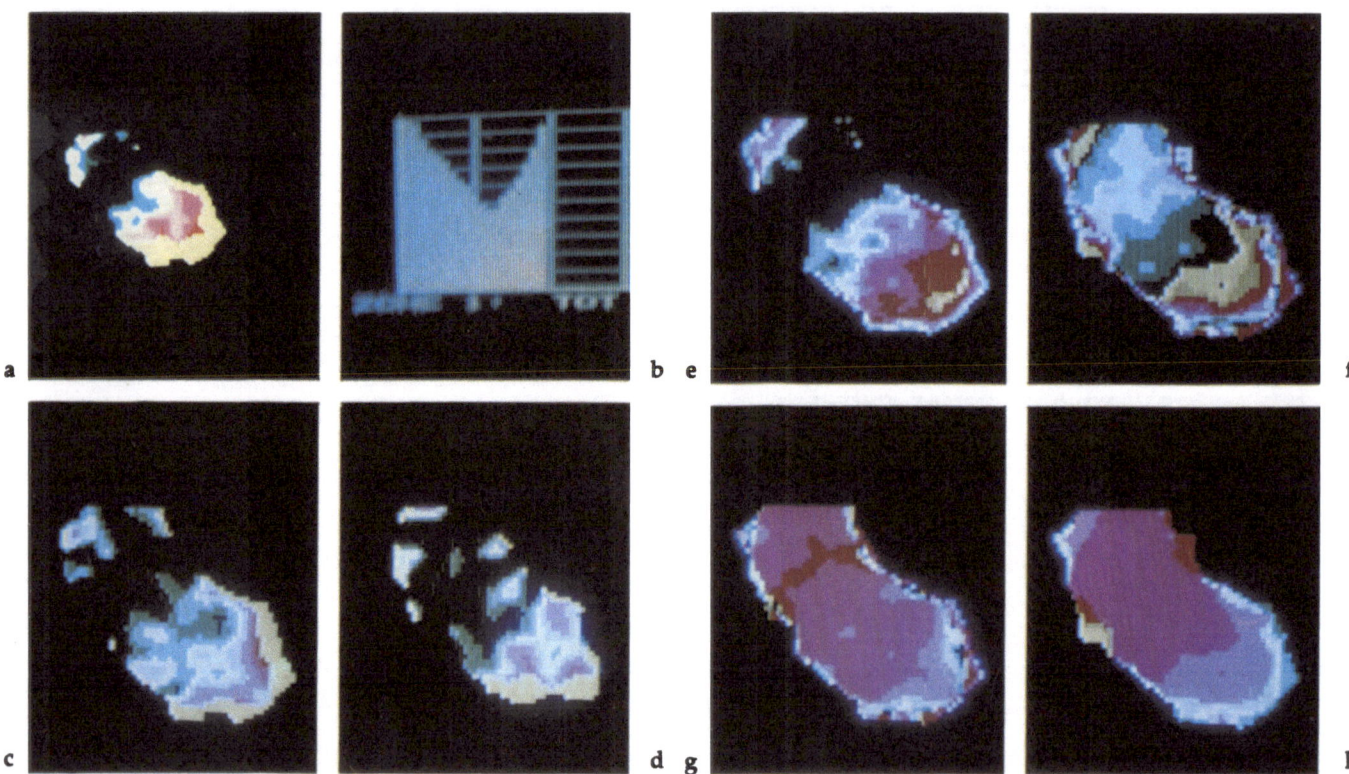

Figure 11.12 *Case 7, Idiopathic cardiomyopathy*. This patient had chest pain and normal coronary arteriograms. Exercise, ANT LVEF was 48% at rest and 35% at exercise. Images show diffuse wall motion abnormality but large yellow crescent of maximum velocity remains central in the rate image closer to the apex. There are no segmental

changes in early systole such as would be expected with ischaemia. The transit and rate images particularly favour cardiomyopathy over ischaemia in this situation. **a**, REFI; **b**, volume curve; **c**, first half REFI; **d**, second half REFI; **e**, ejection rate; **f**, first half ER; **g**, transit; **h**, first half transit.

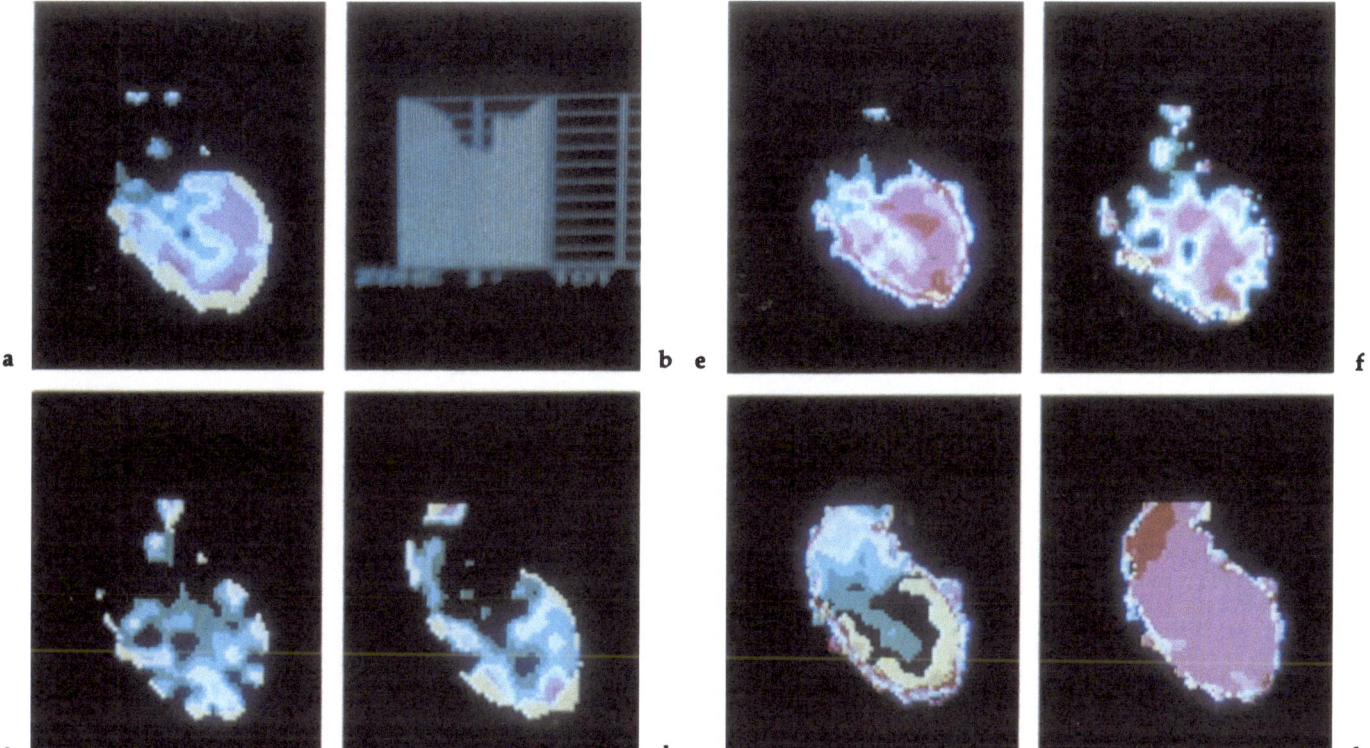

Figure 11.13 *Case 8, Postpartum cardiomyopathy.* This patient had congestive heart failure and rhythm disturbances following pregnancy. Images show marked dilatation of the left ventricle with diffuse wall motion abnormality. LVEF 30%. **a**, REFI; **b**, volume curve; **c**, first half REFI; **d**, second half REFI; **e**, rate; **g**, first half rate; **f**, transit; **h**, first half transit.

12

Functional Imaging in Mitral Valve Prolapse and Non-specific Left Ventricular Dysfunction

J. W. FLEMING AND E. J. ANDREWS, JR.

Mitral valve prolapse may be associated with characteristic patterns of regional wall motion variants as seen in contrast or radionuclide ventriculography. These variants as well as those of non-specific left ventricular dysfunction (NSLVD) are seen frequently in clinical practice and may mimic ischaemic heart disease in radionuclide studies (see Chapters 5 and 11).

Mitral valve prolapse (MVP) or the click-murmur syndrome is a very common clinical entity which is usually benign (Barlow et al., 1968; Towne, 1978). However, some patients have significant cardiac rhythm and conduction disturbances (Gooch et al., 1972; Hancock, 1984). Chest pain is common and usually atypical, but a few patients with MVP have chest pain which can be confused with angina pectoris associated with ischaemic heart disease (Malcolm et al., 1979; Schlant et al., 1980). According to many surveys, signs of MVP occur in 5–10% of the general population (Markiewicz et al., 1976; Savage et al., 1983). Primary, idiopathic MVP is probably a heritable connective tissue disorder in which the mitral valve eventually may develop myxomatous changes (Jeresaty, 1971, 1975, 1978; Devereaux et al., 1976; Chesler et al., 1983). A wide spectrum of aetiologies may be associated with the secondary forms of MVP (Barlow et al., 1979; Naggar and Aretz, 1984).

The presence of mitral valve prolapse may be considered as a normal variant in some individuals, and it has a benign prognosis in the great majority of symptomatic patients with this condition. However, the unique regional as well as global ventricular functional changes occur in many patients with MVP (Gooch et al., 1972; Scampardonis et al., 1973; Liedtke et al., 1973; Mathey et al., 1977; Gibson and Brown, 1979; Cobbs, 1974; Fleming et al., 1980). These changes are sometimes very difficult to differentiate from the wall motion abnormalities (WMA) associated with ischaemic heart disease.

The basic criteria for cineventriculographic diagnosis of MVP (Barlow et al., 1968) are postero-inferior bulging of the scallops of the posterior mitral valve leaflet in the right anterior oblique (RAO) view; bulging of the anterior leaflet or scallops may be visualized in the left anterior oblique view (Barlow and Pocock, 1979; Cohen et al., 1979). Although wall motion in MVP may be normal,

many abnormalities have been described. Scampardonis et al. (1973), using contrast cineventriculography, described five characteristic patterns of regional wall motion in MVP patients, as follows.

(1) *'Ballerina foot'*. This is characterized by indentation of the inferior left ventricular wall, bulging of the free wall and a tapered appearance of the apex. The high lateral bulge of the left ventricle occurs in early diastole and persists into systole resulting in little change in radionuclide ventriculography (RNV) counts in that area. Thus, the apparent decreased motion in this area may be confused with ischaemic WMA (Figure 12.1).

(2) *'Hour glass' contour*. This is similar to the above but with indentation of the high lateral left ventricular wall. The tugging of the leaflets on the anterior and posterior papillary muscles may cause these indentations (Cobbs and King, 1977).

(3) *Failure of long axis shortening*. With this condition, there are few or no diastolic to systolic changes in the RNV apical counts; this mimics apical ischaemia (Figures 12.1–12.3).

(4) *Inferior akinesis*. There are a number of reasons why RNV in patients with MVP give an appearance of hypokinesis or akinesis of the inferior wall and can mimic inferior ischaemia:

   (a) Some patients have, actually, little or no movement of the LV inferior wall, while other portions of the LV wall are contracting moderately or vigorously (Figure 12.1; see also Figures 3.1 and 3.4).

   (b) Some patients have complex, brief, outward and/or inward systolic inferior wall motions which result in a summation effect of decreased inferior wall movement (Figures 12.1 and 12.2).

   (c) A myxomatous mitral valve may remain coved and dilated with blood, even during diastole. In large mitral valve prolapses, some have described 'intravalvular regurgitation' (Cobbs and King, 1977). This miniature blood pool within the coved mitral leaflets may briefly entrap a portion of counts in the region of the mitral valve, resulting in no count difference between diastole and systole, spuriously suggesting no movement. When an anterior view is used, looking at a cross-section of the mitral valve, the miniature pool in the mitral valve area may, in effect, face the camera; persistence of counts and lack of changes from systole to diastole may result in spurious representation of inferior WMA across a wide area adjacent to the inferior margin of the RNV image.

The 'fixed counts' in the region of the mitral valve, as described above, also may account for the contour of the mean transit time image as shown in Figure 12.4. In the RNV there is more or less a vertical line at the base of the LV contour and a rounded area of changes in the region of the mitral valve. Following exercise, this line of delineation of the ventricle may straighten or be replaced by a miniature outline of a 'ballerina foot'.

(d) Counts in the descending thoracic aorta may be registered as no change from diastole to systole and alter wall motion spuriously in the recording (Fleming, 1982). In the anterior (ANT) projection the aorta lies right behind the heart, particularly the inferobasilar region. Rotation of the patient to a shallow RAO may not be enough to rotate the aorta away from the inferior border of the heart. Rotation to more than 20° may be necessary in some patients to clear the image of the aorta from the inferior border of the heart (*see* Chapter 3). Thus, patients with MVP often have a hyperdynamic circulation and counts in the aorta reach the level of the heart base after one or two representative cycles.

(e) With MVP or myxomatous mitral valve disease, endocardial friction rubs occur frequently (Towne, 1978; Chesler *et al.*, 1983). These are due to friction of stretched or thickened chordae over the endocardium, resulting in confluent, subendocardial fibrosis, sometimes with imbedded chordae in the posterobasalar wall of the LV (Chesler *et al.*, 1983). This could contribute to alteration in the inferior wall motion in some patients.

(f) With the anterior view, used by many laboratories to enhance acquisition of the counts from the cardiac blood pool, it is apparent that this tangential projection can result in striking differences in the evaluation of inferior wall motion, as compared to an RAO view (*see* Figures 12.7 and 12.8 showing contrast cineventriculogram outlines in the RAO and ANT views in the same patients. Also *see* Chapter 3, Figures 3.1–3.4).

(5) *Hyperkinetic* ventricle with cavity obliteration pattern.

All of the above contour patterns described by Scampardonis *et al.* (1973) may be recognizable in the RNV of many patients with MVP. These contours may be more apparent at rest in some cases or more apparent with exercise in others. Inferior WMA usually are more pronounced late in systole (and in second half of systole images), but these WMA also may be seen in both the first and second halves of systole.

Many patients with MVP have normal or hyperkinetic resting and exercise global function, reflected in normal or increased ejection fractions (EF) (Newman *et al.*, 1981). In our experience, and in that of other investigators (Gottdiener *et al.*, 1979; Ahmad *et al.*, 1979), from one third to one half of MVP patients studied had no appreciable increase or a fall in EF with exercise.

Some MVP patients may have non-specific myocardial abnormalities or NSLVD of mild to moderate degree. This may represent idiopathic cardiomyopathy or possible transient or residuals of myocarditis in some cases. These myocardial abnormalities may result in varying degrees of diffuse RNV wall motion abnormality in the functional images. Also, in about 10% of our cases of MVP with normal coronary arteriograms there were localized central and apical wall motion abnormalities seen best in the first half regional ejection fraction image (REFI); these were very similar to changes associated with ischaemic heart disease. These types of wall motion abnormality usually do not extend or bisect the perimeter of the images. Sometimes in the latter type of 'ischaemia-like' wall motion abnormality in the REFI, the transit image will be normal, helping to mitigate against the likelihood of ischaemia (Figures 12.13 and 12.14).

Bulging of the mitral valve may be evident in the inferior border in many patients with MVP. A patient with an extremely large myxomatous mitral valve had a large regurgitation of counts into the left atrial area (Figure 12.19). Apparently, intravalvular regurgitation into the left atrial area, as described by Cobbs (1974), is depicted in the rate image showing the rate of increase in counts. This patient's image shows rounded, nodular densities representing intravalvular counts in the dilated scallops of the prolapsed mitral valve. This contrasts with a more diffuse RNV pattern of mitral regurgitation through the valve leaflets into the left atrium.

One of the more common signs of MVP in our functional imaging is the flat bottom of the left ventricular contour, particularly in the anterior view. Often there is a notch in the inferior contour toward the right side of the image and/or varying degrees of bulging in the regions of the mitral valve.

Non-specific left ventricular dysfunction, global and/or regional, may occur in patients with normal coronary arteries without demonstrable MVP at cardiac catheterization. Berger *et al.* (1981), using first pass RNV, reported 31 patients with chest pain, ischaemic-appearing exercise electrocardiograms, angiographically normal coronary arteries, and no demonstrable MVP. An abnormal EF response was noted in 12 of 31 patients. Regional dysfunction was noted in four patients and five had exercise-induced thallium perfusion defects. Gibbons *et al.* (1981) also reported that 60 patients with chest pain, normal coronary angiograms and normal rest EF had wide variations in EF response to exercise (they did not describe wall motion changes or presence or absence of MVP).

SUMMARY

In functional imaging, contours of the 'ballerina foot' and variants as well as inferior wall motion abnormalities are common in MVP. The variants may be miniature contours or may be only reminiscent of the lateral bulge, the tapered apex and the notched inferior border with bulging of the valve area. Many patients with MVP have mild to moderate, nonspecific left ventricular dysfunction manifested by regional WMA or reduction in global function, i.e. a decrease or a failure to increase EF with exercise. The presence of the inferior, apical and high lateral contour changes usually can be recognized as MVP, particularly, in the presence of hyperdynamic ventricles. Some cases have other wall motion abnormalities or regional NSLVD which are virtually indistinguishable from those seen with ischaemic heart disease or significant cardiomyopathy. In our experience, approximately 10% of the patients with MVP fall into this category (i.e., false positive for ischaemia).

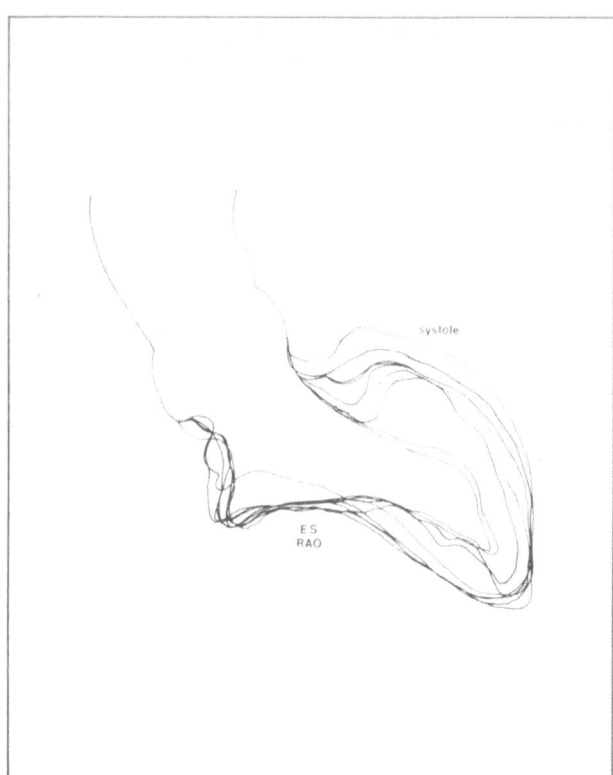

Figure 12.1 *Mitral valve prolapse: RAO projection, contrast left ventriculogram,* frame by frame contour drawings. *Systole* begins at the outer perimeter. In this patient, there is very little inferior wall motion, prominent mitral valve bulging, incomplete long axis shortening, and a lag in the high lateral wall motion. See Figure 12.12 for similar high lateral wall motion abnormality on RNV.

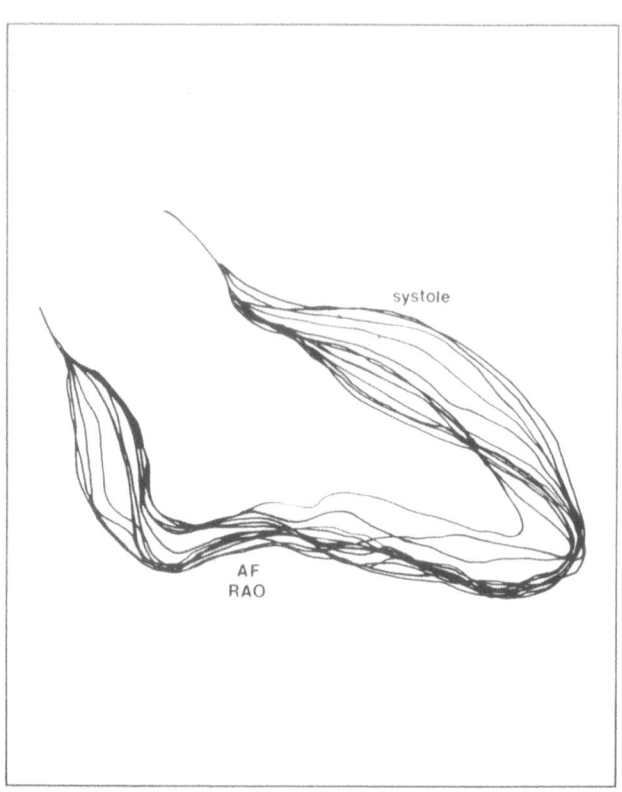

Figure 12.2 *Mitral valve prolapse: RAO projection, contrast left ventriculogram,* frame by frame contours. *Diastole* begins at the inner perimeter. This shows wall motion changes during diastole and relatively small excursion of the inferobasalar segment.

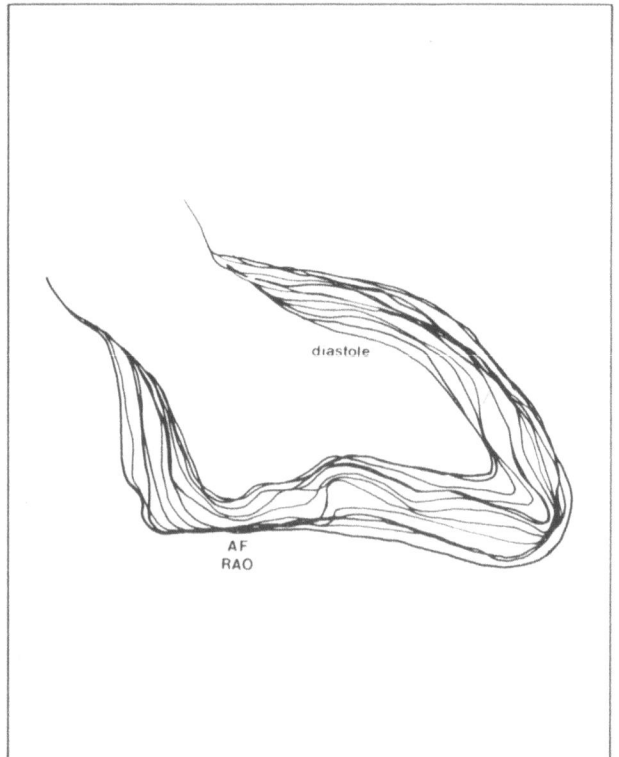

Figure 12.3 *Mitral valve prolapse: ANT projection, contrast left ventriculogram,* frame by frame contours. Systole begins at the outer perimeter. This shows a lag in inferior wall motion during the first half of systole, then more rapid movement in the latter half of systole. Same patient as in figure 12.4.

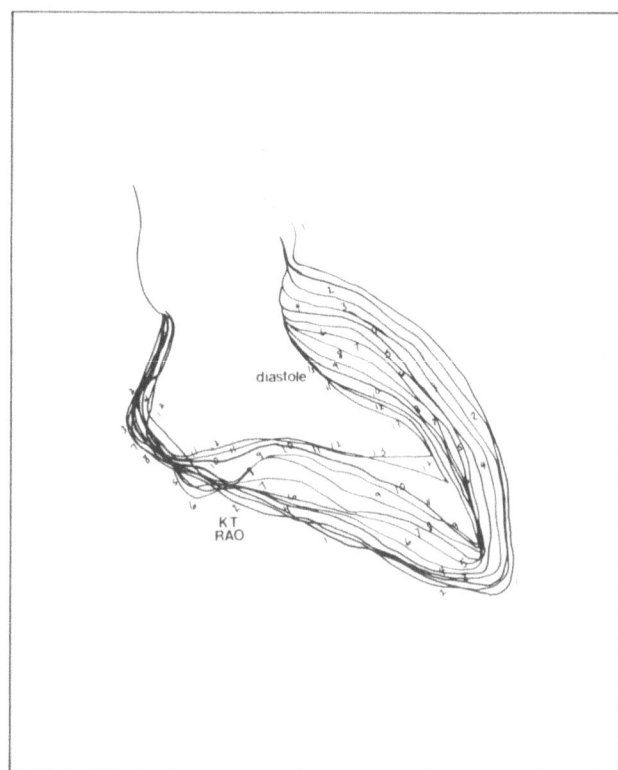

Figure 12.4 *Mitral valve prolapse: RAO projection, contrast left ventriculogram,* frame by frame contours. Systole begins at the outer perimeter. There is a lag of the apical motion and only brief movement in late systole at the apex. Inferior contours shown here account for notching in some RNV and 'flat bottoms' in others.

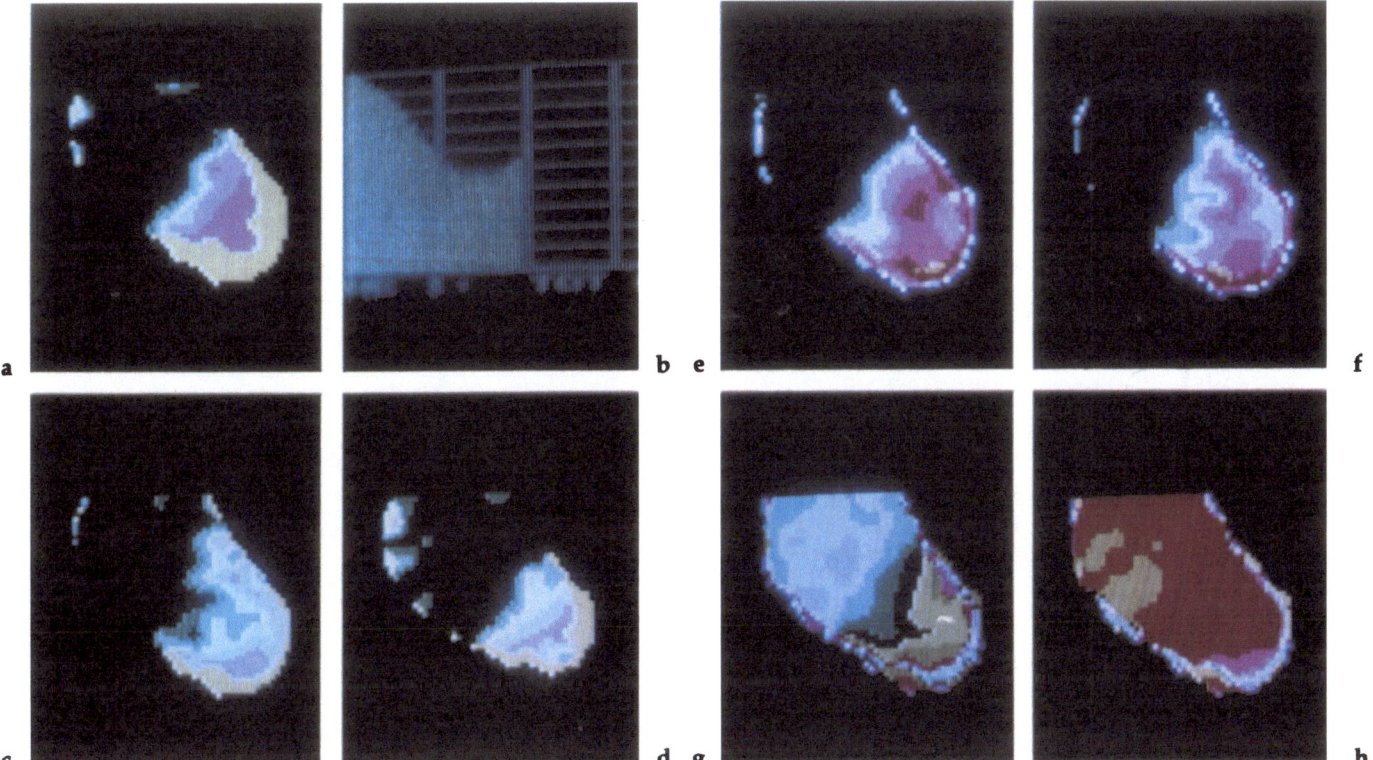

Figure 12.5 *Mitral valve prolapse:* Rest, ANT. (Colour image.) Note the suggestion of MVP configuration in REFI and the second half REFI. The inferior wall image might be confused with ischaemia in the first half images; however, MVP is suggested by the rounded asymmetric countour of the inferobasilar segment. **a**, REFI; **b**, volume curve; **c**, first half REFI; **d**, second half REFI; **e**, rate; **f**, first half rate; **g**, transit; **h**, first half transit.

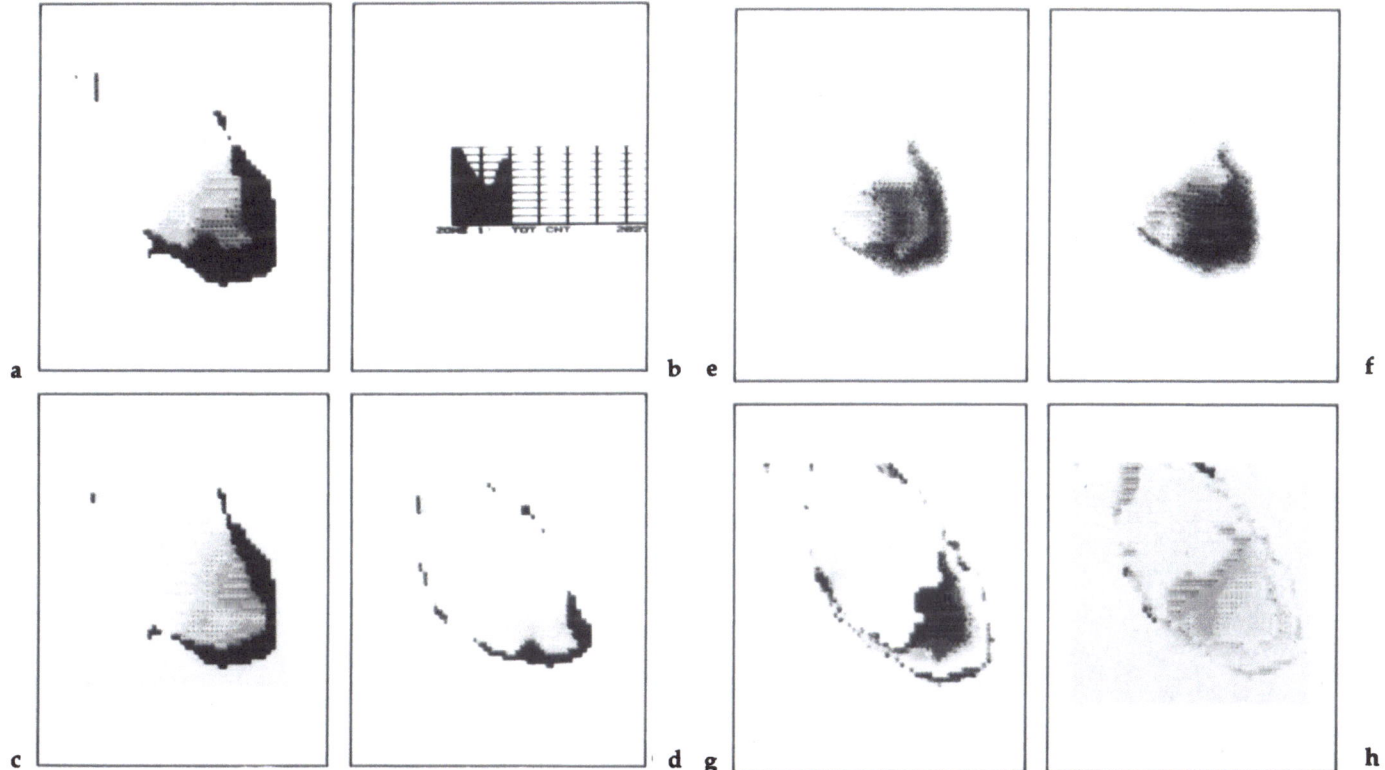

Figure 12.6 *Mitral valve prolapse:* Exercise study on the *same patient as above*. LVEF 57%. Notice the accentuation of the contour and fixed counts in the region of the mitral valve in this black and white study. **a**, REFI; **b**, volume curve; **c**, first half REFI; **d**, second half REFI; **e**, rate; **f**, first half rate; **g**, transit; **h**, first half transit.

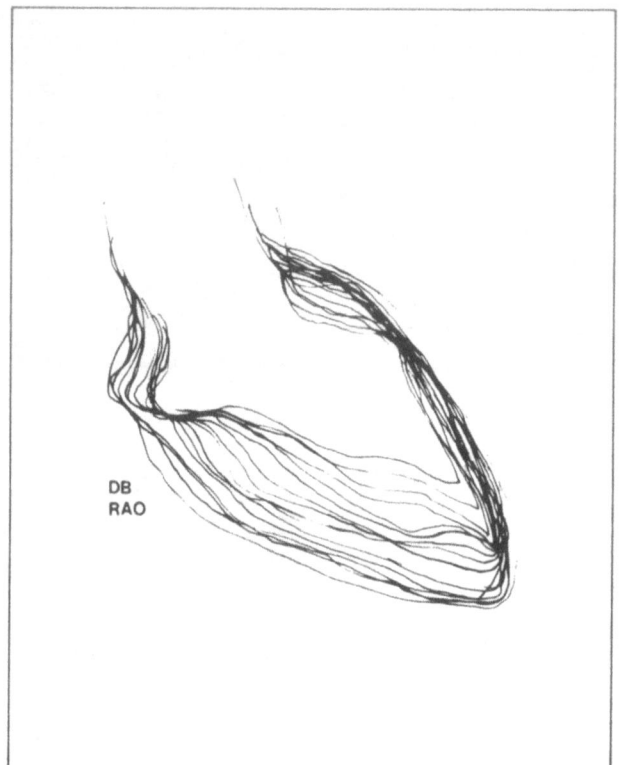

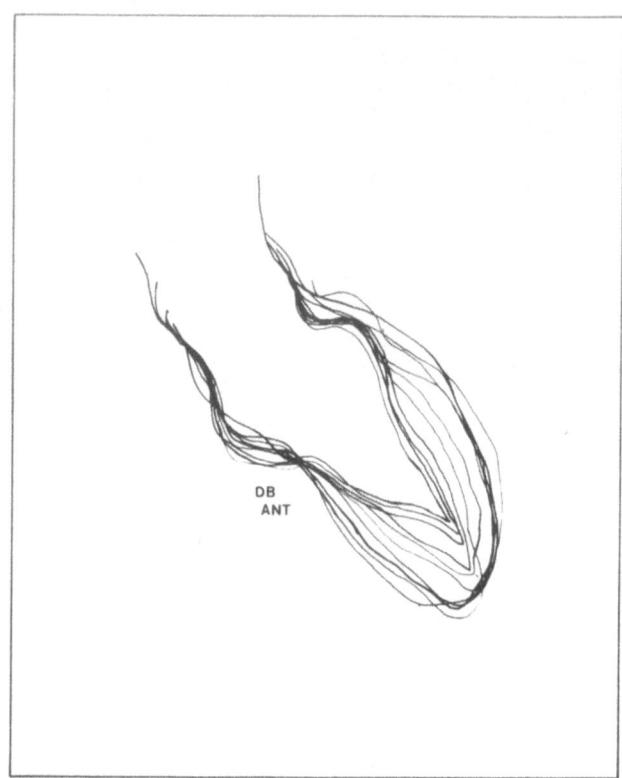

Figure 12.7 *Mitral valve prolapse: RAO projection, contrast left ventriculogram,* frame by frame contour drawing. Systole begins at the outer perimeter. Note lag in high lateral wall with bulge in the contour and excellent inferior wall motion and prominent mitral valve prolapse.

Figure 12.8 *Mitral valve prolapse; ANT projection, contrast left ventriculogram,* frame by frame contours. Systole begins at the outer perimeter. Notice the striking difference in the ventricular contour and the decreased inferior wall motion in this projection. This is the *same patient as Figure 12.7* and also the same patient as depicted in Figures 12.9 and 12.10.

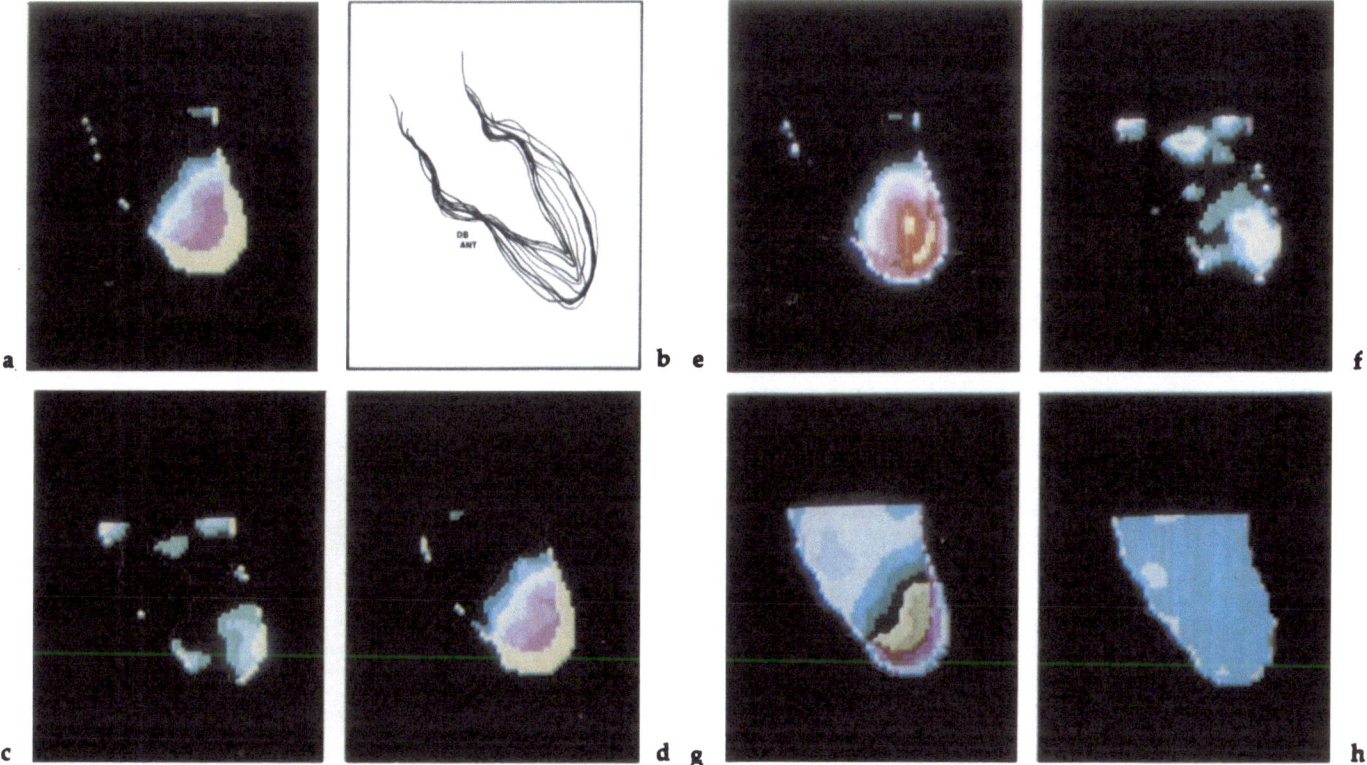

Figure 12.9 *Mitral valve prolapse:* with normal coronary arteriograms. Exercise, ANT. Notice inferior wall motion abnormality in very abnormal first half images with distor-tion of inferior and central wall. **a**, REFI; **b**, contrast LV-gram, anterior; **c**, first half REFI; **d**, second half REFI; **e**, rate; **f**, first half rate; **g**, transit; **h**, first half transit.

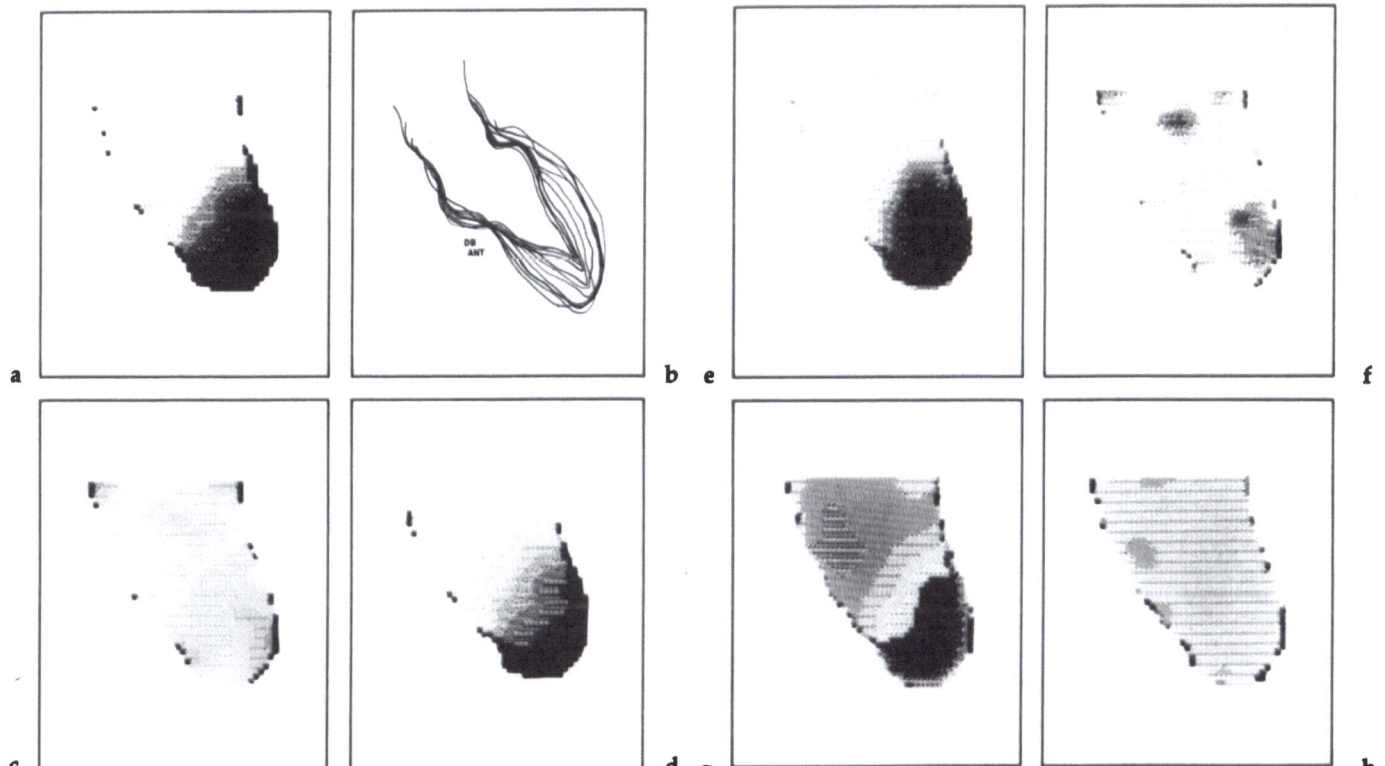

Figure 12.10 *Mitral valve prolapse:* with normal coronary arteriogram. Same patient as in Figure 12.9 with black and white images. **a**, REFI; **b**, contrast LV-gram, anterior; **c**, first half REFI; **d**, second half REFI; **e**, rate; **f**, first half rate; **g**, transit; **h**, first half transit.

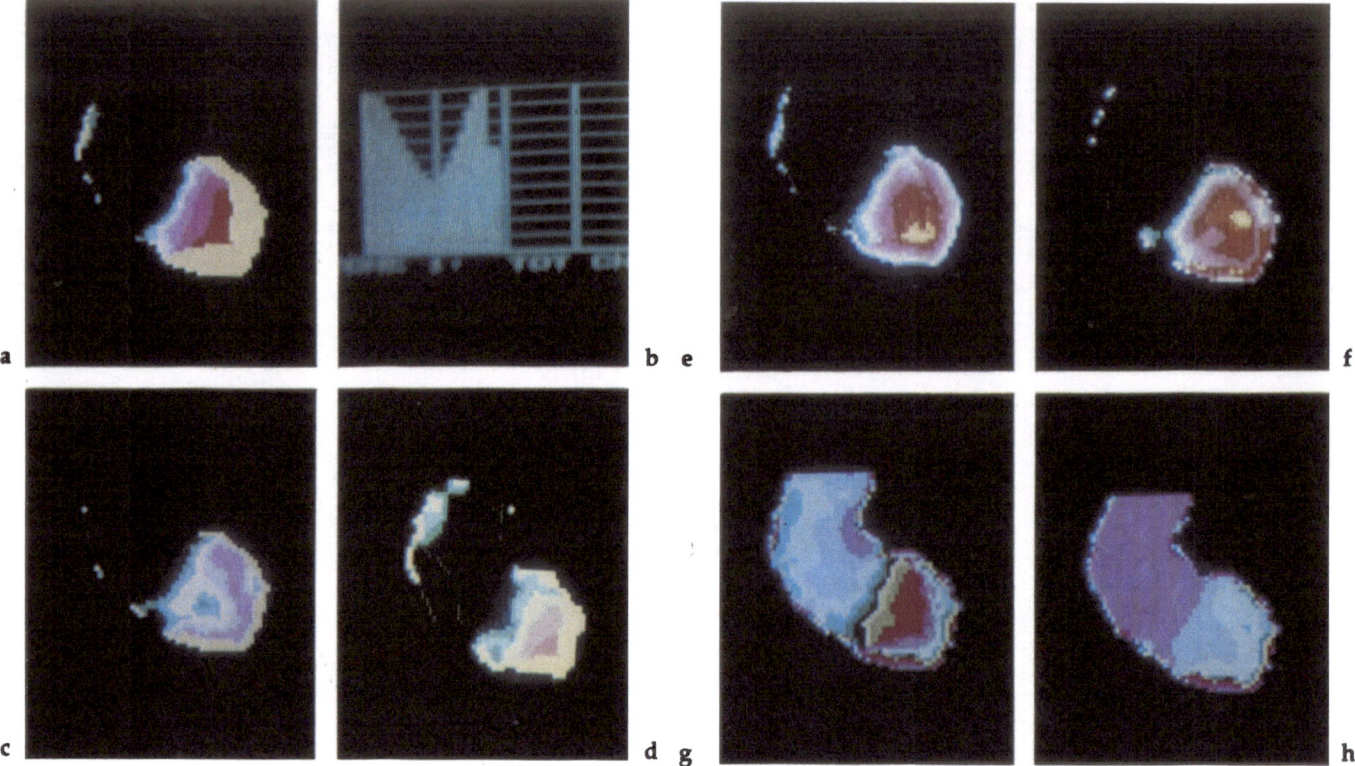

Figure 12.11 *Mitral valve prolapse:* with normal coronary arteriograms. Exercise, ANT. Patient had strongly positive electrocardiographic stress test. There is a configuration of MVP with a lag in the high lateral wall which might be confused with ischaemia but this is typical of patients with MVP. **a,** REFI; **b,** volume curve; **c,** first half REFI; **d,** second half REFI; **e,** rate; **f,** first half rate; **g,** transit; **h,** first half transit.

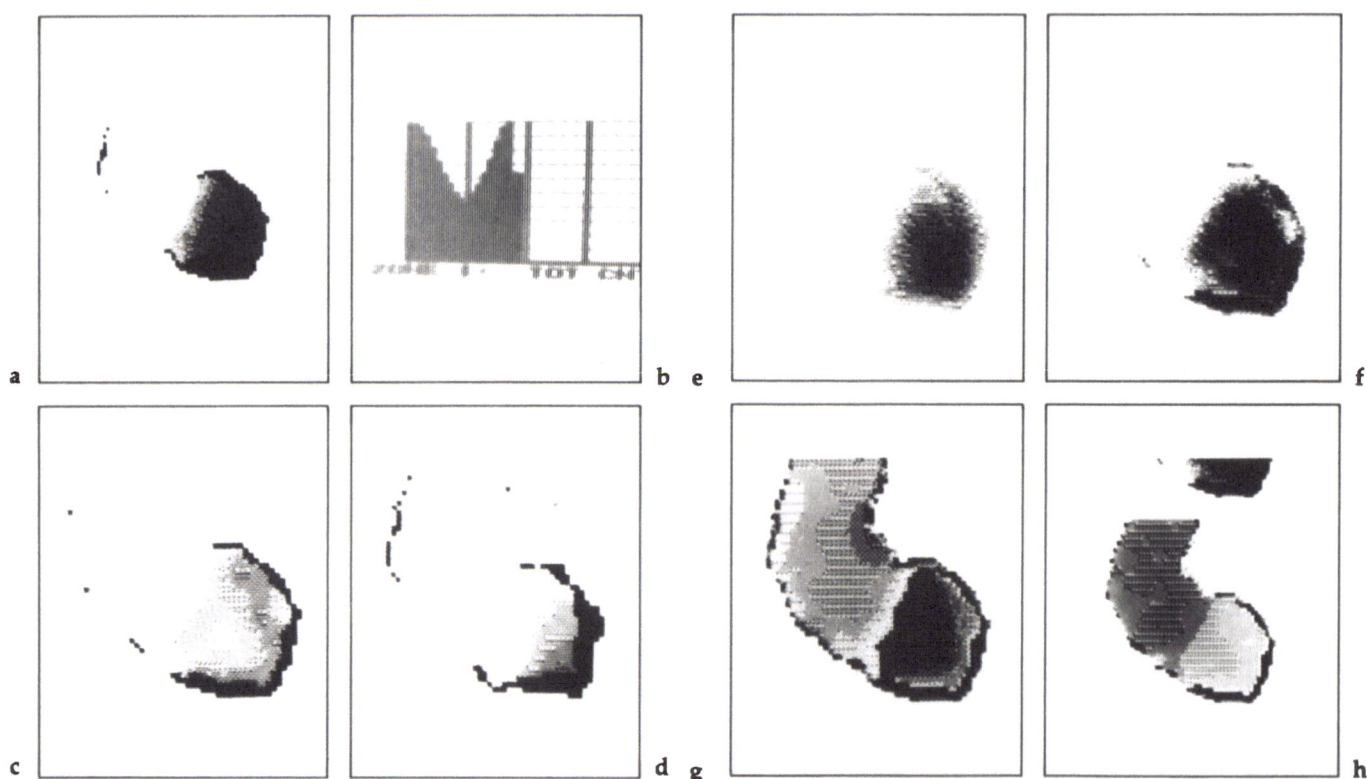

Figure 12.12 *Mitral valve prolapse:* Same patient as in Figure 12.11. Exercise, ANT. LVEF of 55%. **a,** REFI; **b,** volume curve; **c,** first half REFI; **d,** second half REFI; **e,** rate; **f,** first half rate; **g,** transit; **h,** first half transit. The half/half REFI shown here are typical of MVP.

106

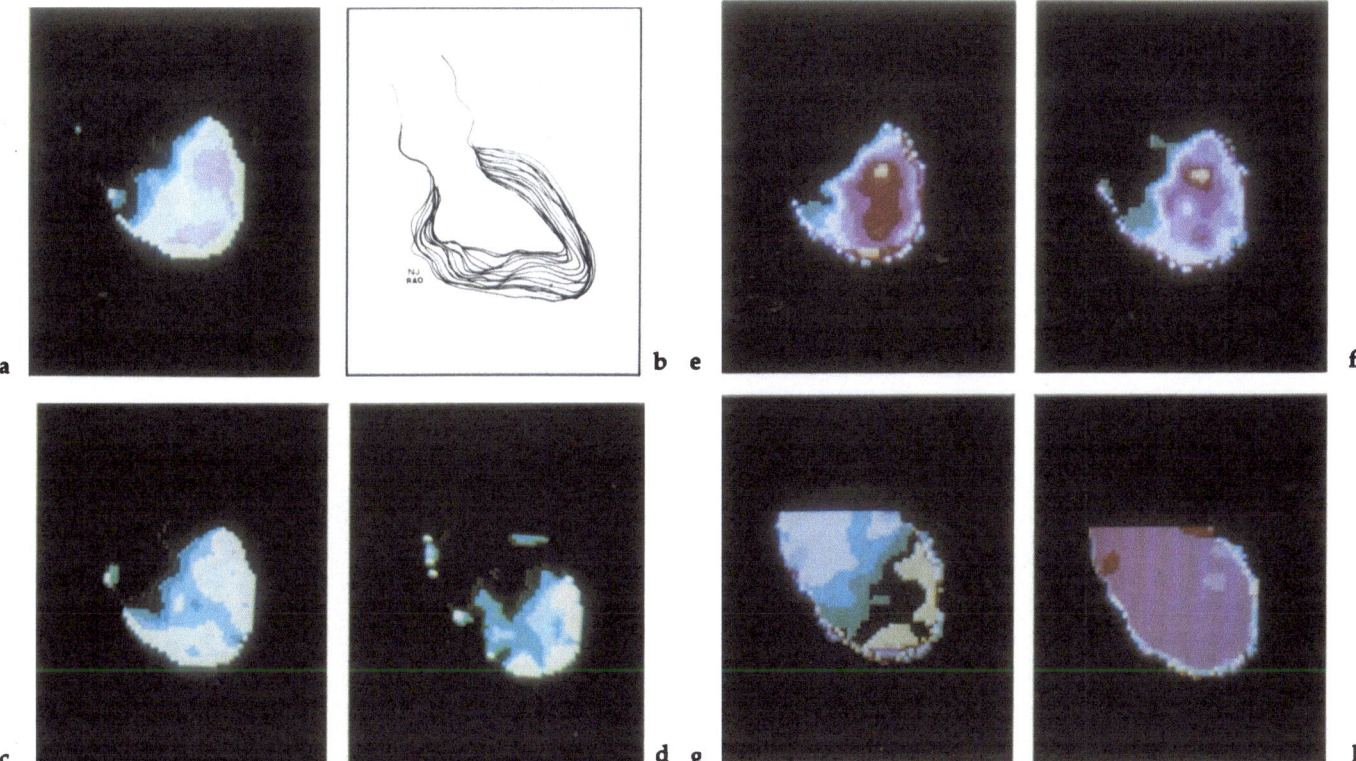

Figure 12.13 *Mitral valve prolapse:* 45-year-old female with normal coronary arteriograms. Exercise, ANT. Notice marked central wall motion abnormality extending toward the apex. This is accentuated during first half of systole and can be confused with ischaemia. **a**, REFI; **b**, contrast LV-gram, RAO; **c**, first half REFI; **d**, second half REFI; **e**, rate; **f**, transit; **g**, first half rate; **h**, first half transit.

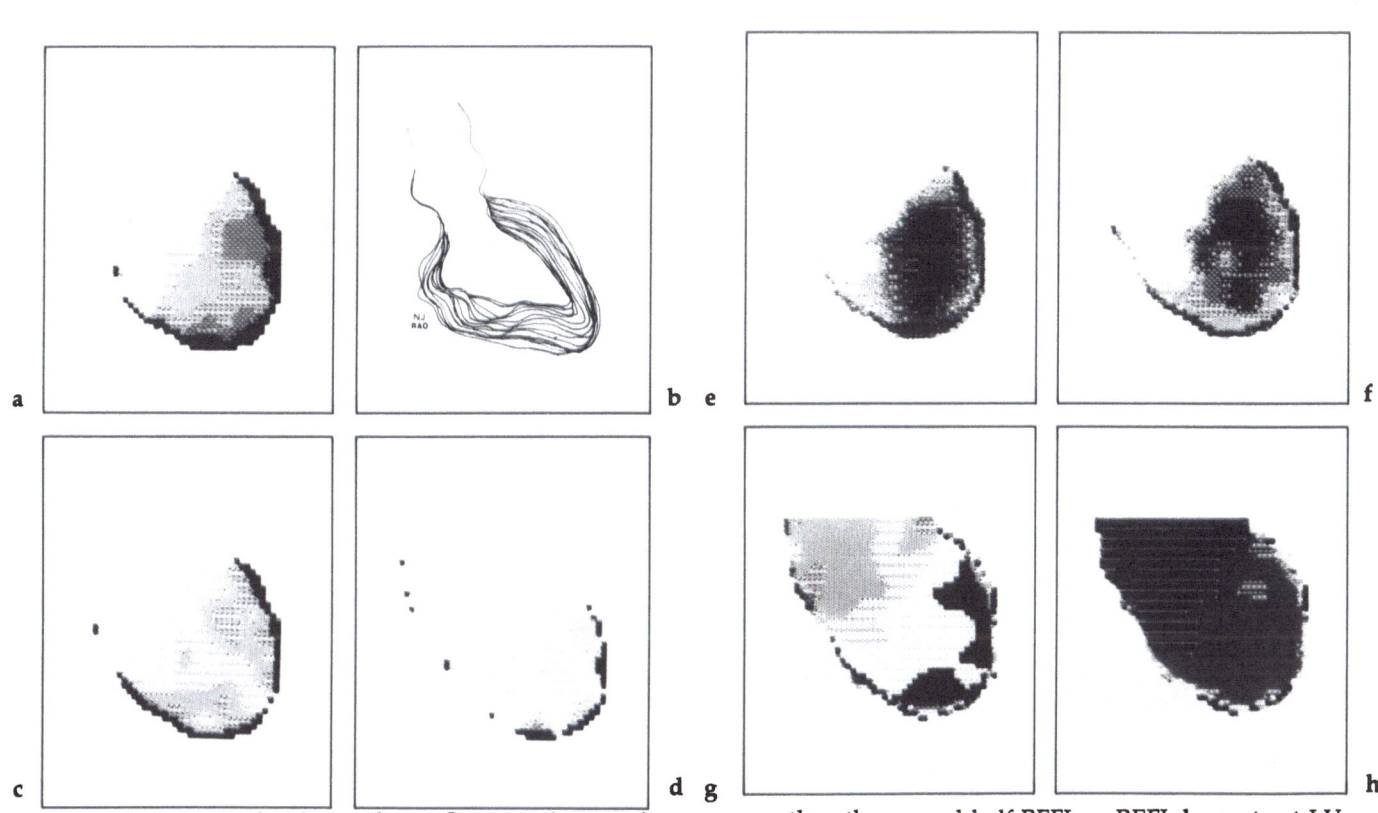

Figure 12.14 *Mitral valve prolapse:* Same patient as in Figure 12.13. There are prominent wall motion abnormalities in both first half and second half. This resembles ischaemia but ischaemia usually affects the first half image more than the second half REFI. **a**, REFI; **b**, contrast LV-gram, RAO; **c**, first half REFI; **d**, second half REFI; **e**, rate; **f**, transit; **g**, first half rate; **h**, first half transit.

107

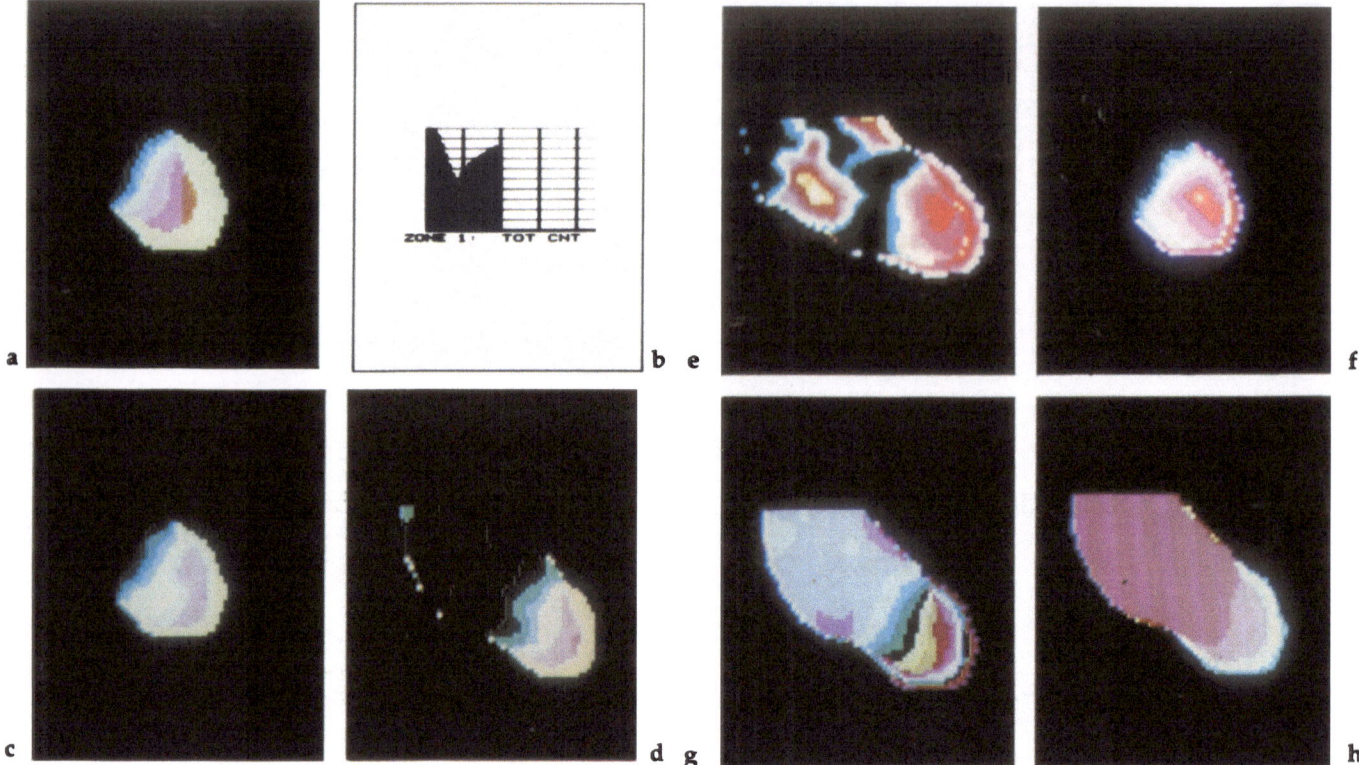

Figure 12.15 *Mitral valve prolapse*, with a very large myxomatous mitral valve. Cardiac catheterization showed normal coronary arteriograms and a huge scalloped mitral valve. Rest, ANT. There is an inferior wall motion abnormality in the first half REFI; a striking representation of the intravalvular regurgitation is depicted in the modified rate image (counts in the ventricular and atrial areas are equalized and presented contiguously). A contrast ventriculogram showed a similar nodular conformity of the huge valve. **a**, REFI; **b**, volume curve; **c**, first half REFI; **d**, second half REFI; **e**, rate; **f**, first half rate; **g**, transit; **h**, first half transit.

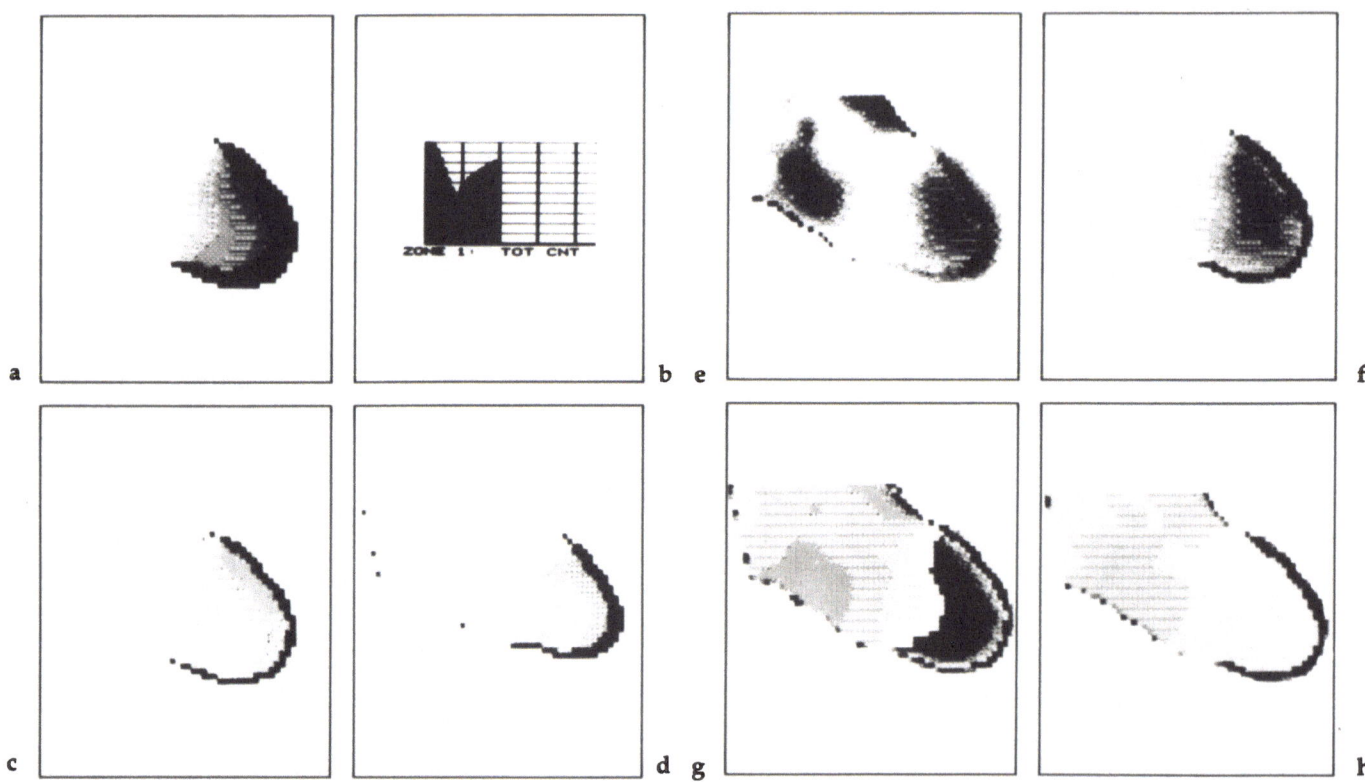

Figure 12.16 *Mitral valve prolapse* with normal coronary angiograms. Same patient as in Figure 12.15. The rate image shows the huge mitral valve outline well in the grey scale. **a**, REFI; **b**, volume curve; **c**, first half REFI; **d**, second half REFI; **e**, rate; **f**, first half rate; **g**, transit; **h**, first half transit.

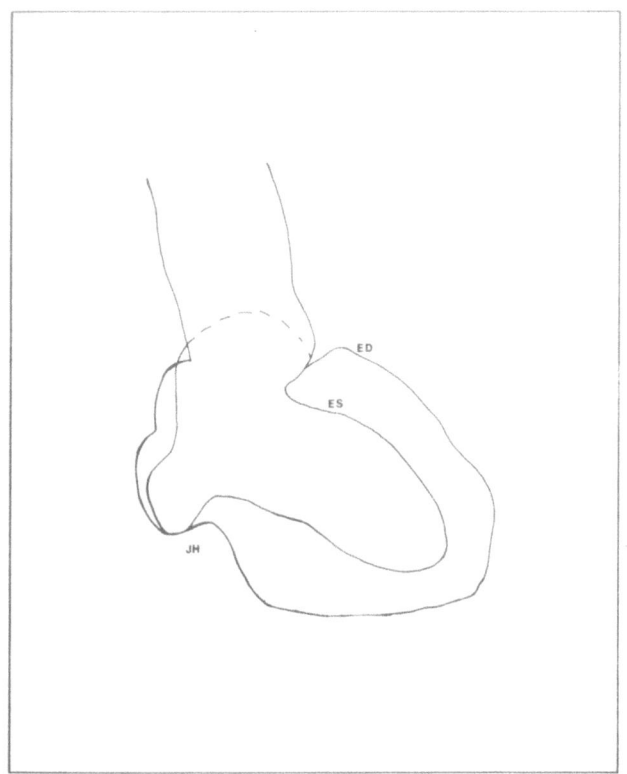

Figure 12.17 *Mitral valve prolapse:* contour drawings of same patient as Figure 12.15.

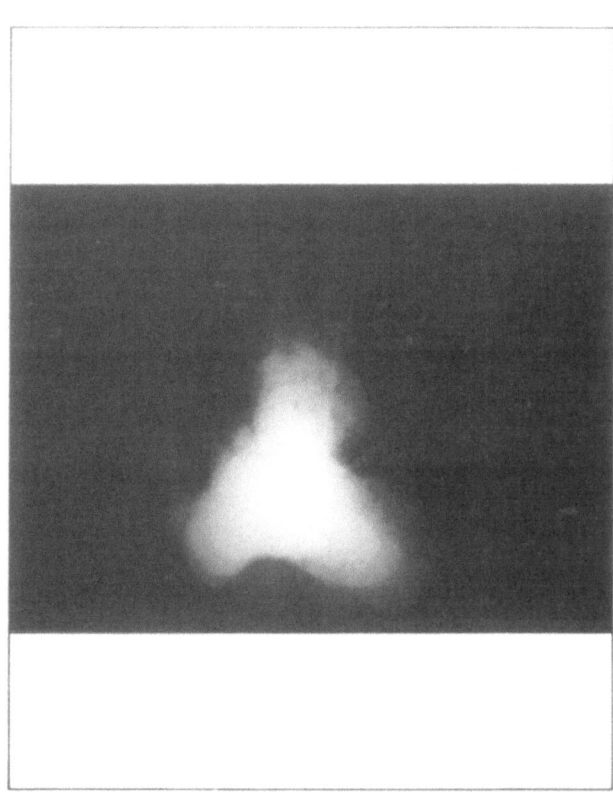

Figure 12.18 *Mitral valve prolapse:* cine angiogram of same patient as Figure 12.17.

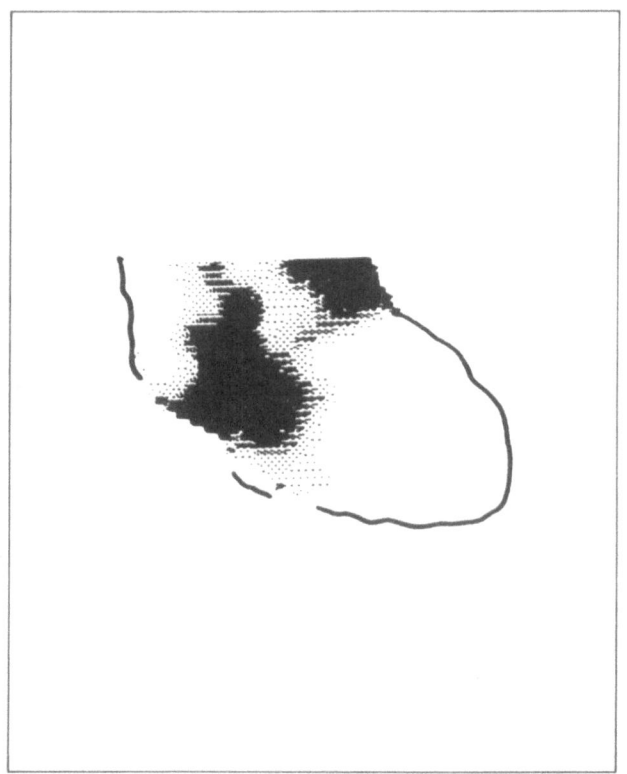

Figure 12.19 *Mitral valve prolapse:* rate image showing activity outlining the large prolapsing valve similar to angiogram (Figure 12.18).

13

Functional Imaging in Aortic and Mitral Valve Disease

E. J. ANDREWS, JR. AND J. W. FLEMING

Valvular heart disease promises to be another area where radionuclide ventriculography (RNV) can be extremely useful in patient management. Although radionuclide studies can often define valvular heart disease, they are not cost-effective tests for diagnostic screening, yielding to the physical examination and ultrasound studies. RNV is helpful, however, in left ventricular (LV) assessment and in evaluation for associated coronary artery disease (CAD). The positive decision, and timing for surgical intervention and valve replacement, are often difficult for the clinician. The optimal time of replacement, particularly for volume overload lesions, should be as late as possible, but *before* irreversible myocardial damage occurs. The situation in valvular stenosis is better defined with valve area measurements, e.c.g. changes, and the clinical picture major determinants for surgical intervention. Two-dimensional echocardiography is a useful non-invasive test in this group. This chapter will briefly discuss application of RNV in valvular heart disease and give case examples.

LEFT VENTRICULAR VOLUME OVERLOAD

Both aortic and mitral regurgitation (AR and MR) are usually well tolerated clinically, but these lesions lead to significant degenerative myocardial changes which may occur even before the patient develops clinical symptoms (Boucher *et al.*, 1981). Johnson *et al.* (1983), suggest that LV volume determination by RNV studies yields more useful information about myocardial functional reserve than the ejection fraction (EF) alone. LV volume can be approximated accurately from first pass RNV studies (Nickel *et al.*, 1982). However, functional imaging adds a new dimension in patient management in that characteristic wall motion changes often are seen even before global parameters become abnormal. RNV studies have been shown to be reproducible (Upton *et al.*, 1980), but it is essential that serial studies be performed with the same patient position (i.e. supine vs erect) as illustrated by Manyari and Kostuk (1983). Exercise tolerance is usually preserved in patients with regurgitant lesions (Levinson *et al.*, 1970) and for this reason there is need for a good non-invasive study which can detect myocardial dysfunction before irreversible symptoms develop.

AORTIC REGURGITATION

Borer *et al.* (1978) and Wexler *et al.* (1981) suggest that surgical intervention for aortic insufficiency should be performed at a time when resting function is normal, but exercise response is diminished. Becoming somewhat disenchanted with EF response to exercise as a reliable indicator of dysfunction, Steingart *et al.* (1983) developed a regurgitant index (LV stroke counts/RV stroke counts) and found this number significantly higher in patients with AR. This index usually decreased with exercise in these patients and may be the mechanism for preservation of exercise tolerance in patients with AR. However, Nicod *et al.* (1982) could not accurately differentiate between 2+, 3+, and 4+ aortic regurgitation using this index. This leaves timing of aortic valve replacement controversial (Selzer *et al.*, 1976; Rahintoola, 1977; O'Rourke and Crawford, 1980).

Wall motion abnormalities are seen by contrast ventriculography in patients with chronic volume overload from either AR or MR with a measurable decrease in velocity of fibre shortening (Osbakken *et al.*, 1981). In all patients, however, global function (EF) was below normal. Wall motion evaluation with functional imaging using RNV reveals characteristic abnormalities which can be followed non-invasively.

Case 1: Figures 13.1 and 13.2

This 58-year-old female presented with palpitations and back pain. RNV shows typical wall motion changes seen in association with AR. There is a central, cone-shaped abnormality seen best in the REFI and mean transit time images which does not extend to the cardiac apex but increases with exercise. End-diastolic volume decreases from 220 ml at rest to 196 ml at exercise and ejection fraction decreases from 49% to 37%. Cardiac output and cardiac index both increase with exercise, accounting for the lack of symptomatology. Associated ischaemia cannot be totally excluded in the presence of valvular heart disease as both conditions lead to similar wall motion changes (Hecht and Hopkins, 1981); however, with ischaemia, functional images usually are less symmetrical and the abnormality may disrupt the apical perimeter during early systole (*see* Chapters 4 and 5).

Case 2: Figures 13.3 and 13.4

This 24-year-old essentially asymptomatic male with known AR presumably due to rheumatic fever underwent RNV as part of a routine evaluation. Studies revealed severe enlargement of the left ventricle (EDV 393 ml) with a central wall motion abnormality which does extend to the apex and which can be confused with ischaemia. Following exercise, wall motion deteriorated further but cardiac output and index were preserved. Because of the severe abnormalities seen by RNV, the patient underwent cardiac catheterization where he was found to have a markedly dilated LV, 4+ AR, and normal coronary arteries. There was no MR. After valve replacement, function and wall motion have improved dramatically.

MITRAL REGURGITATION

Parameters for following patients with MR are more complex than for those with AR because the EF is usually normal and occasionally supernormal because of the decreased resistance created by the incompetent mitral valve (Bolen and Alderman, 1977; Miller *et al.*, 1965; Kennedy *et al.*, 1970). In actuality, EF in this situation is an additive of both forward (aortic) ejection as well as the regurgitant fraction (mitral) which passes back into the left atrium. A more accurate measure of function would be to calculate only the percentage ejected into the aorta with systole, but present methods of calculation (area/length and LV counts) are concerned only with what leaves the ventricle by either direction. Invariably, patients with MR show a significant decrease in EF following surgical valve replacement (Boucher *et al.*, 1981). To date, no method of preoperative evaluation can accurately predict the postoperative EF (Phillips *et al.*, 1981).

Using first pass RNV, a method for determining the 'forward' or true ejection fraction has been developed which in fact adds the regurgitant left atrial counts back to the LV counts before calculation is made. This corrected ejection fraction equals LV end diastolic counts − (LV end systolic counts + left atrial counts) ÷ end diastolic counts (*see* Figure 13.11). After surgery which closes the lower resistance regurgitant pathway, the overall ventricular residual resistance is increased, which results in a lower EF. However, with readjustments in volume (fibre length) in the postoperative period, some improvement in global function can be hopefully expected. In a series of five patients, the corrected ejection fraction correctly predicted the postoperative EF (Table 13.1).

Wall motion changes seen in association with MR are also common and similar to those described with AR, but MR usually produces abnormalities oriented more toward the LV septum.

Table 13.1 Mitral valve replacement. Five patients – RNV prediction of postoperative ejection fraction

| Patient | Preoperative | | Postoperative Ejection fraction |
	Ejection fraction	Corrected ejection fraction	
1	40	19	20
2	44	35	35
3	60	41	45
4	64	49	47
5	58	39	33

Case 3: Figure 13.5

This 74-year-old male with a cardiac murmur since childhood presented with a recent episode of mild congestive failure. Initial RNV study showed good global function (EF = 58% at rest and 52% with exercise) and mild diffuse wall motion changes most pronounced in the septal area. The corrected ejection fraction, however, was calculated to be 39% at rest. Subsequent cardiac catheterization revealed severe MR, trace AR, and normal coronary arteries. He underwent mitral valve replacement and the resting EF immediately after surgery was 33%. This increased to 52% 2 weeks later and at 1 year, function remains normal with EF 55% at rest and 58% with exercise. Wall motion has also returned to normal.

Case 4: Figure 13.6

This 42-year-old female was seen for cardiac evaluation prior to eye surgery. RNV study revealed central wall motion changes similar to those described in association with AR. In this case, EDV was 258 ml, EF 43% at rest and exercise. Enlargement of the left ventricle with associated decrease in velocity of fibre shortening produces the central abnormality.

LEFT VENTRICULAR PRESSURE OVERLOAD

Pressure overload produces a much different effect upon the LV than volume overload and consequently different considerations regarding surgical intervention. Pichard *et al.* (1981) showed a reduction in coronary vascular reserve in patients with LV hypertrophy secondary to hypertension. Rabinowitz and Zak (1975) state that myocardial metabolism is almost exclusively aerobic with substantial quantities of adenosine triphosphate (ATP) supplied by mitochondrial oxidation of fatty acids and carbohydrate substrates. The ATP requirement increases significantly with stress and is usually met by increased mitochondrial synthesis. Attarian *et al.* (1981) have shown that LV hypertrophy results in lower endocardial blood flow, lower subendocardial high-energy phosphate stores, and depressed mitochondrial function. Therefore, the myocardium is more susceptible to ischaemia. Wangler *et al.* (1982) also demonstrated decreased coronary reserve in patients with hypertension and cardiac hypertrophy. RNV with functional imaging can detect wall motion abnormalities which result from increased metabolic demands and decreased coronary reserve in LV hypertrophy. These findings are most pronounced in patients with aortic stenosis (AS) and are often identical to findings seen associated with CAD.

AORTIC STENOSIS

Patients with aortic stenosis (AS) commonly present with angina pectoris not explained by associated coronary artery disease. Several investigators suggest that relative subendocardial ischaemia occurs secondary to myocardial hypertrophy, and that this may be the mechanism for chest pain associated with AS. Rembert et al. (1978) demonstrated, in animal studies, decreased endocardial blood flow associated with concentric LV hypertrophy. Marcus and colleagues (1982) suggest that decreased coronary reserve may be the mechanism for angina pectoris in patients with AS and normal coronary arteries. Kuhajda et al. (1981) described focal replacement fibrosis or subendocardial concentric band necrosis in 13 patients with severe AS and normal coronary arteries at autopsy.

Case 5: Figure 13.7

This 75-year-old female presented with chest pain and exercise intolerance. Cardiac catheterization revealed severe AS and normal coronary arteries with good LV function. RNV studies showed normal global LV function but an anterolateral wall motion abnormality was seen during early systole similar to changes associated with ischaemia.

Case 6: Figure 13.8

This 53-year-old male had previous aortic valve replacement but was studied because of symptoms of valve malfunction. RNV revealed moderately severe LV dysfunction with LVEF decreasing from 55% at rest to 40% at exercise. Rather severe wall motion abnormalities also developed with exercise. Cardiac catheterization revealed stenotic as well as insufficient prosthetic valve. Gradient was 63 mm of mercury. Valve replacement was recommended.

Longstanding systemic arterial hypertension and obstructive cardiomyopathy may produce a similar effect upon LV related to myocardial hypertrophy (see Chapter 11, Cardiomyopathy).

MITRAL STENOSIS

Curry and colleagues (1972) described LV wall motion abnormalities observed by cineventriculograms in patients with mitral stenosis (MS). They postulated that RV enlargement associated with MS may produce secondary abnormalities of LV contractility. Mitral stenosis is also commonly associated with AI which may additionally affect contractility. RNV studies often demonstrate LV wall motion abnormalities in the absence of associated CAD.

Case 7: Figure 13.9

This 38-year-old female was found to have severe MS, mild AI, and normal coronary arteries at cardiac catheterization. Because of the symptoms of congestive failure she underwent valve replacement. There was a return to LV function to normal 3 years following surgery (LVEF 53%). Wall motion of the left ventricle is relatively well preserved but the inflow image (diastolic) is abnormal (not shown).

Case 8: Figure 13.10

This 26-year-old male presented with signs and symptoms of valve malfunction 3 years after mitral valve replacement. RNV studies showed severe LV dysfunction with severe wall motion abnormalities in contrast to the previous case. Severe functional stenosis of the prosthetic valve was found at cardiac catheterization and replacement was recommended.

SUMMARY

Valvular heart disease commonly produces LV contraction abnormalities in the absence of associated CAD (Hecht and Hopkins, 1981). The pressure overload lesions with associated LVH may have early systolic wall motion abnormalities indistinguishable from ischaemia. Volume overload lesions usually are less confusing and may produce diagnostic RNV functional images. For example, a central cone-shaped central wall motion abnormality with an enlarged LV is highly suggestive of aortic insufficiency. However, early systolic wall motion abnormalities extending to the periphery of the left ventricle in patients with valve disease should at least raise the question of associated CAD.

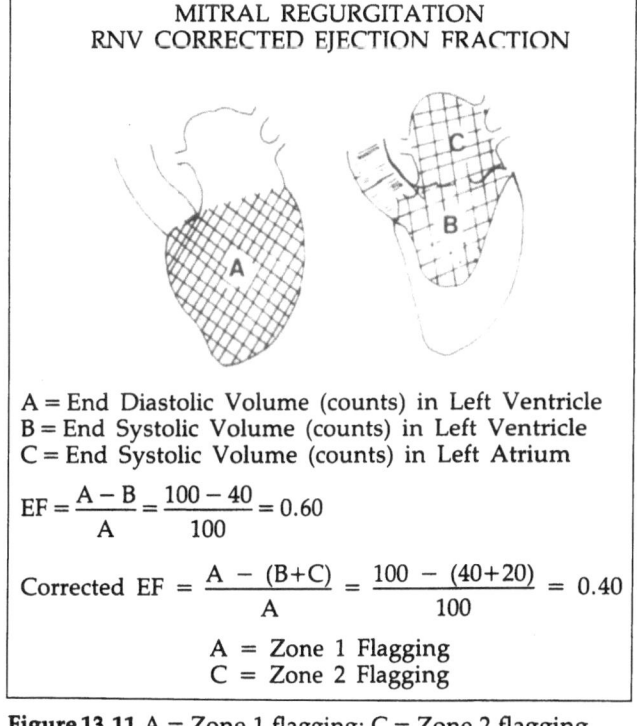

MITRAL REGURGITATION
RNV CORRECTED EJECTION FRACTION

A = End Diastolic Volume (counts) in Left Ventricle
B = End Systolic Volume (counts) in Left Ventricle
C = End Systolic Volume (counts) in Left Atrium

$$EF = \frac{A - B}{A} = \frac{100 - 40}{100} = 0.60$$

$$\text{Corrected } EF = \frac{A - (B+C)}{A} = \frac{100 - (40+20)}{100} = 0.40$$

A = Zone 1 Flagging
C = Zone 2 Flagging

Figure 13.11 A = Zone 1 flagging; C = Zone 2 flagging.

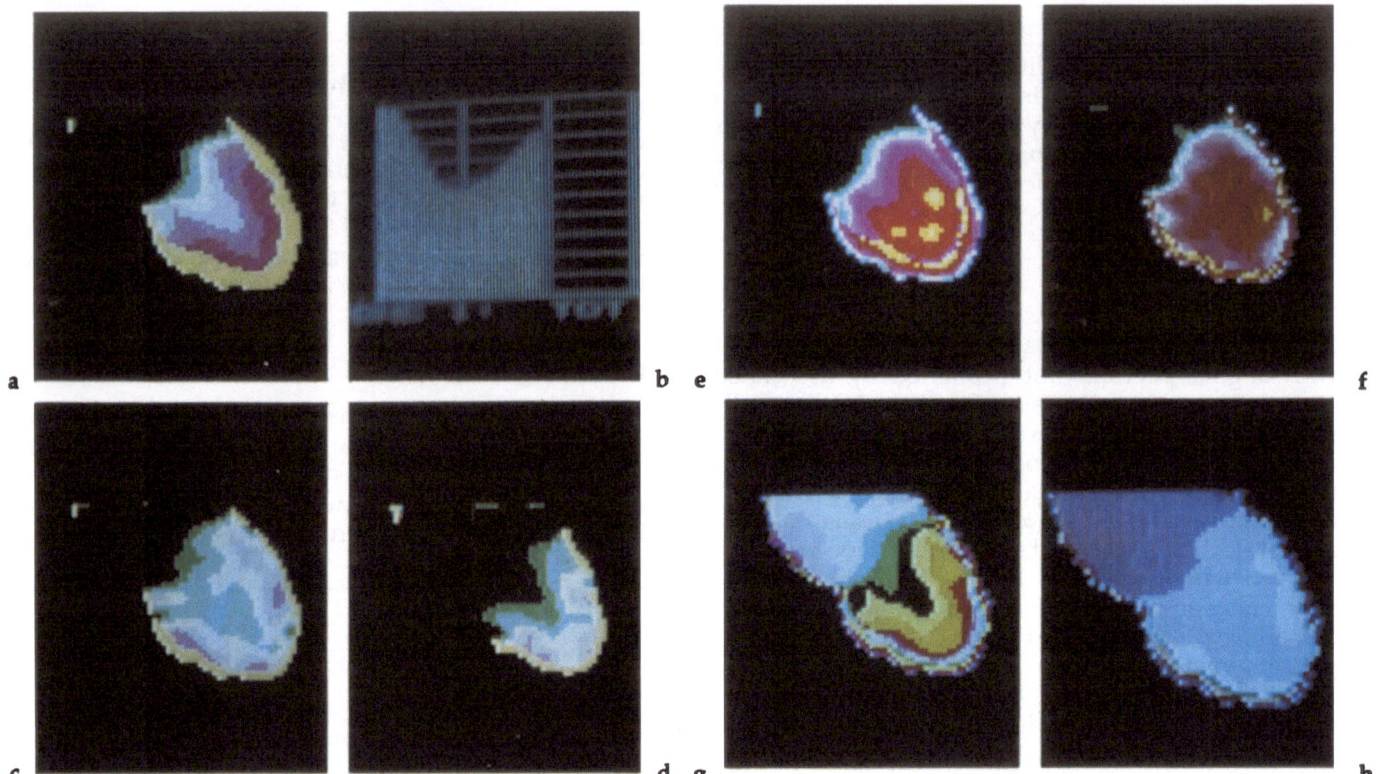

Figure 13.1 *Case 1. Aortic insufficiency.* Normal coronary arteries, palpitations and back pain. 3+ aortic regurgitation, rest anterior LVEF 49%. Images show a cone shaped central wall motion abnormality which is commonly seen with elongation of the left ventricle associated with aortic insufficiency. The apex is preserved. **a**, REFI; **b**, volume curve; **c**, first half REFI; **d**, second half REFI; **e**, ejection rate; **f**, first half ER; **g**, transit; **h**, first half transit.

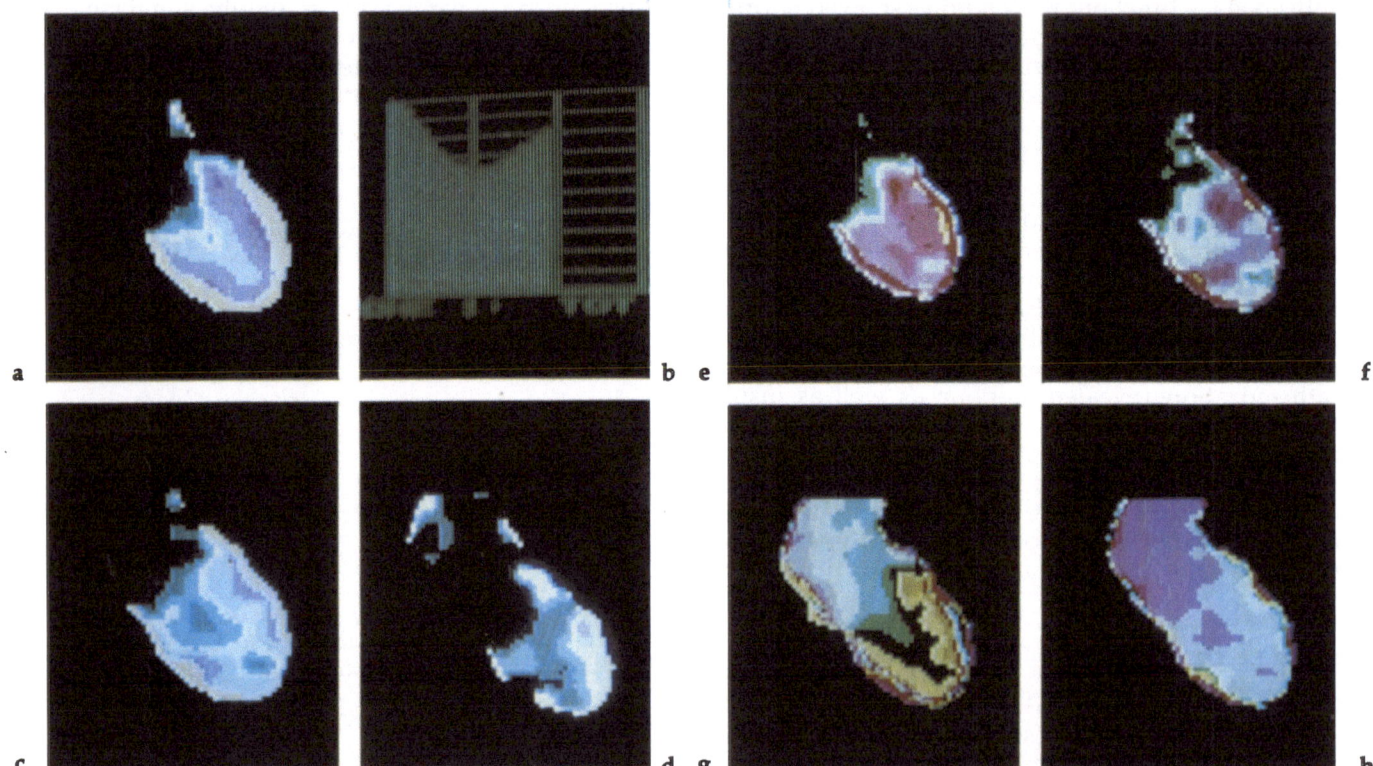

Figure 13.2 *Case 1. Aortic insufficiency,* anterior, exercise LVEF 37%, global function decreases with exercise and the central wall motion abnormality extends further toward the apex. The septal abnormality also develops late in systole on the second half REFI image. **a**, REFI; **b**, volume curve; **c**, first half REFI; **d**, second half REFI; **e**, ejection rate; **f**, first half ER; **g**, transit; **h**, first half transit.

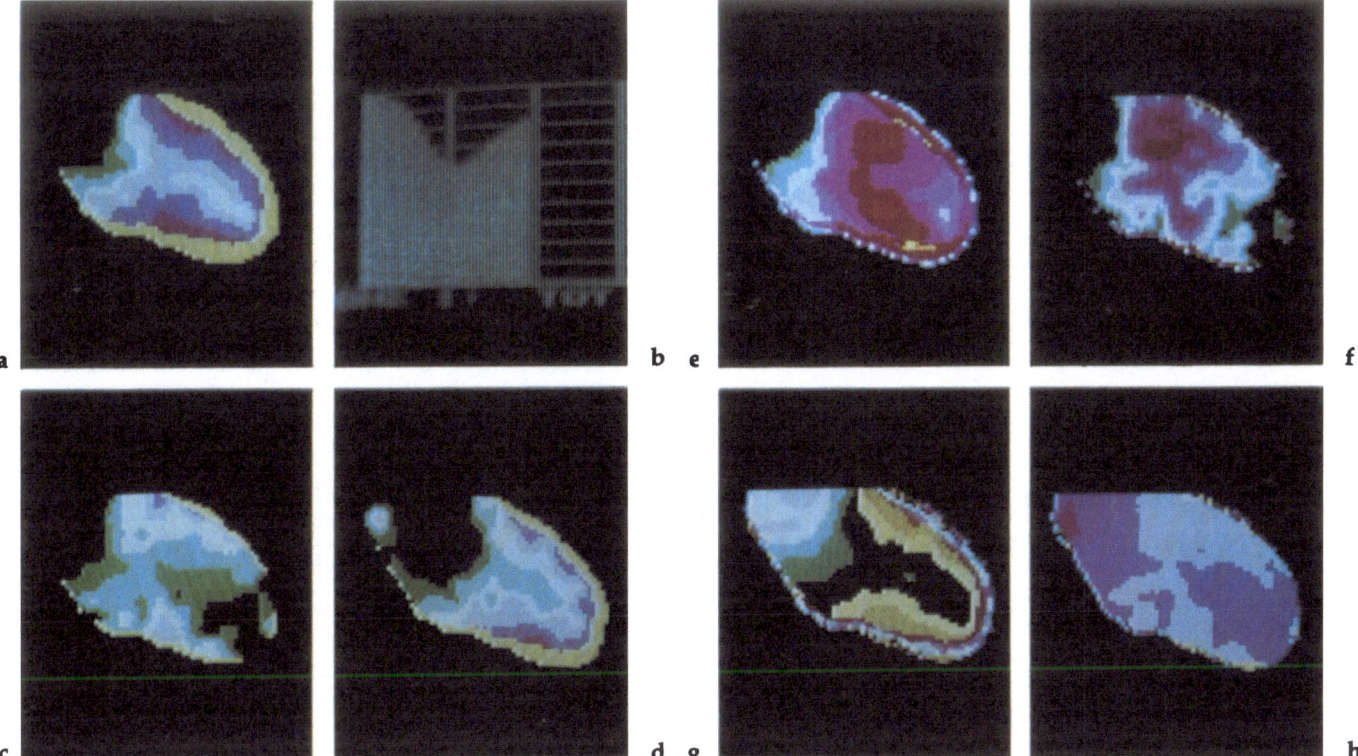

Figure 13.3 *Case 2. Aortic insufficiency.* Asymptomatic, rest anterior RVEF 35%. Images show central wall motion abnormality which extends to the apex on the first half REFI, mean transit and rate images. This pattern is indis-

tinguishable from ischaemia. **a**, REFI; **b**, volume curve; **c**, first half REFI; **d**, second half REFI; **e**, ejection rate; **f**, first half ER; **g**, transit; **h**, first half transit.

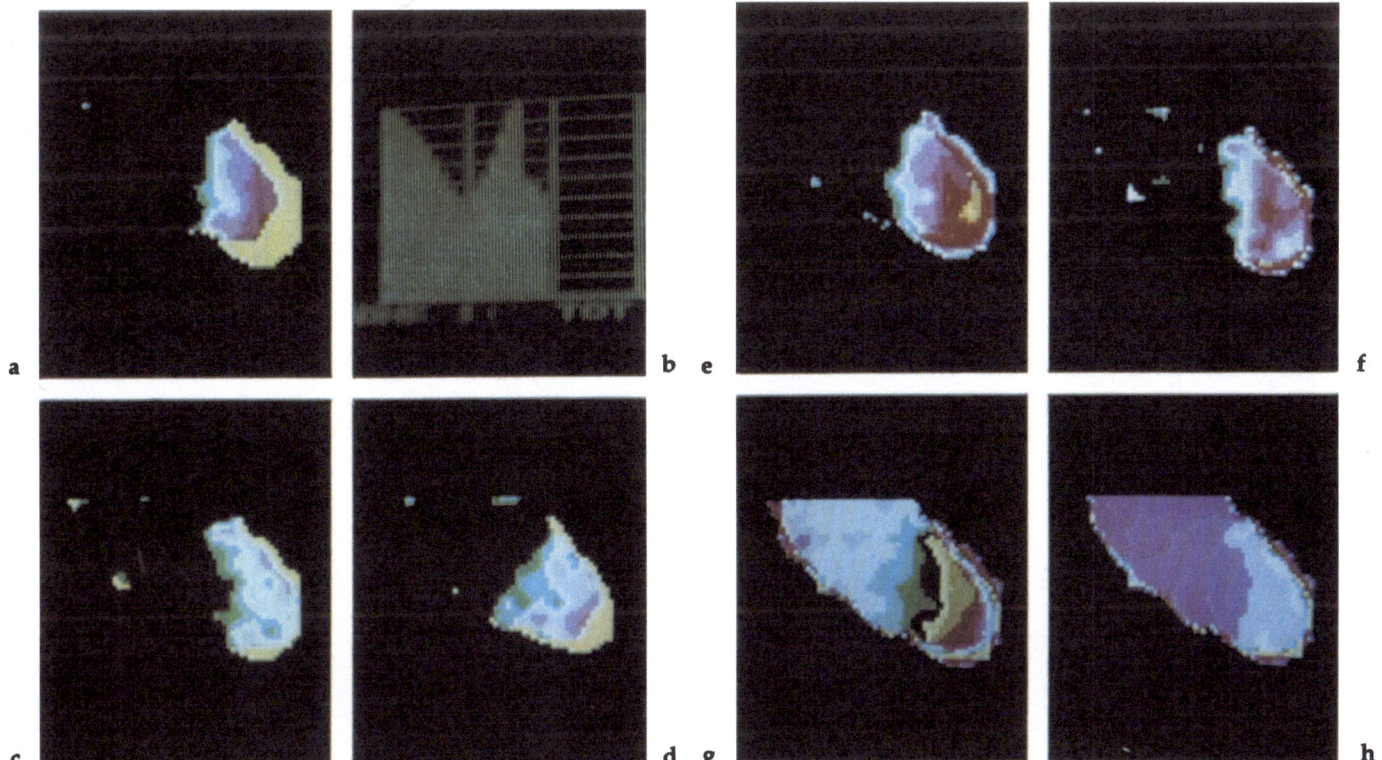

Figure 13.4 *Case 2. Aortic insufficiency*, postoperative, rest anterior LDEF 48%, global function has improved and wall motion has returned nearly to normal following aortic valve replacement. The elongated appearance of the

ventricle has also diminished. **a**, REFI; **b**, volume curve; **c**, first half REFI; **d**, second half REFI; **e**, ejection rate; **f**, first half ER; **g**, transit; **h**, first half transit.

115

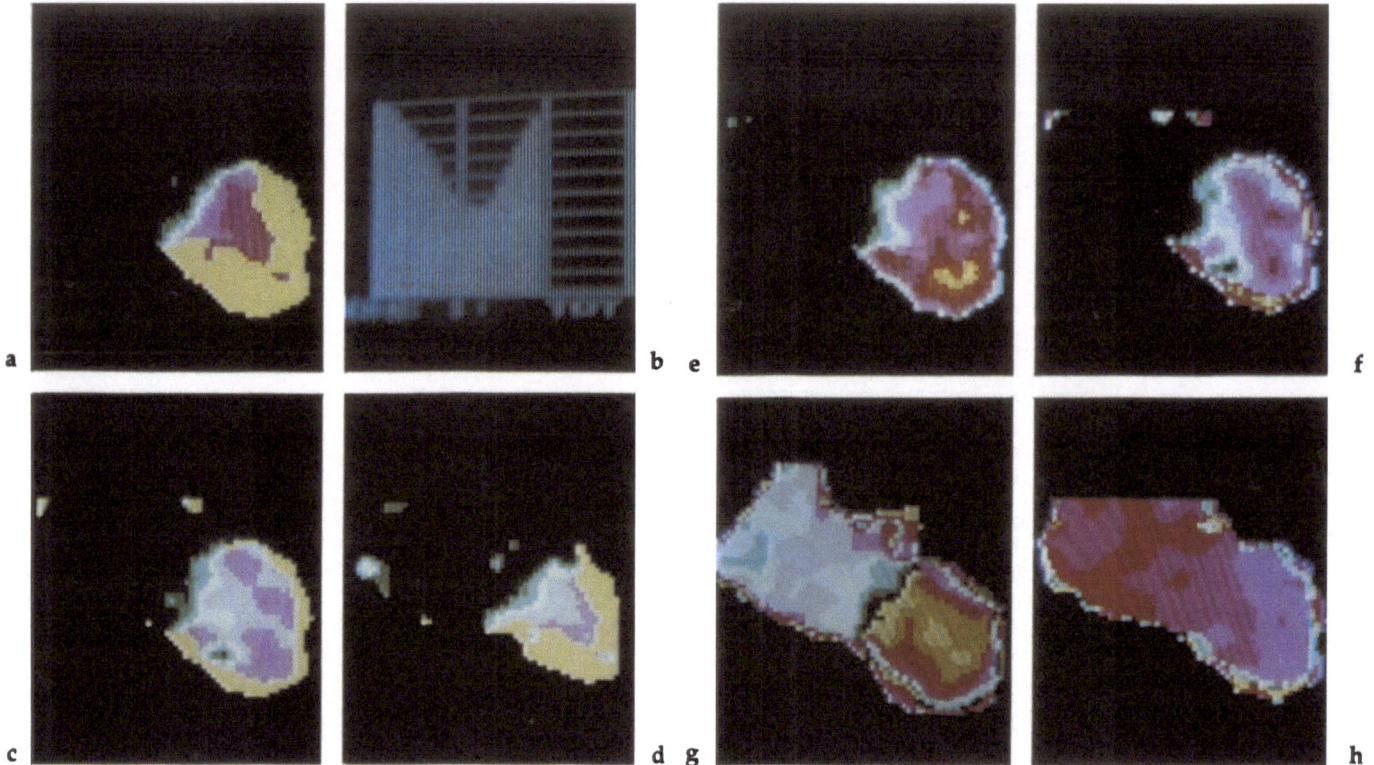

Figure 13.5 *Case 3. Mitral regurgitation*, normal coronary arteries. Congestive failure. Rest anterior LVEF 58%. Images show diffuse wall motion changes most pronounced in the septal region of the LV, best seen on the second half REFI and first half transit images. These findings are non-specific. **a**, REFI; **b**, volume curve; **c**, first half REFI; **d**, second half REFI; **e**, ejection rate; **f**, first half ER; **g**, transit; **h**, first half transit.

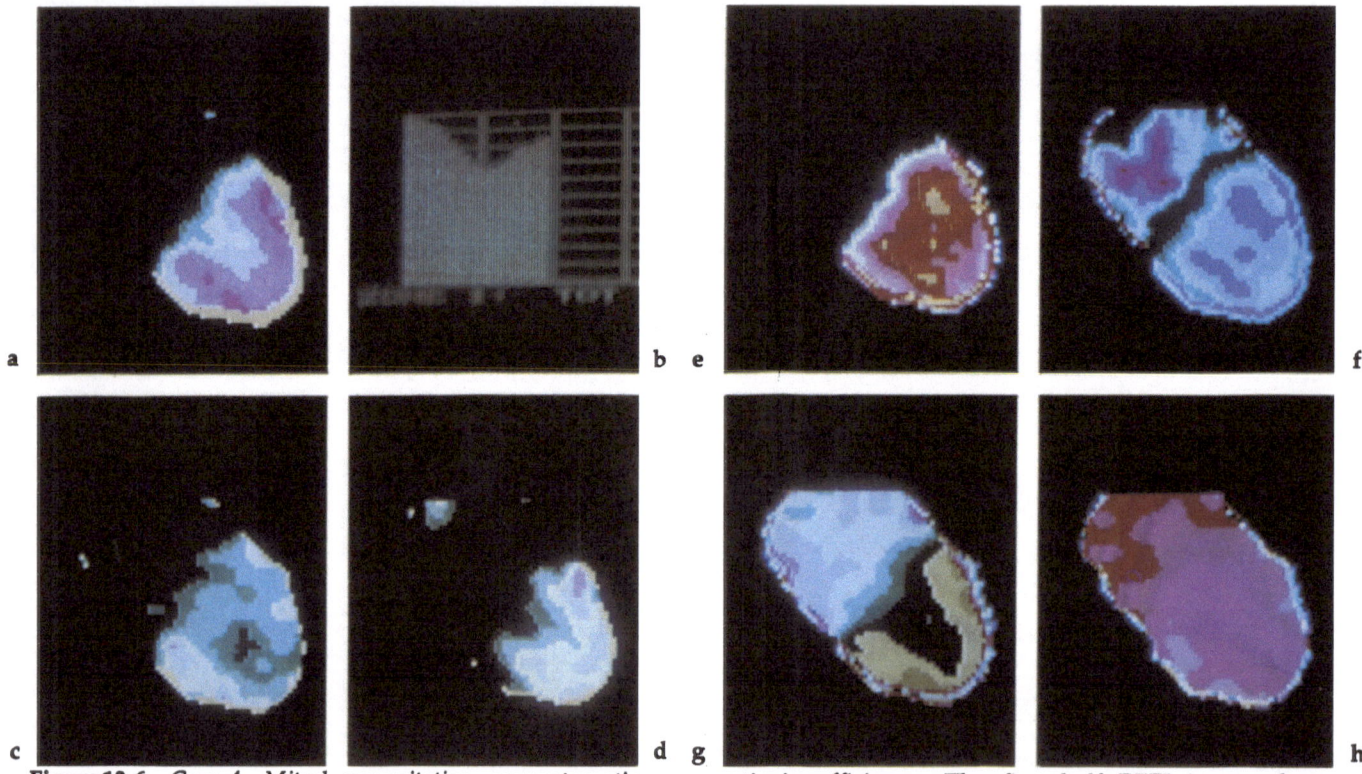

Figure 13.6 *Case 4. Mitral regurgitation*, asymptomatic, 4+ mitral regurgitation, normal coronary arteries, moderate LV dysfunction. Rest anterior LVEF 43%. Images showed diffuse wall motion changes more pronounced than the previous case. A central cone shaped abnormality is seen on the mean transit image similar to aortic insufficiency. The first half REFI image shows abnormality of the anterior lateral wall which could be confused with ischaemia. LA activity is shown in f. **a**, REFI; **b**, volume curve; **c**, first half REFI; **d**, second half REFI; **e**, ejection rate; **f**, first half ER; **g**, transit; **h**, first half transit.

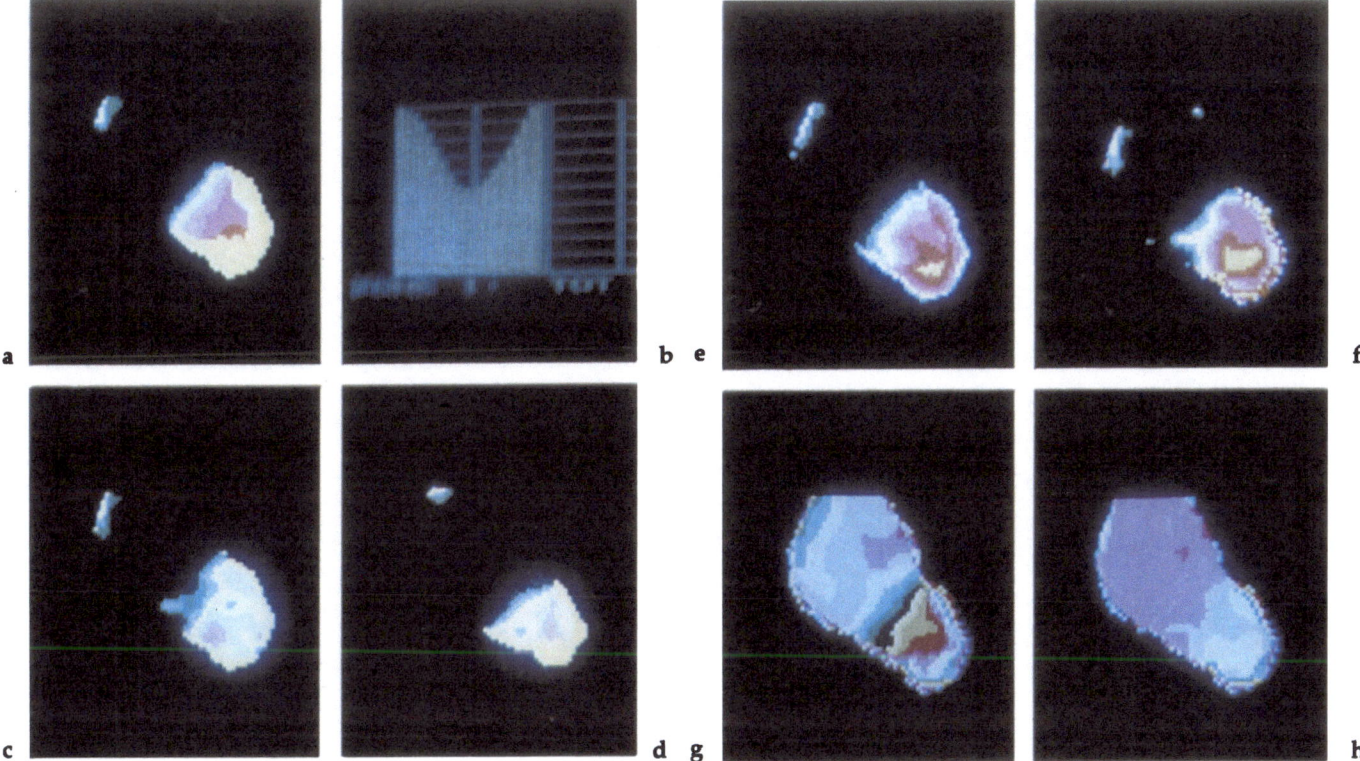

Figure 13.7 *Case 5. Aortic stenosis*, normal coronary arteries, chest pain, exercise anterior LVEF 60%. There is preservation of wall motion except for a focal antero lateral abnormality which is similar to ischaemia. **a**, REFI; **b**, volume curve; **c**, first half REFI; **d**, second half REFI; **e**, ejection rate; **f**, first half ER; **g**, transit; **h**, first half transit.

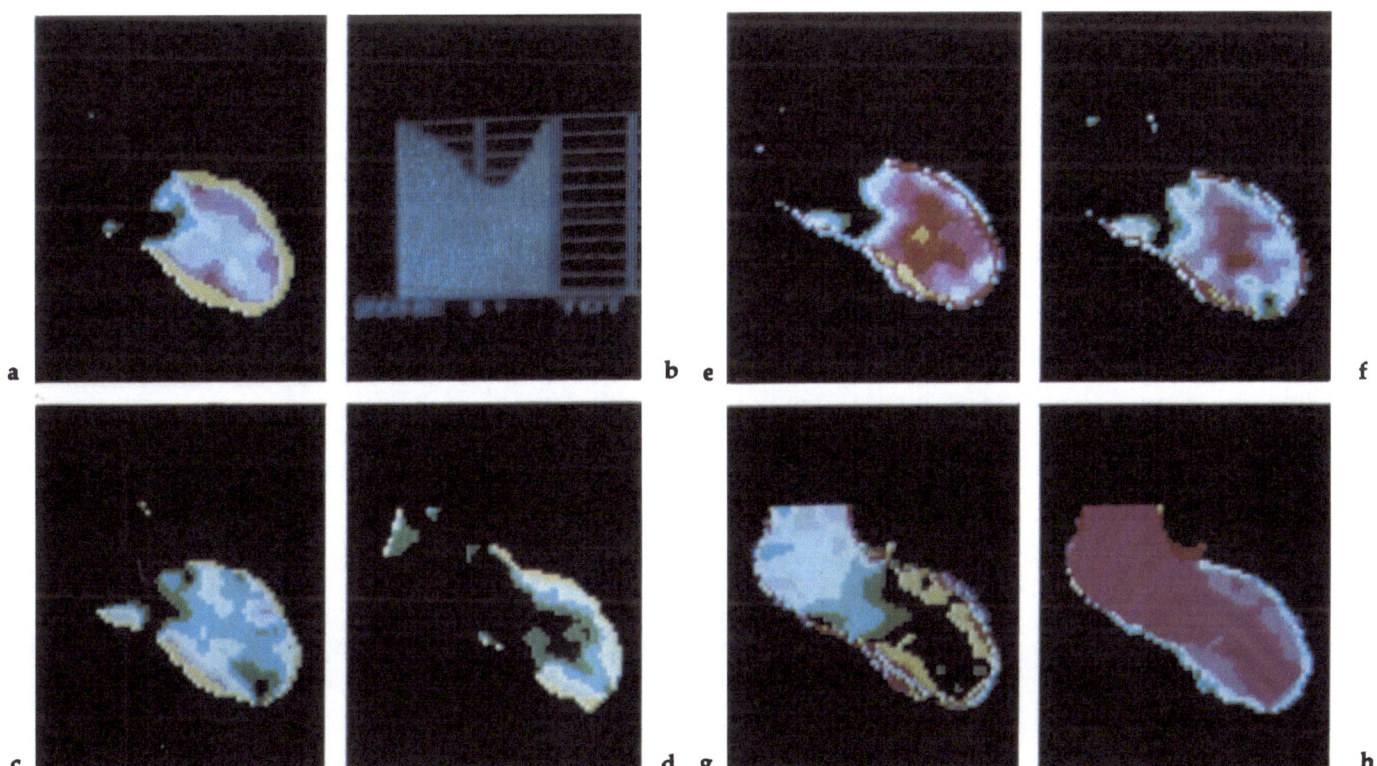

Figure 13.8 *Case 6. Aortic stenosis*. Normal coronary arteries, previous aortic valve replacement, recent symptoms of valve malfunction, exercise anterior LVEF 45%. Images show diffuse wall motion changes extending to the apex contributed to by aortic insufficiency as well as stenosis. **a**, REFI; **b**, volume curve; **c**, first half REFI; **d**, second half REFI; **e**, ejection rate; **f**, first half ER; **g**, transit; **h**, first half transit.

117

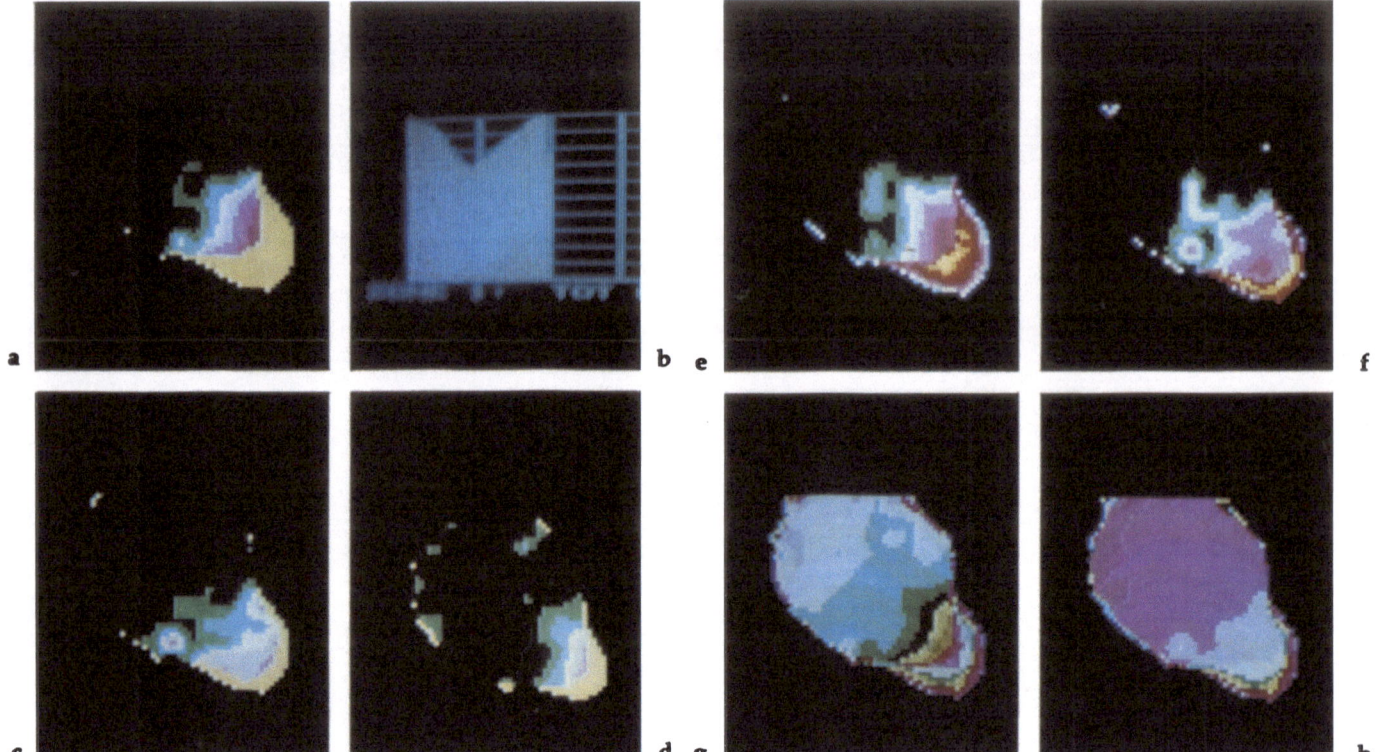

Figure 13.9 *Case 7. Mitral stenosis*, normal coronary arteries, moderate aortic regurgitation, rest anterior. **a**, REFI; **b**, volume curve; **c**, first half REFI; **d**, second half REFI; **e**, ejection rate; **f**, first half ER; **g**, transit; **h**, first half transit.

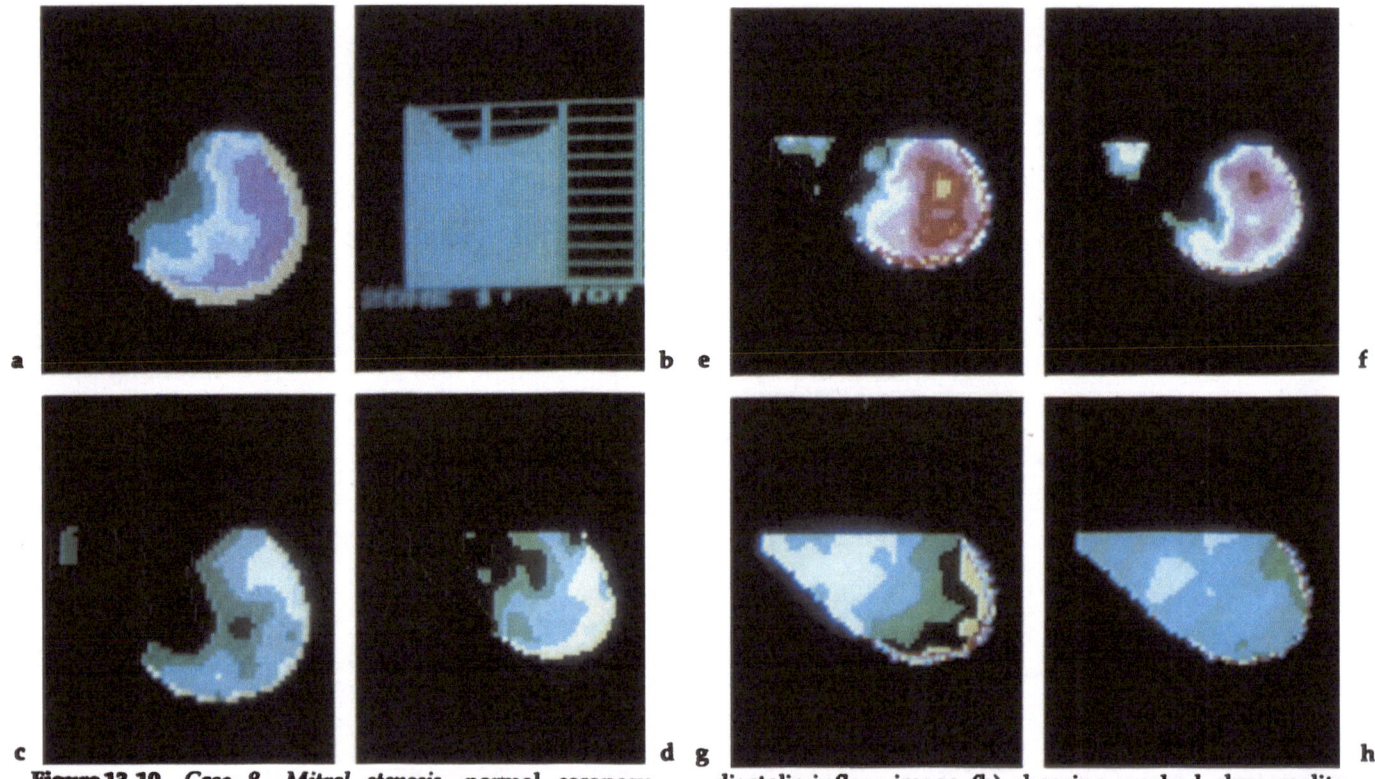

Figure 13.10 *Case 8. Mitral stenosis*, normal coronary arteries, previous mitral valve replacement, recent symptoms of valve malfunction, rest anterior LVEF 39%, moderate diffuse wall motion changes are seen with the diastolic inflow image (b) showing marked abnormality due to the stenotic prosthetic valve. **a**, REFI; **b**, volume curve; **c**, first half REFI; **d**, second half REFI; **e**, ejection rate; **f**, first half ER; **g**, transit; **h**, first half transit.

14

First Pass Radionuclide Studies in Evaluation of Mitral Valve Replacement in Chronic Insufficiency Using Björk–Shiley Tilting Disc Valves

B. REICHART, N. SCHAD, G. BOUGIOUKAS, R. HATZ, E. KREUZER AND M. LUTHER

Operations of the mitral valve comprise a vast field of heart surgery. Unlike aortic valvular disease which may be due to both congenital and acquired defects, mitral valve disease is more frequently acquired. A common cause of mitral valve destruction is rheumatic endocarditis. The three dominant changes produced by mitral stenosis as well as by mitral insufficiency are an increase in left atrial pressure, reduction in cardiac output and an increase in pulmonary vascular resistance. Two other significant events occur at a later stage of the disease in most patients: atrial fibrillation and its associated risk of systemic embolization.

The indication for mitral valve replacement depends upon the severity of congestive heart failure according to the New York Heart Association (NYHA) classification. Patients in categories II, III or IV are usually considered for operation. Also, right and left heart catheterization play an important role in accurately assessing cardiac output, left atrial and pulmonary pressures, the extent of atrial regurgitation, left end-diastolic and systolic volumes and, finally, the left ventricular ejection fraction.

Surgical therapy usually consists of replacing the valve with a mechanical or biological prosthesis. Some examples are the Björk–Shiley disc valve, the St Jude double-disc valve and the Hancock bioprosthetic valve (porcine valve). Each valve type has its advantages and its disadvantages. For example, patients with a mechanical prosthesis must receive anticoagulant medication permanently because of the high risk of thromboembolism. On the other hand bioprosthetic valves show less durability than mechanical ones.

However, mitral valve replacement particularly for mitral insufficiency presents one dilemma that concerns many heart surgeons throughout the world: it has the highest peri- and postoperative mortality rate of all valve implantations, ranging from 10 to 20% in recent years. In 95% of the cases this high mortality rate is due to the low-cardiac-output syndrome which might appear as an acute or chronic complication. This phenomenon causes a remarkable rise in left atrial and pulmonary pressures and lowers cardiac output.

Therefore, it is necessary to obtain an accurate long term prognosis in patients with valve replacement for chronic mitral incompetence. Up to now postoperative evaluation of cardiac status has been based mostly on clinical examination and grading of disability according to the criteria of the NYHA classification. These do not reflect accurately enough the haemodynamic situation. Additional information may be obtained from the e.c.g. and chest X-ray. Exact data of right and left ventricular performance are assessed only by cardiac catheterization. However, this invasive method is inconvenient for the patient, is not without risk, and cannot be frequently repeated.

Unlike cardiac catheterization, technetium 99m pertechnetate first pass scintigraphy is a non-invasive procedure which is easy to carry out and yields objective information on right and left ventricular performance and on the implanted mitral valve prosthesis at rest and during exercise. This procedure can be performed repeatedly in patients post operatively, making possible long-term observations. This chapter deals with 12 patients who had undergone valve replacement for chronic mitral insufficiency and were examined on a long term basis, using first pass radionuclide ventriculography (of a technetium 99m pertechnetate bolus).

Nine males and three females underwent operation between January 1977 and December 1980. The age of the patients varied between 23 and 70 years, the mean age being 48.3 ± 13 years. Preoperatively three patients were in clinical stage II, eight in stage III and one in stage IV. The reason for operating on stage II patients was recurrent arterial embolism.

Preoperative left heart catheterization revealed normal systolic (129.9 ± 19 mmHg) and elevated end diastolic pressure (18 ± 9 mmHg). Left ventricular volumes were calculated from angiograms according to the formula of Sandler and Dodge (1968). The left ventricles elevated end diastolic and end systolic volumes (230.9 ± 66 ml and $73.5 \pm$

26 ml respectively). The total stroke volume was 157.5 ± 47 with $49.4 \pm 9\%$ regurgitating into the left atrium. The left ventricular ejection fraction proved normal in all patients ($67.6 \pm 6\%$).

Right heart catheterization revealed normal mean pulmonary pressure (< 20 mmHg) in two cases. Seven patients had slightly (20–35 mmHg) and three moderately (35–60 mmHg) elevated pulmonary pressures.

According to patient histories, intraoperative findings and histological examination of the resected valve tissue, mitral insufficiency was due to bacterial endocarditis in five cases, rheumatic heart disease in four and degenerative changes in three.

All of the implanted valves were mechanical Björk–Shiley tilting disc valves (Figure 14.1), the diameters ranging from 27 mm to 31 mm.

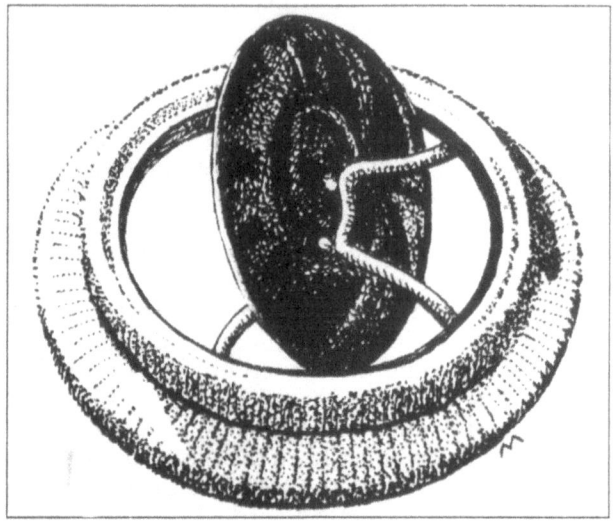

Figure 14.1 Drawing of a mechanical tilting disc valve (Björk–Shiley).

The patients were studied 19.8 ± 11 months (range 9–42 months) postoperatively both at rest and during age-related maximum exercise on a bicycle ergometer. During both parts of the study, *radionuclide ventriculograms* were done in the RAO position of the heart with the patients sitting on the bicycle. For the technique of injection, data acquisition and processing, *see* Chapters 1 and 2.

The end-diastolic volume (EDV) was calculated by a formula experimentally derived by O. Nickel (1982):

$$EDV = CF \cdot [K_1 \times NTC - K_2 \times (1 + K_3 \times Z)^2]$$

(NTC = normalized total count rate, calculated as the count integral of the ventricle divided by the maximum count density; Z = distance collimator/left ventricle; K_1, K_2, K_3 and CF are constants: $K_1 = 11.5$ ml $-$ cm^{-2}; $K_2 = 60.8$ ml; $K_3 = 0.051$ cm^{-1}; CF $= 0.81$ without dimension).

The end-systolic volume (ESV) and the ejection fraction (EF) were calculated as follows:

$$ESV \text{ (ml)} = \frac{\text{end-systolic counts}}{\text{end-diastolic counts}} \times EDV$$

$$EF \text{ (\%)} = \frac{\text{end-diastolic counts} - \text{end-systolic counts}}{\text{end-diastolic counts}} \times 100.$$

Stroke volume (SV) and cardiac output (CO) were calculated in the usual manner.

The function of the prosthesis implanted in the mitral position was assessed by the rapid filling rate of the left ventricle (RFR) and the mean pulmonary transit time (PTT).

The rapid filling rate was calculated as the volume of the rapid diastolic filling divided by its duration (Figure 14.2; normal values: 207.8 ± 54 ml/s at rest and $411 \pm$ ml/s during maximum exercise).

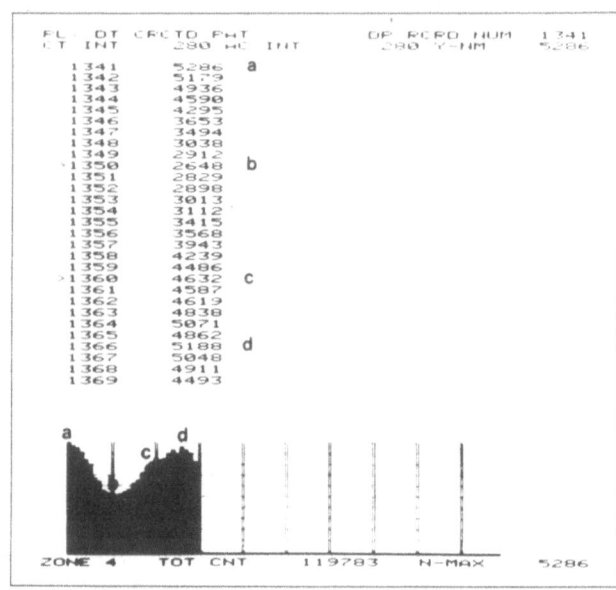

Figure 14.2 Time–activity curve of the left ventricle at rest: at **a** and **d** diastole is terminated at **b** systole; point **c** marks the end of the rapid diastolic filling of the left ventricle. The rapid diastolic filling rate arises from the counts during rapid diastolic filling divided by the corresponding time. (Figure 14.2 and all other figures in Chapter 14 by permission of the Thieme Verlag, Stuttgart.)

The mean pulmonary transit time was defined as the time a radionuclide bolus needed to travel from the pulmonary artery to the left atrium. According to Upton and co-workers (1980) 5.8 ± 1 s is normal at rest and 2.5 ± 0.4 s during maximum exercise.

Data were averaged and statistical differences obtained by the paired Student's t-test using a Hewlett Packard Computer 67.

In Figure 14.3 the preoperative functional grading (NYHA classification) is compared with the postoperative one. On an average the patients improved from preoperative class 2.6 to 1.8 postoperatively.

Left and right ventricular function: the end-diastolic volumes of the left ventricles measured postoperatively 121.8 ± 38 ml at rest and 122 ± 29 ml during exercise (Figure 14.4). The end-systolic volumes decreased after exercise from 52.8 ± 35 ml to 37.6 ± 22 ml ($p < 0.05$). Whereas the heart rate increased during peak exercise from 78 ± 14 to 149 ± 23 s^{-1}, cardiac output nearly doubled: 6.5 ± 2 l/min and 10.3 ± 2.8 l/min respectively ($p < 0.05$).

Exercising ejection fraction increased from $57.7 \pm 12\%$ to $69.7 \pm 10\%$ ($p < 0.05$).

Postoperative volumes and ejection fractions of the right ventricle were within normal ranges

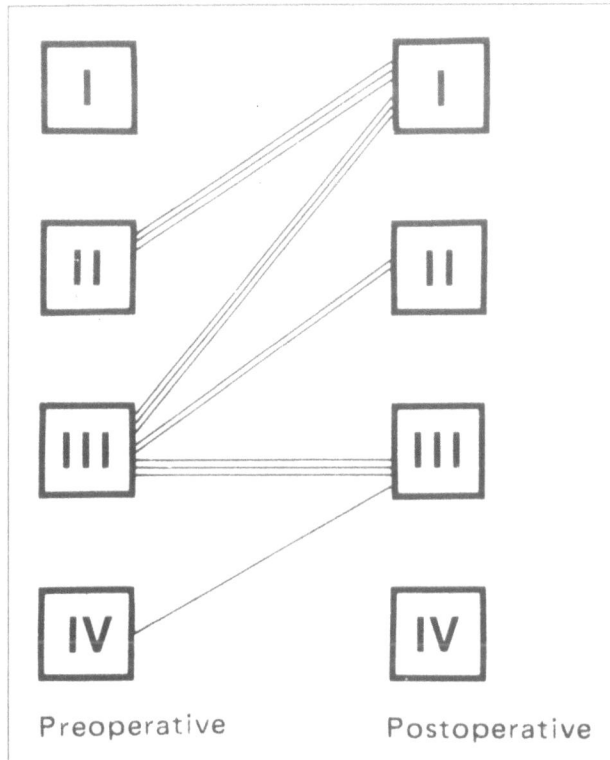

Figure 14.3 Pre- and post- (19.8 ± 11 months) operative New York Heart Association classification.

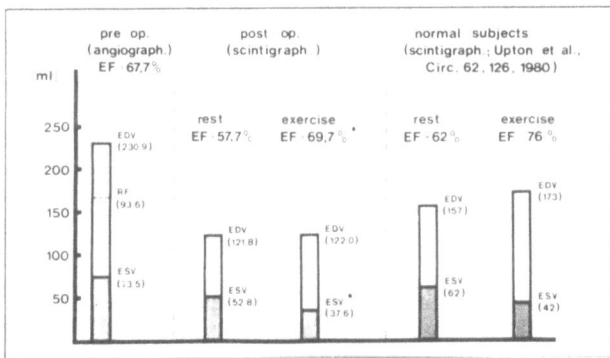

Figure 14.4 Postoperative left ventricular volumes as assessed by first pass radionuclide ventriculography (between the two dashed lines). To the left: data derived from preoperative angiogram; to the right: data issued by Upton *et al.* on normal subjects. EDV = end-diastolic volume; ESV = end-systolic volume; EF = ejection fraction; RF = regurgitation; * = f < 0.05.

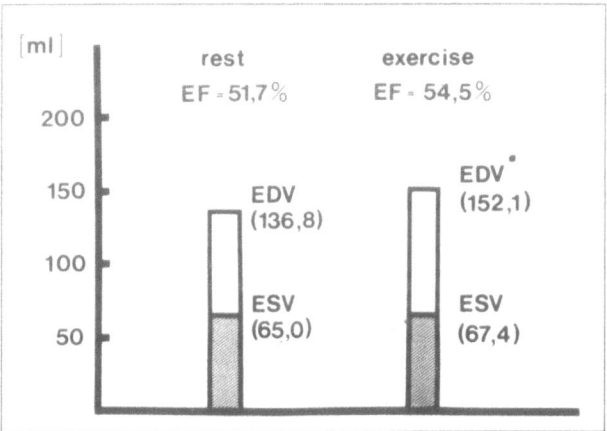

Figure 14.5 Postoperative mean right ventricular volumes at rest and during maximum exercise. EDV, ESV = end-diastolic and end-systolic volumes, respectively; EF = ejection fraction.

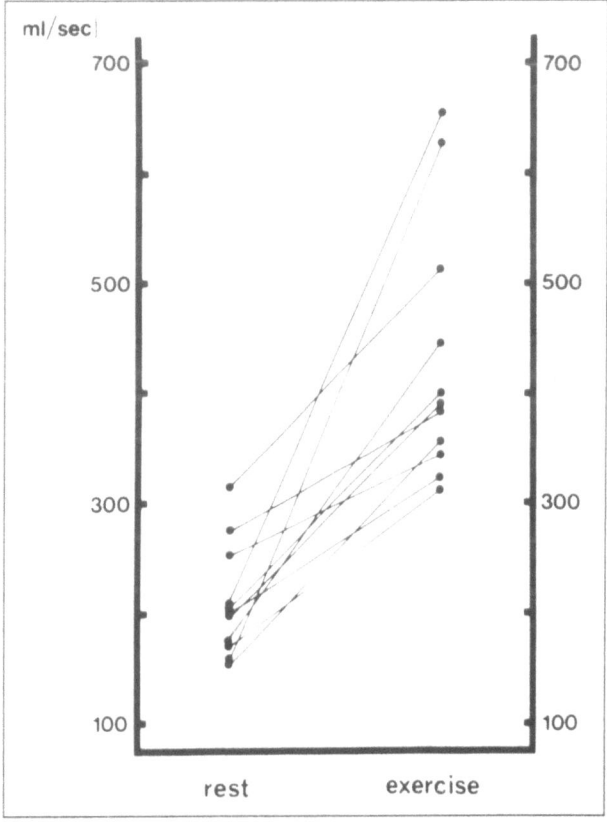

Figure 14.6 Rapid filling rates at rest and following age-related maximum exercise after valve replacement for chronic mitral insufficiency.

(Figure 14.5): the end diastolic volumes increased from 136.8 ± 15 at rest to 152.1 ± 120 ml during exercise ($p < 0.05$); the end systolic volumes remained unchanged: 65.0 ± 12 ml at rest and 67.4 ± 11 ml during exercise. The ejection fractions of the right ventricles measured $51.7 \pm 8\%$ and $54.5 \pm 4\%$.

Function of the implanted valve prosthesis: the rapid filling rate averaged postoperatively 211.9 ± 50 ml/s at rest and was doubled during maximum exercise (433.4 ± 118 ml/s, $p < 0.05$). Figure 14.6 illustrates all values at rest and during exercise.

The mean pulmonary transit time was significantly reduced by exercise, from 7.3 ± 1.2 s to 4.4 ± 1 s ($p < 0.05$). In Figure 14.7 each value is shown both at rest and during exercise.

Chronic mitral insufficiency affects the left ventricular function by volume overload due to systolic regurgitation into the low pressure left atrium in combination with afterload reduction (Braunwald, 1969; Wong and Spotnitz, 1979). Longstanding malfunctions initiate structural changes within the left ventricular myocardium. These include myocardial hypertrophy, development of new sarcomeres, displacement of myofibrils, myocardial fibrosis and, finally, ventricular dilatation which is characterized by a reduced ventricular wall stiffness as visualized by a flattened volume pressure curve (Rankin *et al.*, 1975; Ross *et al.*, 1971; Wong and Spotnitz, 1979). At

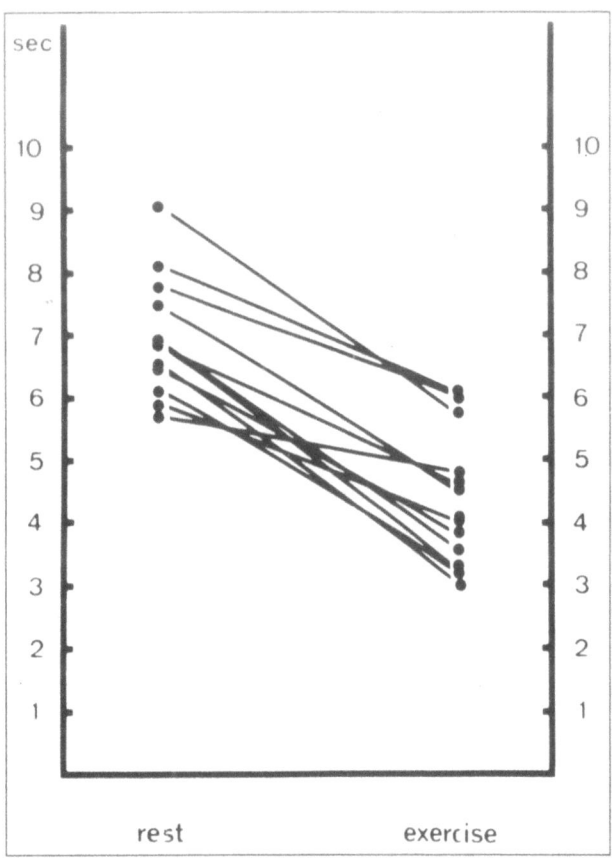

Figure 14.7 Mean pulmonary transit times at rest and following age-related maximum exercise after valve replacement for chronic mitral insufficiency.

this point the ventricles have become dependent upon systolic afterload reduction; mitral valve replacement abruptly eliminates afterload reduction, causing severe postoperative impairment of left ventricular function and low cardiac output syndrome in some cases. Using M-mode echocardiography Schuler *et al.* (1979) noted a clear correlation between preoperative left ventricular diameters and postoperative haemodynamic changes in patients with valve replacement for chronic mitral insufficiency; when end systolic and end diastolic diameters preoperatively exceeded 5 cm and 7 cm respectively, there was poor left ventricular function postoperatively, documented by increased ventricular diameters.

Classifying left ventricular function after mitral valve replacement applying radionuclide ventriculography: the grading of a patient's condition by NYHA classification, clinical investigation, e.c.g. and chest X-ray are all useful in evaluating the postoperative result. Nevertheless, all these parameters give only an indirect indication of ventricular function. Furthermore, NYHA classification relies, to a high degree, on the patient's subjective report (compare the scattered postoperative NYHA classification of Figure 14.3 with the uniform haemodynamic improvements displayed in Figures 14.5 and 14.6).

By contrast, radionuclide ventriculography, like heart catheterization, gives objective information concerning right and left ventricular function, and assessment of the haemodynamic effects of the implanted valve prosthesis is possible. First pass

scintigraphy is non-invasive, convenient for the patient, without major risks and may be performed repeatedly (Schad, 1976, 1977, 1983; Upton *et al.*, 1980). Furthermore, cardiac functional imaging represents not only a two-dimensional projection of the ventricular bolus but provides also a three-dimensional access to the distribution of the radioactivity within the left and right ventricle. Consecutively, volume measurements can be performed. The validity of the experimentally derived equation has been proven in 71 patients whose scintigraphically and angiographically measured end diastolic volumes revealed a close correlation ($r = 0.95$; Nickel *et al.*, 1982).

In Figure 14.4 preoperatively angiographically assessed end-diastolic left ventricular volumes are compared to values measured postoperatively using radionuclide ventriculography. To facilitate classification, data from normal persons – drawn from Upton and co-workers using a similar technique (1980) – are added. The left ventricular volumes which were enlarged preoperatively clearly normalized 19.8 ± 11 months after surgery. This illustrates that valve replacement for chronic mitral insufficiency in these patients improved left ventricular function.

In addition, left ventricular performance of all 12 patients studied by technetium 99 m pertechnetate scintigraphy revealed a near physiological response to age-related maximum exercise: end diastolic volumes remained unchanged, and end systolic volumes decreased by 27%. According to these findings exercise initiated an increase of the stroke volume by 25% and the ejection fraction by 21%. Cardiac output was nearly doubled.

Our data – uniform postoperative decrease of left ventricular volumes at rest – disagree with the results from the Durham group which also studied 18 patients with valve replacement for chronic mitral insufficiency using first pass technique radionuclide ventriculography. Peter and co-workers (1981) were unable to find any postoperative reduction of left ventricular volumes. However, a closer look at their individual patients shows that only three had unchanged elevated end diastolic and end systolic left ventricular volumes postoperatively, causing wide standard deviations of the mean values. According to Schuler and co-workers (1979) those ventricles had obviously become dependent upon preoperative systolic afterload reduction.

Assessment of prosthetic function of the Björk–Shiley mitral valve: the ventricular rapid filling rate aided in evaluation of the prosthetic function. A significant increase during maximum exercise demonstrates adequate function even under high cardiac output situations. Without exception the rapid filling rate of the left ventricles increased in all cases and, on an average, doubled (Figure 14.6).

A prolonged pulmonary transit time which does not decrease during exercise is considered an indicator of poor mitral valve function. Schad *et al.* (1982) found unmeasurable pulmonary transit times in two patients with bioprostheses implanted in the mitral position indicating long term risk. Accordingly, both prostheses had to be replaced because of severe stenosis due to calcification. However, pulmonary transit time may be modified by disease of the lungs or right ventricular dysfunction. Since none of our patients showed markedly elevated pulmonary mean pressures preoperatively, severe postoperative pulmonary hypertension should be ruled out.

In our patients pulmonary transit time was found normal: 7 ± 1 s at rest, a value which decreased physiologically to 4.4 ± 1 s during maximum exercise. These values are in accordance with the findings of Scholz et al. (1980) and Rerych et al. (1978a) obtained in healthy persons.

SUMMARY

First pass radionuclide ventriculography is a non-invasive, convenient and safe procedure which may be performed repeatedly. Like invasive heart catheterization it yields objective data on both right and left ventricular performance as well as on implanted valve function. Therefore, this method can be used to obtain long term follow-up controls in patients with mitral prosthesis. Very important is the technique's objectivity as opposed to the method of classification according to the NYHA. Furthermore, first pass radionuclide ventriculography helps to demonstrate that valve replacement for chronic mitral insufficiency may lead to restoration of normal left ventricular function in many cases.

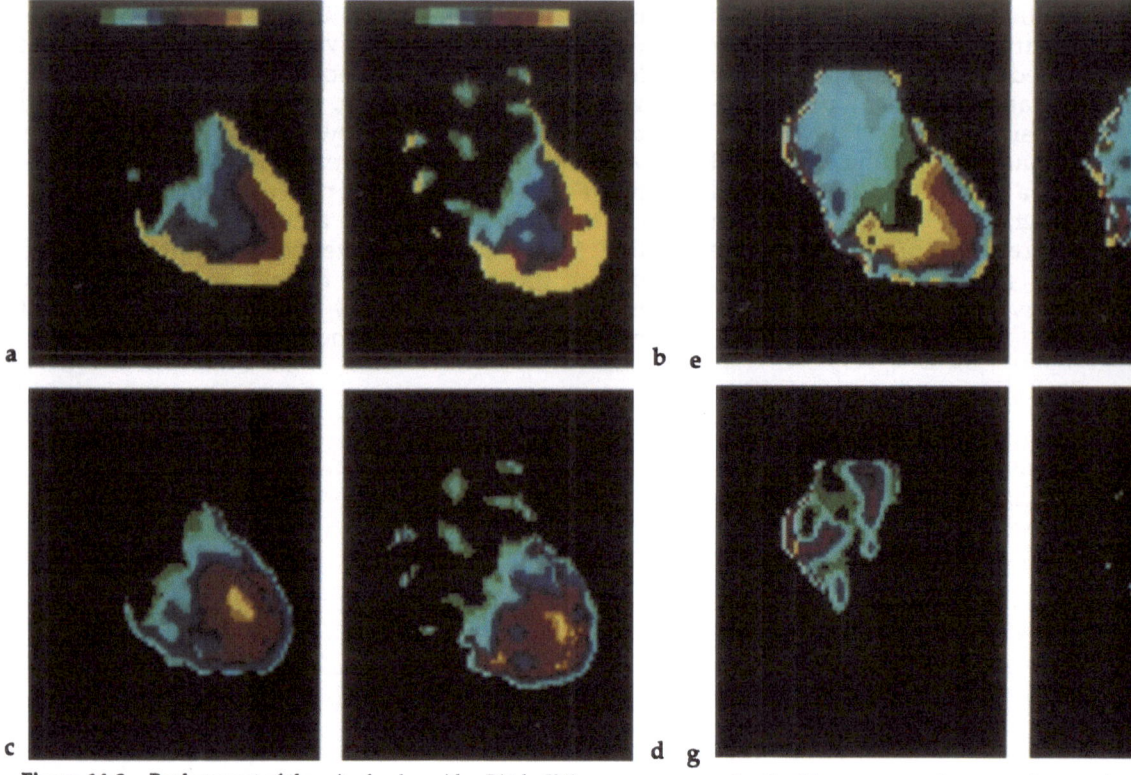

Figure 14.8 *Replacement of the mitral valve with a Björk–Shiley prosthesis. Follow-up after 12 months NYHA: pre op IV, post op III*
a,b,c,d, Partial improvement of function from rest (left) to exercise (right) on REFI (**a,b**) and REjR (**c,d**). Only a small posterior region presents reduced function. Global ejection rate at rest 178 ml/s, under stress 288 ml/s. Lung mean transit time 6.6 s at rest, 3 s under stress.

e,f,g,h, Short mean times at the parietal zone, somewhat prolonged times at the base at rest (**e**) and under stress (**f**). Minimal reflux into the left atrium on the systolic increase image (**g**). High rapid filling rates directed to the apex only slightly deviated, small zone with low rapid filling rates immediately below the prosthesis (**h**).

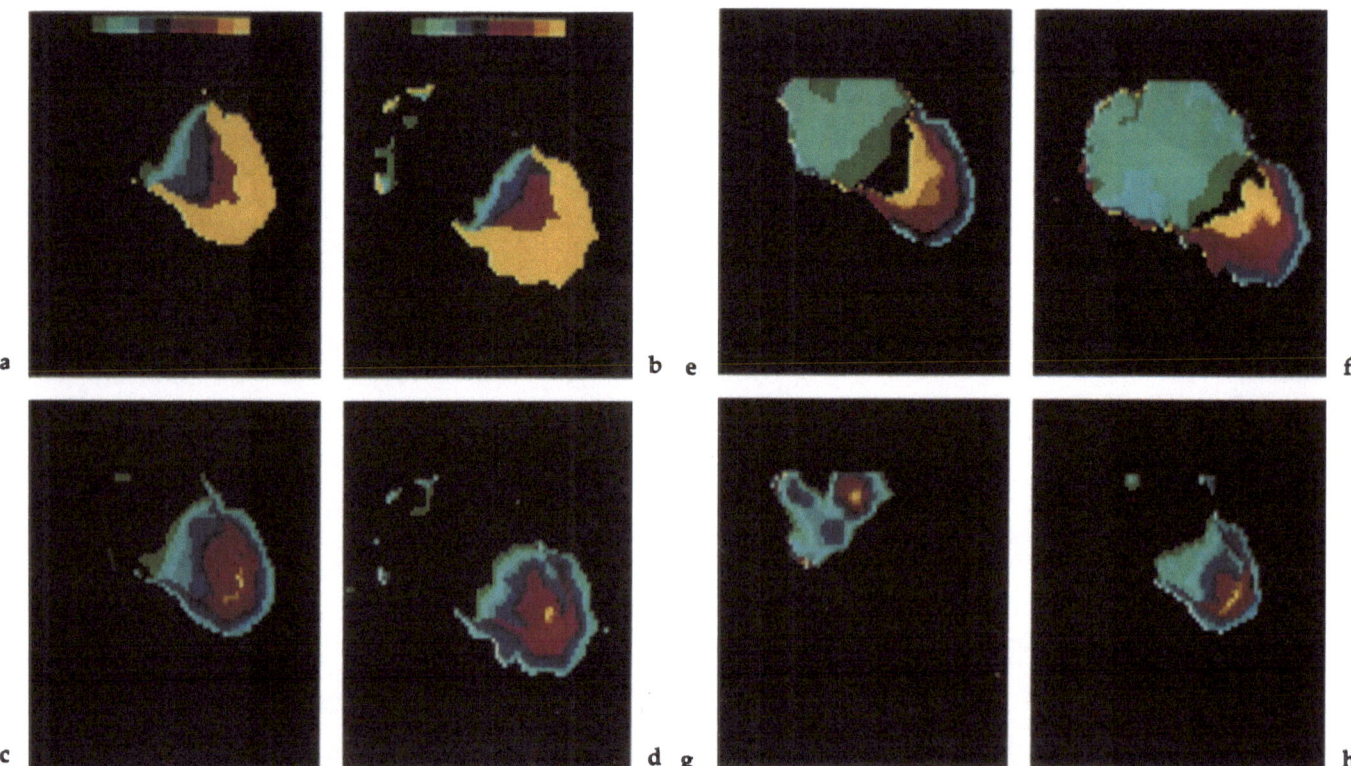

Figure 14.9 *Replacement of the mitral valve with a Carpentier–Edwards prosthesis. Follow-up after 14 months. NYHA: pre op III, post op I*
a,b,c,d, Significant improvement of function from rest (left) to exercise (right) on REFI (**a,b**) and REjR (**c,d**). Only a small posterior zone with reduced function immediately under the prosthesis. Global ejection rate at rest 163 ml/s, under stress 445 ml/s. Lung mean transit time 6.2 s, under stress 3.1 s.

e,f,g,h, Short mean times at the parietal zone, somewhat prolonged times at the base at rest (**e**) and under stress (**f**). Mild reflux into the left atrium on the systolic increase image (**g**). High rapid filling rates slightly deviated to the anterior wall with reduced rates immediately below the prosthesis (**h**).

15

First Pass Radionuclide Studies in Evaluation of Left and Right Ventricular Function in Patients with Bioprosthetic Mitral Valve Replacement after 9–11 years

B. REICHART, N. SCHAD, R. HATZ, G. BOUGIOUKAS, V. GALLUCCI, U. BORTOLOTTI AND A. MILANO

In Chapter 14 it was shown what contributions first pass radionuclide ventriculography can make in the accurate non-invasive assessment of left ventricular function following the implantation of a *mechanical* mitral valve prosthesis. However, as mentioned earlier, mechanical valves have certain disadvantages such as the necessity of permanent anticoagulant medication. This and many other problems compelled researchers to develop valves consisting of biological materials, usually of xenogenic origin (bovine or porcine). Compared to mechanical valves, these prostheses provide low rates of thromboembolism and hæmorrhage secondary to anticoagulation. Also cases of postoperative endocarditis have a better prognosis.

Besides these advantages, the main drawback in bioprosthetic valves is that they show less durability than mechanical ones. This concern is based on ultrastructural results (Ferrans *et al.*, 1978), on reports dealing with bioprostheses in juveniles in whom the rates of dysfunction seems to be accelerated (Kutsche *et al.*, 1979; Geha *et al.*, 1979; Backet *et al.*, 1979) and on long term – 5–8 years – follow-up studies reporting a primary tissue failure rate which is approximately tenfold greater than during the initial 5 postoperative years (Oyer *et al.*, 1980).

As reported by several authors (Casarotto *et al.*, 1979; Cohn *et al.*, 1981; Magilligan *et al.*, 1980; Oyer *et al.*, 1980; Hancock Laboratories, 1980) tissue valve failure almost always occurs gradually. Although changes in symptomatology might require surgery within a month, sudden catastrophes, well known in disc valve patients, are uncommon. Therefore, decision-making for reoperation requires clinical examination, invasive studies in the catheterization laboratory and reproducible and quickly available non-invasive methods.

Scintigraphic evaluation of left and right ventricular function may be performed under nearly physiological conditions with a patient in an upright sitting position both at rest and during peak exercise; these situations are difficult to obtain when applying echocardiographic or phonocardiographic techniques. This chapter summarizes our experiences with 15 patients who received porcine mitral valve replacement at the University of Padua between April 1970 and May 1972. Cardiac performance and valve function were assessed using technetium 99m pertechnetate scintigraphy at rest and at peak exercise.

The mean age at operation of the seven men and eight women was 37.9 ± 10 years, ranging from 29 to 69 years. According to the NYHA classification, 12 patients belonged to class III preoperatively and three to class IV. Ventriculography verified pure mitral stenosis in three patients and pure regurgitation in one case. In 11 cases combined disease was present. The preoperative cardiac index was 2.61 ± 0.5 l/min per m^2. The mean pulmonary wedge pressure measured 28.3 ± 10 mmHg. The average pressure gradient across the mitral valve was 13.3 ± 8 mmHg. Pulmonary artery pressure was 20–35 mmHg (mean) in five patients, 35–50 mmHg in four and $\geqslant 50$ mmHg in five cases. One patient had no preoperative catheterization.

All porcine Hancock® valves were glutaraldehyde fixed and mounted on rigid frames covered by Dacron (Figure 15.1). The following valve sizes were implanted: numbers 27 and 29, six each; one number 31 and two number 33.

At the time of this study (123 ± 8 months postoperatively) most of the patients were still improved (Figure 15.2). According to the NYHA classification seven were class II and eight class III. Thirteen patients were in atrial fibrillation and two in sinus rhythm. Eight patients received anticoagulation and seven did not. There were no thromboembolic events.

The scintigraphic ventriculograms were performed in the same manner as described in Chapter 14. The following parameters were measured: global ejection fraction (EF), stroke volume (SV), end-diastolic volume (EDV), end-systolic volume (ESV), cardiac output and cardiac index (CI), volume of the rapid filling rate, rapid filling rate (RFR), and mean pulmonary transit time (PTT).

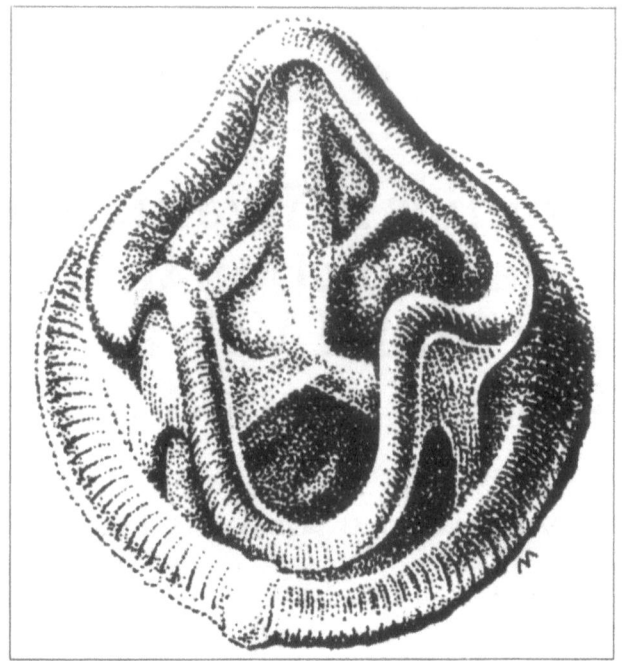

Figure 15.1 Representation of a bioprosthetic heart valve with glutaraldehyde fixed leaflets mounted on a rigid frame covered by Dacron.

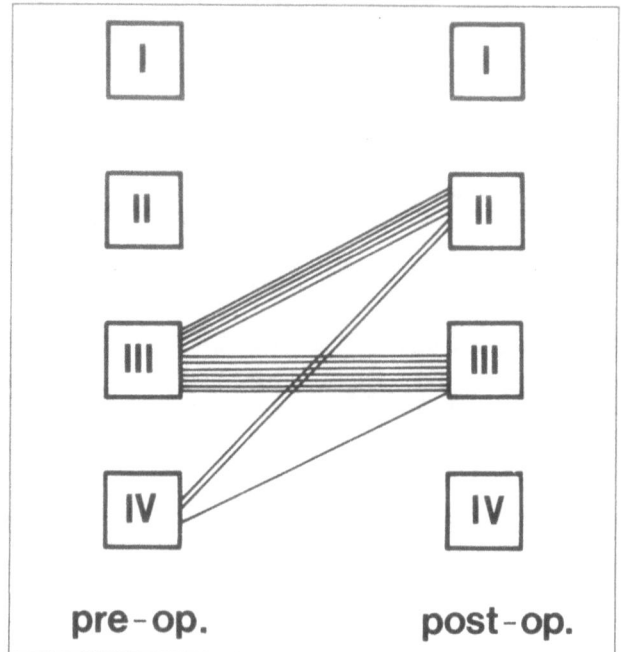

Figure 15.2 Pre- and postoperative (123.8 ± 8 months) classification according to the New York Heart Association. (All figures with permission of Yorke Medical Books, New York.)

Table 15.1 Postoperative left ventricular volumes assessed by scintigraphic technique

	Rest	*Exercise*	*Statistics*
HR (min^{-1})	85.1 ± 16	150.5 ± 24	$p < 0.05$
EDV (ml)	130.6 ± 44	130.6 ± 46	NS
ESV (ml)	64.8 ± 38	67.7 ± 42	NS
SV (ml)	63.3 ± 15	61.2 ± 17	NS
CI (litres/min per m^2)	3.29 ± 1.04	5.50 ± 1.45	$p < 0.05$
EF (%)	51.4 ± 13	50.3 ± 14	NS

HR = heart rate; EDV = end-diastolic volume; ESV = end-systolic volume; SV = stroke volume; CI = cardiac index; EF = ejection fraction.

Table 15.2 Postoperative right ventricular volumes

	Rest	*Exercise*
EDV (ml)	129.7 ± 22	126.9 ± 19
ESV (ml)	63.8 ± 22	59.5 ± 15
EF (%)	50.5 ± 12	50.9 ± 10

For abbreviations, see Table 15.1.

Table 15.3 Comparison of left ventricular data

	Normal volunteers	*Pts. with mitral valve replacement*	*Statistics*
HR (min^{-1})	79.6 ± 16	85.1 ± 16	NS
EDV (ml)	121.0 ± 21	130.6 ± 44	NS
ESV (ml)	45.0 ± 20	64.8 ± 38	NS
SV (ml)	77.0 ± 20	63.3 ± 15	NS
CI (litres/min per m^2)	3.3 ± 0.8	3.29 ± 1.04	NS
EF (%)	65.0 ± 7	51.4 ± 13	NS

The normal mean values of 19 subjects were presented by Scholz *et al.* (1980).
For abbreviations, see Table 15.1.

Table 15.1 summarizes the *left ventricular volumes:* at a resting heart rate (HR) of 85.1 ± 6 min^{-1} EDV and ESV measured 130.6 ± 44 and 64.8 ± 38 ml, SV was 63.3 ± 15 ml, and EF was 51.4 ± 13%. The CI was 3.29 ± 1.04 l/min per m^2.

At peak exercise the HR increased to 150.5 ± 24 min^{-1} and the CI increased accordingly.

EDV, ESV and EF remained unchanged.

Right ventricular volumes are listed in Table 15.2.

As in the left ventricular studies, there were no changes of EDV, ESV and EF during peak exercise.

The left ventricular volumes of 14 of our patients are compared in Table 15.3 with the mean values of 19 healthy volunteers presented by Scholz *et al.* (1980). Only measurements at rest are presented since Scholz *et al.* did not perform exercise tests. The HR (79.6 ± 16 vs 85 ± 16 min^{-1}) of both groups at rest are comparable. Also there are no statistical dif-

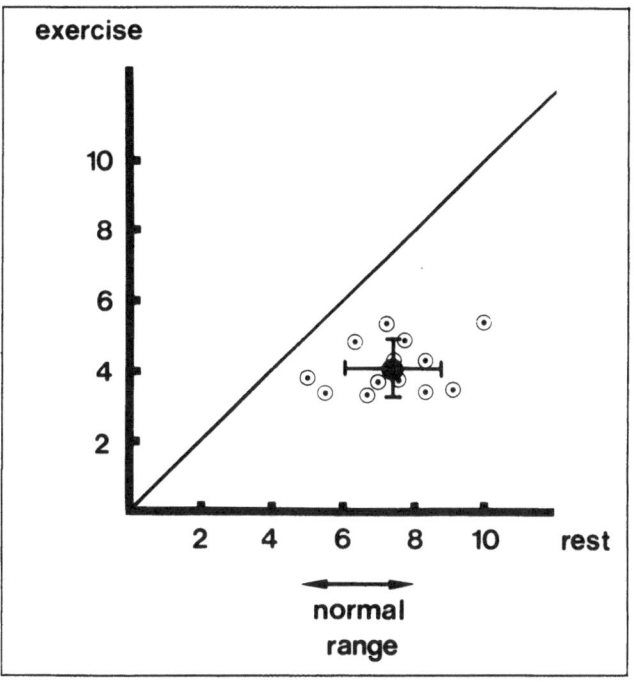

Figure 15.3 Mean pulmonary transit time (PTT) of 13 patients. PTT was 7.4 ± 1.4 s at rest and decreased in each case on an average of 4.2 ± 0.8 s. In two other patients PTT was unmeasurable, in one patient at peak exercise, in the second at both rest and peak exercise.

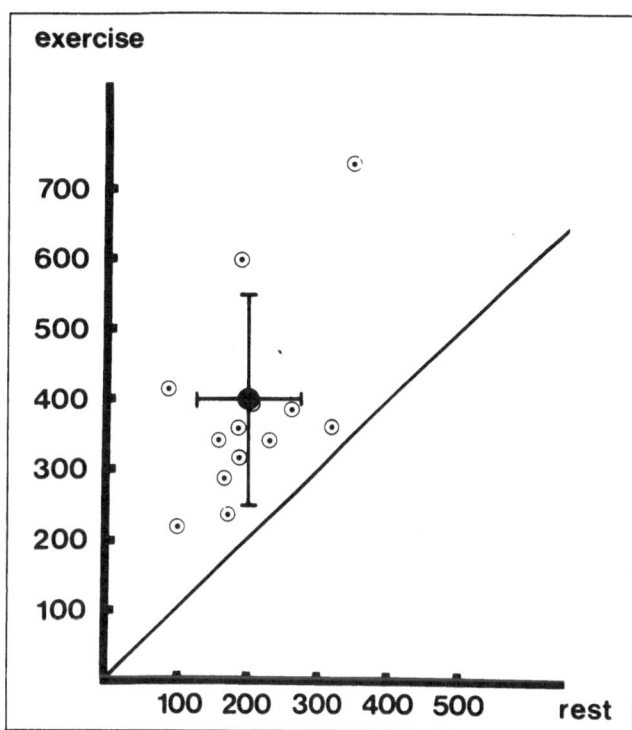

Figure 15.4 Rapid filling rate (RFR; ml/s) of 13 patients increased at peak exercise from 201.9 ± 76 to 400.2 ± 148 ml/s; RFR was unmeasurable in two patients (see Figure 15.3).

Table 15.4 Comparison of mean pulmonary transit time at rest

	Normal volunteers	Pts. with mitral valve replacement	Statistics
Rest	6.5 ± 1.2	7.4 ± 1.4*	NS
Exercise	—	4.2 ± 0.8*	—

The pulmonary transit time was not measurable in 2 patients.
The normal mean values of 10 subjects are derived from the study of Scholz et al. (1980).
*PTT rest/exercise $p < 0.05$.

ferences in any of the rest data presented including EDV, ESV, SV, CI, or EF. In our exercise studies EDV and ESV as well as SV and EF did not change at peak exercise (Table 15.1). Compared with the physiological response of healthy volunteers at peak exercise (Upton et al., 1980) in whom EDV would be expected to increase by 10%, ESV to decrease by 32% and the SV to rise by 36%, our patients had a limited reaction to physical activity depending upon the heart rate. This may be explained by an increased left ventricular wall stiffness since right ventricular volumes remained unchanged at the same time.

The function of the bioprosthesis was assessed applying the mean pulmonary transit time (PTT) and the rapid filling rate (RFR). In two patients we found evidence suggesting that the implanted valve might be severely stenosed, since PTT and RFR were prolonged and unmeasurable: in one case, at rest and at peak exercise; in the other, during exercise only. Degenerated and heavily calcified mitral bioprostheses were replaced in both cases, 112 and 136 months, respectively, after the first operation. In the remaining 13 patients PTT significantly decreased at peak exercise in all cases (7.4 ± 1.4 vs 4.2 ± 0.8 s), which was compatible with adequate mitral valve function (Figure 15.3). PTT at rest was not signifi-

cantly different from the mean values of the 19 volunteers by Scholz et al. (1980): 7.4 ± 1.4 vs 6.5 ± 1.2 s (Table 15.4).

The RFR measured 201.9 ± 76 ml/s at rest in 13 patients. In these patients during maximum exercise RFR increased to 400.2 ± 148 ml/s (Figure 15.4). In the two patients with the stenosed valves the RFR was prolonged and unmeasurable.

SUMMARY

The results presented here show that first pass scintigraphy is an effective diagnostic tool in evaluating tissue valves at long term risk. At 123.8 ± 8 months postoperatively, 13 out of 15 patients with porcine valves in the mitral position showed normal PTT, RFR, and clinical function. Two patients with bioprostheses proven to be stenotic had abnormal PTT and RFR. Valve replacement was required in these patients. In 14 patients, left and right ESV and EDV were normal at rest. Left and right ventricular responses to exercise were abnormal since ESV and EDV did not change, possibly due to decreased ventricular compliance.

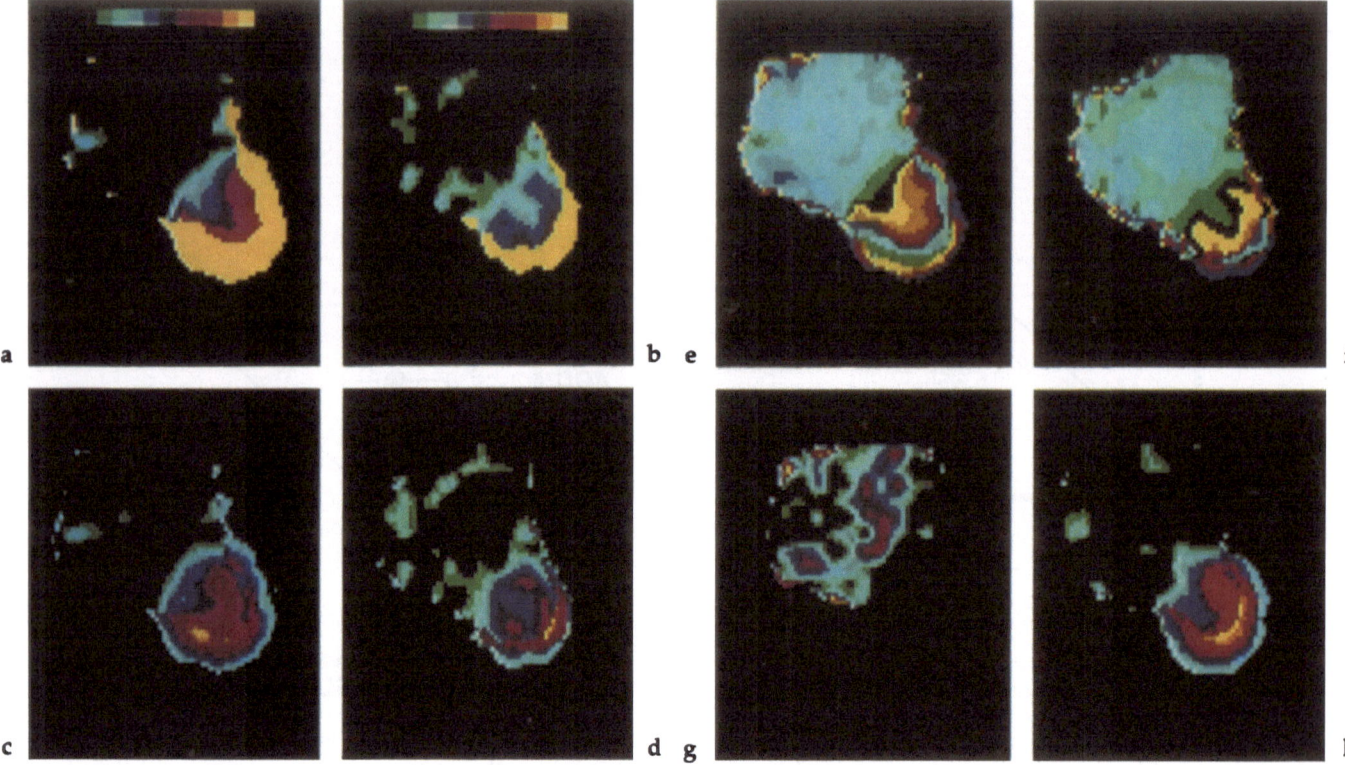

Figure 15.5 *Replacement of the mitral valve with a Hancock bioprosthesis. Follow-up after 9 years – NYHA: pre op IV, post op II*
a,b,c,d, At rest (left) adequate function that somewhat deteriorates under stress (right) on the REFI (**a,b**) and REjR images (**c,d**). Under stress no enlargement of the LV. Global ejection rate 216 ml/s at rest, under stress 262 ml/s. Lung mean transit time 7 s at rest, under stress 3.7 s.

e,f,g,h, Short parietal mean times under stress only slightly prolonged at the base (**e,f**). No significant reflux into the left atrium in the systolic increase image (9). High parietal rapid filling rates, only a small zone with lower rapid filling rates immediately below the prosthesis (**h**)

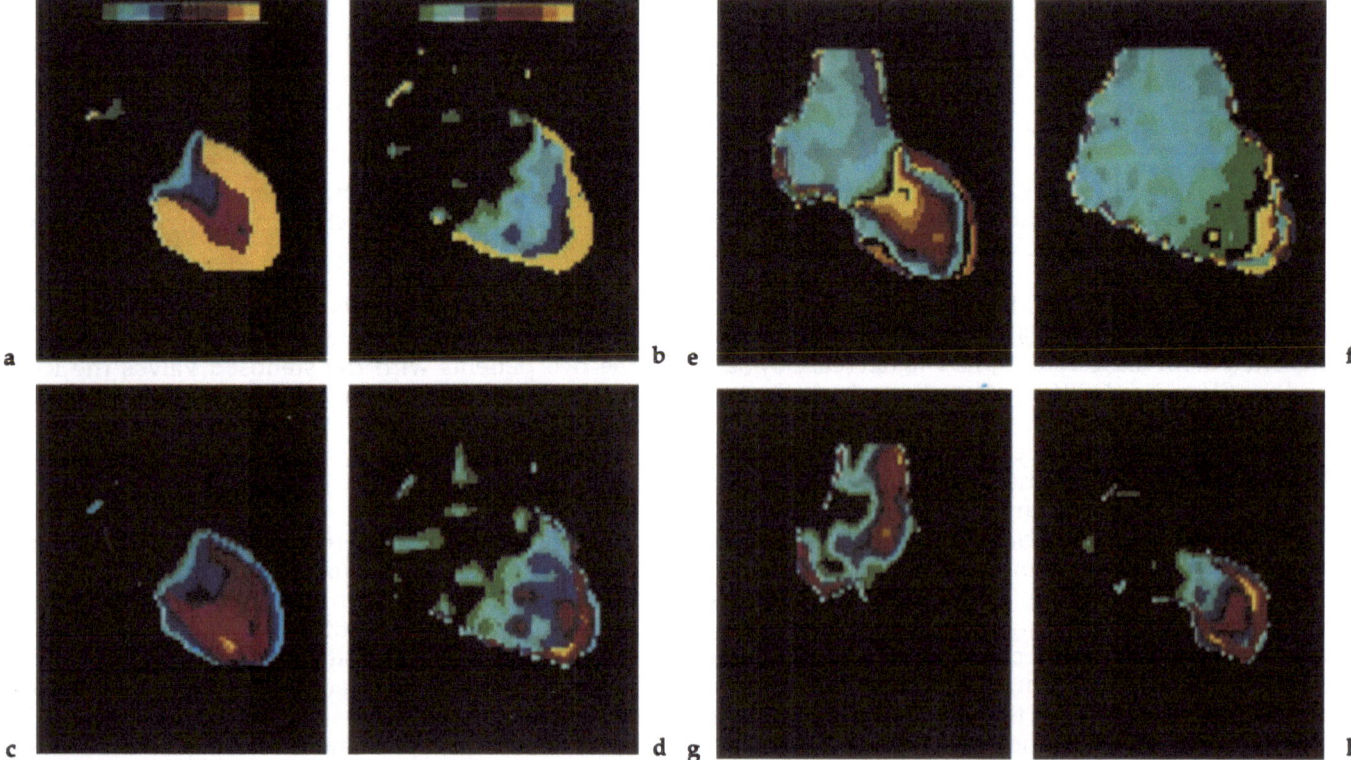

Figure 15.6 *Replacement of the mitral valve with a Hancock bioprosthesis. Follow up after 10 years. NYHA: pre op III, post op III*
a,b,c,d, At rest (left) adequate function that deteriorates under stress (right) on the REFI (**a,b**) and REjR images (**c,d**). Enlargement of the LV. Global ejection rate 256 ml/s at rest, under stress 315 ml/s. Lung mean transit time 6.3 s at rest, 4.8 s under stress.

e,f,g,h, Adequate mean times at rest (**e**), prolonged mean times advancing from the base to the apex under stress (**f**). No significant reflux into the left atrium at rest on the systolic increase image (**g**). At rest high rapid filling rates at the periphery, only a small zone with low rates immediately below the prosthesis (**h**).

16

Functional Imaging of the Rapid Filling Phase and Regional Systolic Motion of the Left Ventricle after Mitral Valve Reconstruction

E. KREUZER, N. SCHAD, B. REICHART, D. PETERS AND R. HATZ

Besides the development and consistent improvement of mitral valve replacement using mechanical prostheses during the past 20 years a different operative approach also evolved – plastic reconstructive surgery of the mitral valve. The main objective of this technique is to conserve the valve and reestablish its function. The first attempts were made by Merendino and Bruce (1957), Lillehei *et al.* (1958), McGoon (1960) and Wooler *et al.* (1962). A systematic classification of indication and surgical techniques is an achievement of A. Carpentier (1969, 1983; Carpentier *et al.* 1980).

ANATOMY

The mitral valve represents a pressure barrier between the left atrium and the left ventricle. The entire valve consists of six anatomical elements: the left atrium, the valve ring, both valve leaflets, the chordae tendineae, both papillary muscles and the left ventricular wall.

The mitral valve is attached to the fibrotic annulus of the heart which holds the four heart chambers, the aorta and the pulmonary artery together. Its central portion joins both atrioventricular valve rings. The aorta is connected to the anterior part of the fibrotic annulus. The mitral valve consists of an anterior and posterior leaflet. The chordae tendineae join the muscular elements of the mitral valve apparatus – the papillary muscles and the left ventricular wall – to both leaflets. On an average, both valve leaflets have 25 chordae: nine are attached to the anterior leaflet of which seven belong to the rough zone and two are supporting chordae, and 14 to the posterior leaflet – ten belonging to the rough zone, with two supporting chordae and two basal chordae. The last two chordae are chordae commissurales which are fixed to the valve commissures (Figure 16.1) (Carpentier *et al.*, 1976).

The mitral valve is egg-shaped *in vitro*. *In vivo* when the aortic root is filled the mitral orifice is kidney-shaped. During systole, the cross-sectional area of the normal mitral valve decreases by 25% due

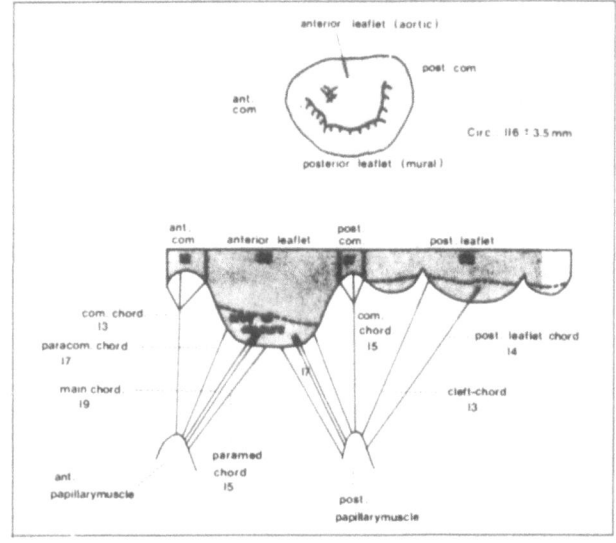

Figure 16.1 Anatomy of mitral valve (diagrammatic representation).

to active contraction of the muscular elements surrounding the valve.

Mitral insufficiency is defined as the incomplete closure of the mitral valve with its characteristic changes in haemodynamics. Its causes are listed in Table 16.1. Often both mitral insufficiency and mitral stenosis are present.

Fundamental knowledge of the physiological and pathological changes of the mitral valve are needed for each operative reconstruction of the valve. One has to differentiate very carefully between the various lesions of the valve, intraoperatively, so that the best possible reconstructive technique can be chosen. Of utmost importance is to find out which functional abnormality is present in each case. This depends upon the mobility of the valve leaflets (Figure 16.2). These results are then correlated with intraoperative pathological findings of the valve when the heart is open. Type I mitral insufficiency shows normal valve leaflet mobility. Regurgitation is caused by dilatation of the valve ring or by perforation or laceration of the leaflet. Type II mitral

Table 16.1 Nosologic Classification of mitral valve insufficiency

Mitral Leaflets
Rheumatic fever
Endocarditis: bacterial, viral, mycotic
External traumas (ruptures)
Systemic lupus erythematosus
Whipple's disease
Periarteriitis nodosa
Defects of tissue
   Barlow's disease
   Ehlers–Danlos syndrome
   Marfan syndrome

Annulus of mitral valve
Dilatation
Calcification
Destruction (rheumatic, infectious, rheumatoid)

Chordae tendineae
Rupture (rheumatic, infectious, idiopathic, traumatic)
Marfan's syndrome
Idiopathic subvalvular aortic stenosis
Myocardial infarct
Carcinoid syndrome

Papillary muscle
Dysfunction or rupture
Myocardial infarct
Myocarditis
Polyarthritis
Aortic stenosis
Sarcoidosis, amyloidosis
Anomalia of coronary arteries
Ventricular aneurysms
Traumas

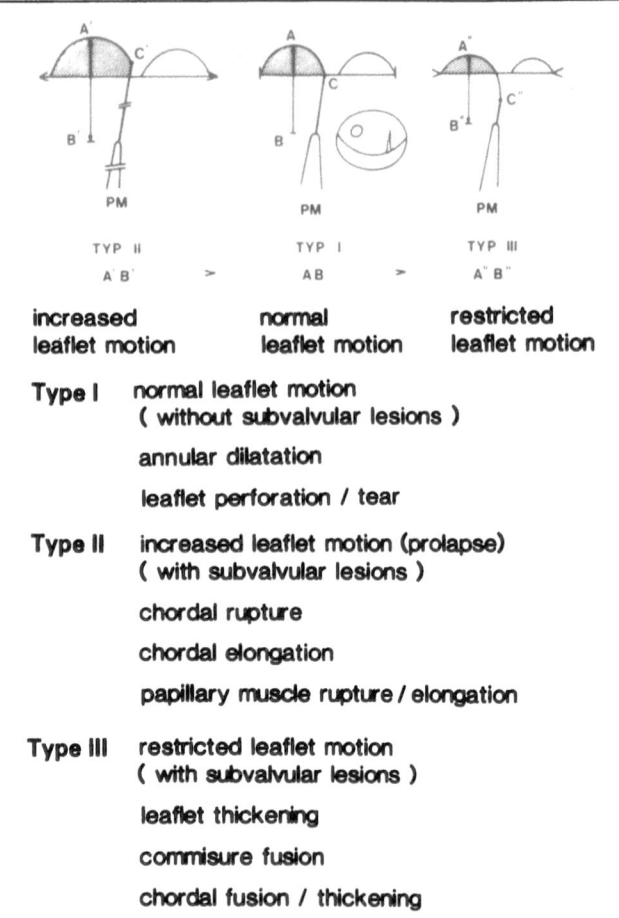

Figure 16.2 Mitral valve insufficiency – pathophysiological classification.

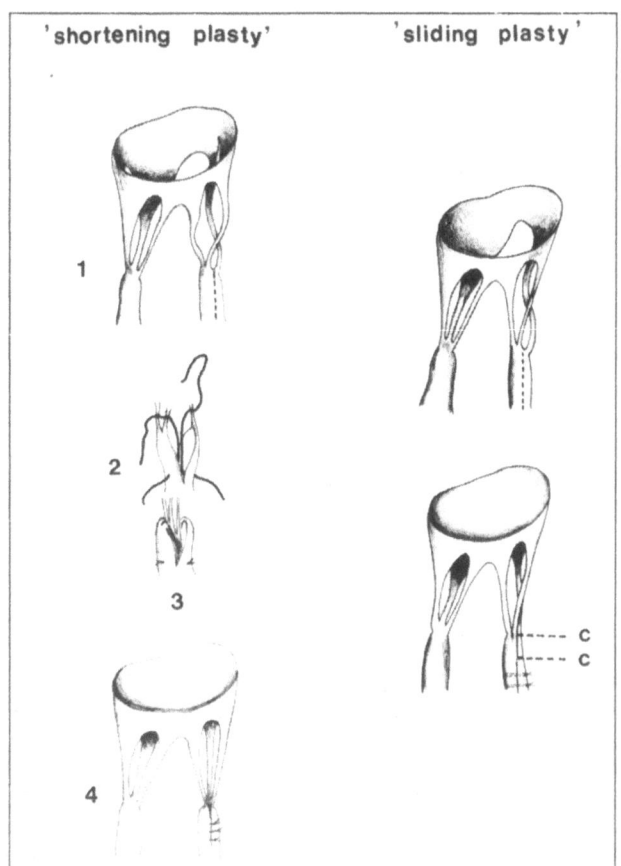

Figure 16.3 Repair of leaflet prolapse due to chordal elongation.

insufficiency presents increased valve leaflet mobility. Either one or both leaflets protrude into the left atrium above the valve ring during systole. Type III insufficiency shows reduced valve leaflet mobility caused by fusion of the commissures and the chordae tendineae beneath the valvular plane. The valve's ability to open in diastole and to close in systole is incomplete (Carpentier, 1983).

OPERATIVE TECHNIQUE

The main goal of reconstructive procedures of the mitral valve is to re-establish its normal function for as long as possible. Pathological changes in each of the components of the mitral valve may cause malfunction. Therefore, various reconstructive techniques were developed. Those used in this study were first described by A. Carpentier (1980; 1983). Two examples are the sliding and shortening plasty (Figure 16.3). These are used to shorten chordae which are too long so that the mitral valve leaflets do not prolapse back into the left atrium above the valvular ring. No matter what reconstructive technique is employed, a Carpentier ring is always implanted which stabilizes the valve annulus and brings both commissures closer together.

Table 16.2 Postoperative volume data at rest and during exercise for nine patients after mitral valve reconstruction, in comparison with same data for normal adults

	Preoperative Angiography		Postoperative Scintigraph. first pass techn.		Normal adults Scintigraph. first pass techn.	
			Rest	Exercise	Rest	Exercise
EDVI (ml/m²)	153.93 ± 34.7		84.6 ± 23.7 10.2% ↓	75.44 ± 21.9	61.6 ± 15.7 10.8% ↑	69.0 ± 15.0
ESVI (ml/m²)	69.56 ± 19.3		40.56 ± 27.5 15.4% ↓	34.33 ± 21.56	21.5 ± 8.1 35.0% ↓	14.6 ± 6.0
SVI (ml/m²)	84.39 ± 25.00		41.52 ± 14.13 6.6% ↑	44.44 ± 17.13	40.2 ± 9.3 26.9% ↓	55.0 ± 13.0
CI (l/m²)	2.82 ± 0.93		3.39 ± 1.01 20.1% ↑	4.24 ± 2.0	3.25 ± 0.75 65.5% ↑	9.4 ± 2.9
EF (%)	56.3 ± 12.9	RF 51.56 ± 6.43	53.56 ± 16.39 7.9% ↑	58.11 ± 16.74	0.66 ± 0.07 11.5% ↑	0.8 ± 0.07
PTT (ml/s)			6.16 ± 1.97 32.8% ↓	4.14 ± 1.03	6.5 ± 1.09 57.0% ↓	2.8 ± 0.7

[1] Right column: same data for normal persons (Rerych et al., 1978; Scholz et al., 1980; Upton et al., 1980)

[2] EDVI = end-diastolic volume index; ESVI = end-systolic volume index; SVI = stroke volume index; CI = cardiac index; EF = ejection fraction; PTT = pulmonary transit time; ↑ = increase (%); ↓ = decrease (%)

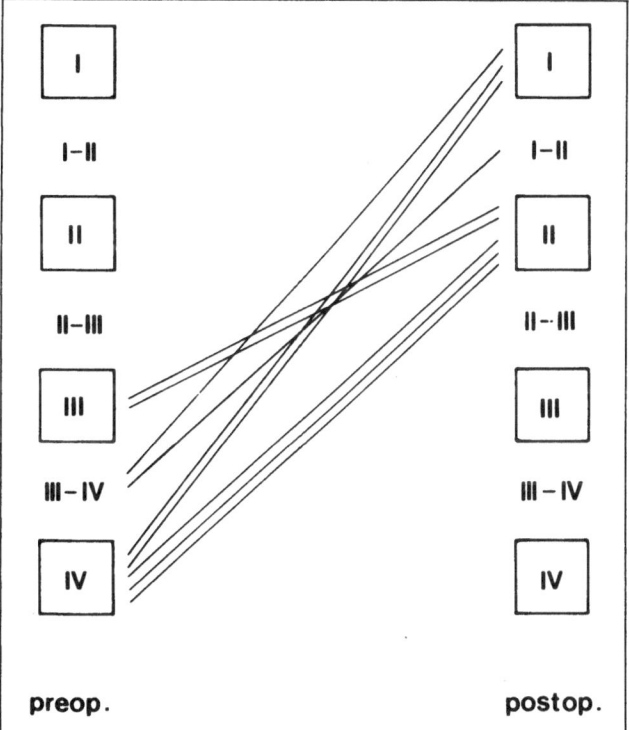

Figure 16.4 NYHA classification for nine patients after mitral valve reconstruction.

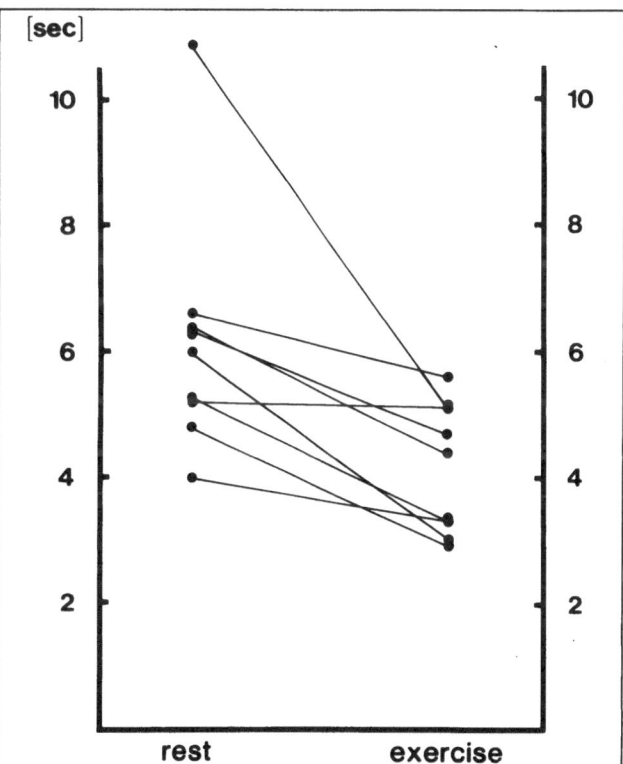

Figure 16.5 Mean pulmonary transit time (ml/s) at rest and during exercise for nine patients after mitral valve reconstruction.

Other surgical procedures for each possible lesion are described and explained by A. Carpentier in the cited papers (1969, 1983).

OBJECTIVES

The main objective of this pilot study was to compare the mechanical function of the reconstructed mitral valves with normal valves and with valve prosthesis. Two phases of the cardiac cycle characterize the function of the reconstructed valves: the rapid filling rate during diastole and the regional myocardial function during systole.

A total of nine patients (with a mean age of 54.5 ± 0.7 years) were studied 15.4 ± 7.5 months after reconstructive surgery of the mitral valve (Figure 16.4). The usual evaluation of transit curves, the mean lung transit time (Figure 16.5), ejection fractions of the right and left ventricles (Table 16.2), and calculations of the regurgitation fractions – all these parameters reflect global myocardial function (Kreutzer *et al.*, 1984). However, after mitral valve surgery the following two parameters are particularly interesting: the rapid filling volumes and the rapid filling rates (Figure 16.6), whereby the rapid filling rate corresponds to the initial upstroke of the volume curve of the left ventricle. These values were derived from the representative cycle, a sum of five to seven cycles during left ventricular washout. In addition, the regional left ventricle function was determined.

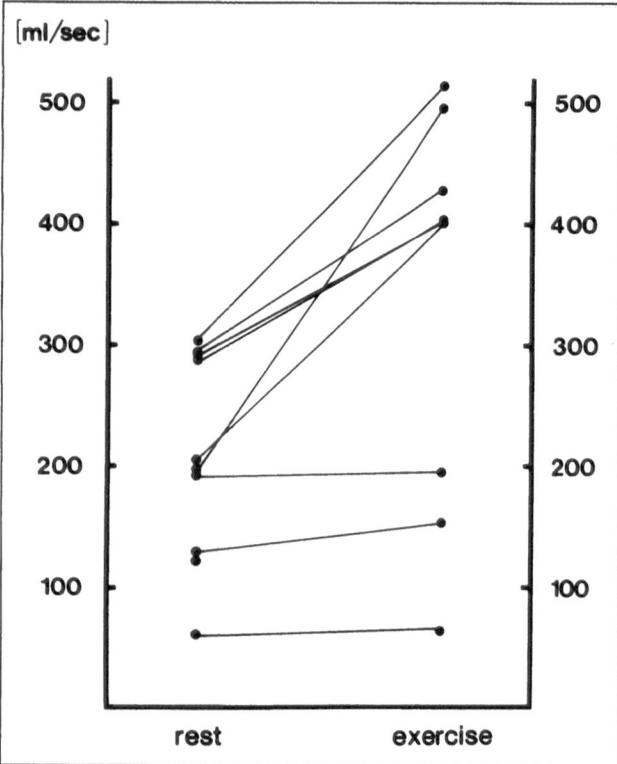

Figure 16.6 Mean inflow velocities (ml/s) during rapid filling phase at rest and during exercise for nine patients after mitral valve reconstruction.

Functional imaging as described in this book shows regional distribution of inflow rates during the rapid filling phase as well as the direction of maximum inflow velocities.

In a normal heart (*see* Chapter 2) maximum rapid filling rate (yellow) is seen near the apex. There is symmetrical distribution parallel to the ventricle's long axis (from the base to the apex). The ventriculogram shows the direction of maximum blood flow towards the apex.

The image of regional mean transit times exhibits the distribution of times at which the centre of gravity of each individual pixel-histogram during the rapid filling occurs. It practically represents the regional persistence of blood.

In healthy individuals, at rest and during exercise, blood flow into the left ventricle and its spreading pattern are symmetrical. After mitral valve reconstruction we find the same symmetrical spreading pattern of the maximum filling rates near the apex at rest and during exercise as seen in normal hearts. The mean transit time of the rapid filling phase and the symmetrical rapid filling pattern demonstrate the unrestricted opening of the corrected mitral valve.

In contrast, the Starr–Edwards valve prosthesis in mitral position shows significant deviation of high inflow rates towards the anterior wall of the ventricle. This pattern was seen in the majority of our patients with a Starr–Edwards valve. The regional mean transit times of the rapid filling and the rapid filling rates in these patients were much lower than in our patients whose mitral valve was reconstructed. Furthermore, we discovered that the posterior wall area of the ventricular cavity shows a remarkable decrease in the inflow filling velocity and an asymmetrical distribution of the rapid filling volume. Abnormalities were similar to the above in regard to the distribution and direction of inflow rates after mitral valve replacement with a Björk–Shiley prosthesis, i.e. deviation towards the anterior wall and loss of symmetry. Also, the rapid filling velocity at the posterior wall region is decreased (green colours). Besides studying the rapid filling phase during diastole we examined the regional systolic function of the left ventricle after the filling phase. The findings seen on normal systolic functional images are described in Chapter 2. During systole the left ventricular wall contracts symmetrically in the direction of the outflow tract. Therefore, the highest blood flow velocities are found in the centre of the left ventricle and the outflow tract regions.

Regional systolic function in patients after mitral valve reconstruction was also studied on an average of 15.4 months after surgery. Again, no differences between these patients and normal individuals were found during the entire systole as well as the first and second half of systole. An initial decrease in global function is usually seen in the early postoperative period (*see* Chapter 13). In the second half of the ejection phase the mean transit time and the ejection rate reach maximum values in all areas of the left ventricle except at the base of the heart. There are no differences between symmetrical regional systolic function patterns at rest and during maximum exercise.

Besides these physiological considerations – i.e. the regional rapid filling phase and the regional systolic function after mitral valve reconstruction – it is important to turn one's attention to the fact that no regurgitation into the left atrium after mitral valve reconstruction could be seen in these patients. The reconstructed mitral valve was absolutely competent.

In contrast, the implantation of a Starr–Edwards valve prosthesis alters ventricular function during the first half of the systolic ejection phase considerably. Only the anterior wall contracts and shows a high regional ejection fraction. The systolic function of the posterior wall area is very low (green and light blue colours). We can speculate with caution that in this region reduction of wall compliance is evident as a result of inflow disturbance or as a consequence of the rigid annulus of the prosthesis.

After the implantation of a Björk–Shiley prosthesis a certain amount of blood may regurgitate into the left atrium. The left ventricle can be enlarged. Posterior wall movement is reduced. As in hearts with a Starr–Edwards prosthesis the highest systolic ejection rate may be found in the anterior wall regions.

CONCLUSION

We conclude that mitral valve reconstruction offers an excellent possibility of obtaining normal diastolic inflow patterns into the left ventricle without alteration of regional systolic function. Mechanical valves cause considerable deviations of diastolic inflow rapid filling volumes which may contribute to the deterioration of regional systolic function. This means that it must be our goal to operate physiologically as far as possible. In other words, in order to obtain a normal regional systolic function it is necessary to re-establish normal physiological inflow patterns. Functional imaging with first pass radionuclide ventriculography is an excellent method to demonstrate the effects of mitral valve reconstruction and especially the improvement of left ventricular function.

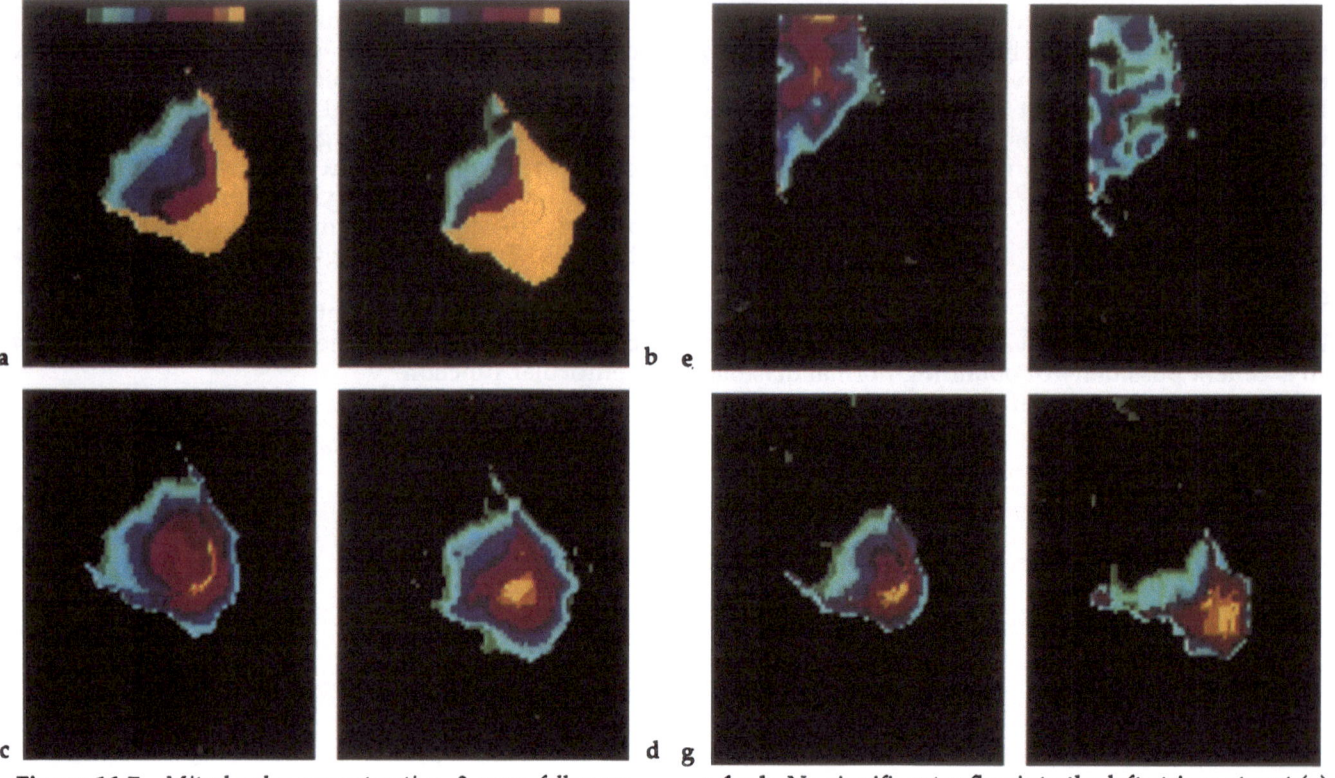

Figure 16.7 *Mitral valve reconstruction. 2 years follow-up. NYHA: pre op IV, post op I*

a,b,c,d, Significant improvement of function from rest (left) to exercise (right) on REFI (**a,b**) and REjR (**c,d**). Global ejection rate at rest 213 ml/s, under stress 527 ml/s. Lung mean transit time 6.0 s at rest, under stress 3.0 s.

e,f,g,h, No significant reflux into the left atrium at rest (**e**) and exercise (**f**). High rapid filling rates symmetrically directed toward the apex at rest (**g**) and under stress (**h**).

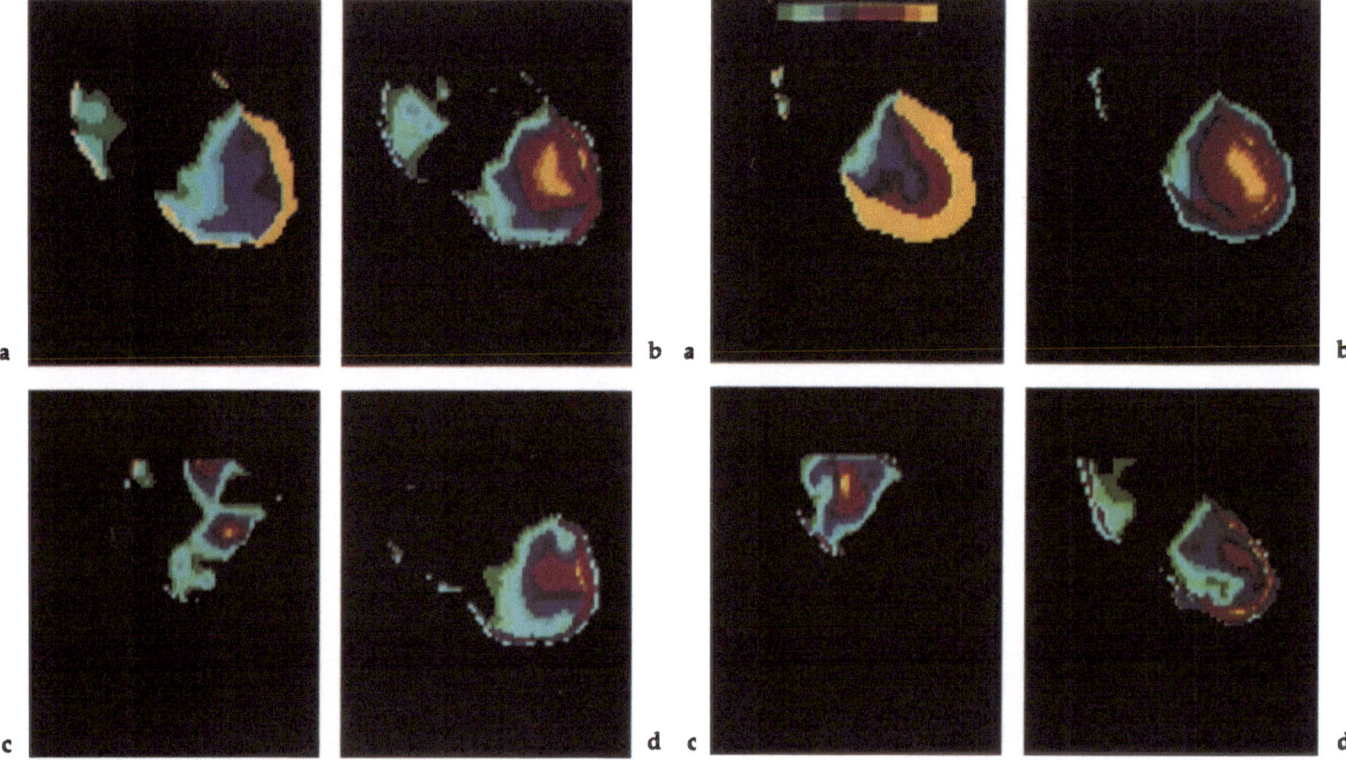

Figure 16.8 *Replacement of the mitral valve with a Starr-Edwards Ball prosthesis. Long term follow-up after 16 years. NYHA: pre op IV, post op II*

a,b,c,d, Reduced function at the infero-posterior wall extending laterally on REFI (**a**) and REjR image (**b**). Mild mitral reflux (**c**). High rapid filling rates displaced anteriorly, low rates posteriorly and inferiorly (**d**). Compare with Figure 16.7 g. Global ejection rate at rest 213 ml/s, under stress 259 s. Lung mean transit time 5.3 s at rest, under stress 4.2 s.

Figure 16.9 *Replacement of the mitral valve with a Björk–Shiley prosthesis. Follow-up after 8 months. NYHA: pre op III, post op II*

a,b,c,d, Somewhat reduced EF's (**a**) and ER's (**b**) posteriorly. No significant reflux (**c**). High rapid filling rates displaced anteriorly (**d**). Compare with Figure 16.7 g. Global ejection rate at rest 200 ml/s, under stress 320 ml/s. Lung mean transit time 6.6 s at rest, under stress 3 s.

17

First Pass Radionuclide Studies in the Evaluation of Long Term (up to 15 Years) Follow Up of Aortic Valve Replacement Using Starr–Edwards Ball Prosthesis

B. REICHART, N. SCHAD, W. HEMMER, E. KREUZER AND R. HATZ

Unlike the mitral valve, reconstructive procedures of the aortic valve are very limited. Therefore, almost all surgical procedures aim at replacing the valve with a mechanical or biological prosthesis. The indications for surgery reflect the extent of the disease: symptoms and physical signs together with additional clinical data including evidence of cardiac hypertrophy by X-ray and e.c.g., and information from echocardiography, nuclear medicine studies and catheterization are utilized to make the decision. Division into four classes of severity by the New York Heart Association is standard. Classes III and IV generally have indications for surgery, and earlier classes may also in some settings.

Aortic stenosis with pressure gradients of 50 mmHg and more usually should have surgery because of the expected progression of the disease. Also, it is important to note that misleading low pressure gradients may exist if the cardiac output had diminished. For this reason, valve area calculations are often utilized to assess disease severity.

The standard surgical therapy of chronic grades III and IV aortic regurgitation is valve replacement. Acute insufficiency is caused by bacterial or fungal infection of the valve, resulting in perforation and destruction of the semilunar leaflets. The operation is performed if the insufficiency leads to cardiac failure or if the infection cannot be treated conservatively.

In many patients, combined stenosis and insufficiency coexist as the consequence of rheumatic endocarditis. The semilunar valve leaflets shrink and calcareous infiltrates develop. The leaflets do not oppose completely and in addition their immobility prevents normal free systolic flow.

The oldest artificial design used for clinical aortic valve replacement is the Starr–Edwards caged ball prosthesis type 1000 introduced in 1963 (Starr *et al.*, 1963). The modified 1200 model consisted of a silicon ball which rested on a metal ring when closed (Figure 17.1) and restrained at the apex of the cage when open. Due to its simple construction, there are few cases of mechanical malfunction or material fatigue. Patients with a Starr–Edwards valve, as with all mechanical prostheses, must take anticoagu-

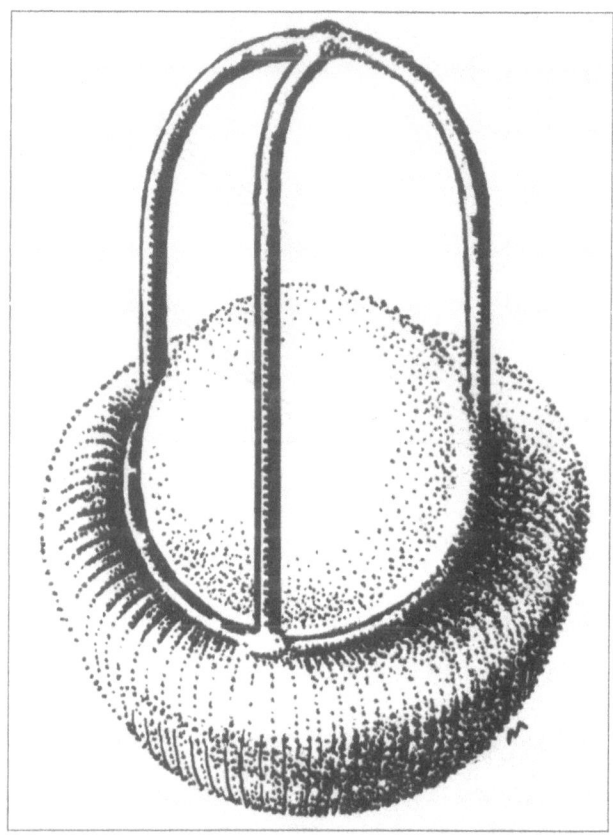

Figure 17.1 Starr–Edwards ball valve prosthesis in the closed position. Silicon ball rests on the ring at the bottom of the metal cage.

lant medication permanently and are thus prone to the associated risks. The haemorrhagic risk is from three to six events per 100 patient years. This complication is fatal in about 5% of all cases.

This study presents an *almost 15-year follow-up of implanted Starr–Edwards prostheses in patients with severe aortic valve disease*, thus covering one of the longest postoperative time periods ever reported for this valve. Our main interest was whether or not the Starr–Edwards prostheses in aortic position functioned properly and what changes, if any, in ventricular dynamics had occurred throughout the years.

Eight men and two women with a mean age of 55.0 ± 7.0 years (ranging from 30 to 51 years) were studied 14.9 ± 2.4 years on an average after aortic valve replacement. Five patients had a combined aortic stenosis and insufficiency, two had pure aortic stenosis and three aortic insufficiency. All patients were assessed preoperatively according to the New York Heart Association classification: eight patients were in clinical stage III and two in stage IV.

Preoperative right and left heart catheterization was performed in eight cases. The left ventricles showed elevated end-diastolic and end-systolic pressures (18 ± 10 mmHg and 184 ± 31 mmHg respectively). Pulmonary pressures were normal except in one patient. In stenotic valves the pressure gradients measured 83 ± 19 mmHg on an average. Mean cardiac output was 4.5 ± 1.0 l/min.

According to case histories and microscopic evaluations of the resected tissue valve destruction was due to rheumatic endocarditis in four cases and bacterial endocarditis in one. In the remaining five patients the primary cause of the aortic valve disease could not be determined.

During surgery the following valve sizes were implanted: one number 9, 13 times; four number 11, 12 times; valve type 1200 was used 6 times, valve type 2300 and 2310 in 4 cases.

At the time the postoperative radioactive studies took place our patients had improved on the New York Heart Association grading scale from a mean preoperative class 3.2 to a mean postoperative class 1.7 (Figure 17.2).

All technetium 99m pertechnetate ventriculograms were done in the same manner as described in the previous two chapters on mitral valve replacement. 14.9 ± 2.4 years after surgery the following parameters were measured at rest as well as during maximum exercise: the end-diastolic and end-systolic ventricular volumes (EDV and ESV), the ejection fraction (EF), the stroke volume (SV), the cardiac output (CO) and index (CI), the mean pulmonary transit time (PTT), the rapid filling rate (RFR) and the systolic ejection rate (SER).

Assessing the *left ventricular volumes* our patients still showed an increased EDV (171 ± 39 ml) and ESV (78 ± 29 ml) as compared to normal. Also, the stroke volume was still elevated, measuring 93 ± 26 ml. A comparison of ventricular volumes at rest and at peak exercise revealed no significant differences (Table 17.1). Correspondingly, the global ejection fraction did not change significantly: from 57 ± 10% to 60 ± 13%. On the other hand, cardiac output and cardiac index increased significantly during maximum exercise: from 7.0 ± 1.9 to 10.9 ± 3.1 l/min and from 3.9 ± 1.2 to 5.9 ± 1.5 l/min per m² ($p = 0.001$ and $p = 0.005$ respectively).

Very important for the *evaluation of aortic valve function* are the rapid filling rate (RFR), the mean pulmonary transit time (PTT) and especially the systolic ejection rate (SER). RFR did not change significantly during peak exercise: 285 ± 123 ml/s at rest and 460 ± 324 ml/s at maximum exercise ($p = 0.1$; Table 17.2). But the mean PTT did show a marked decrease from 5.8 ± 0.7 to 3.9 ± 0.9 s ($p = 0.001$).

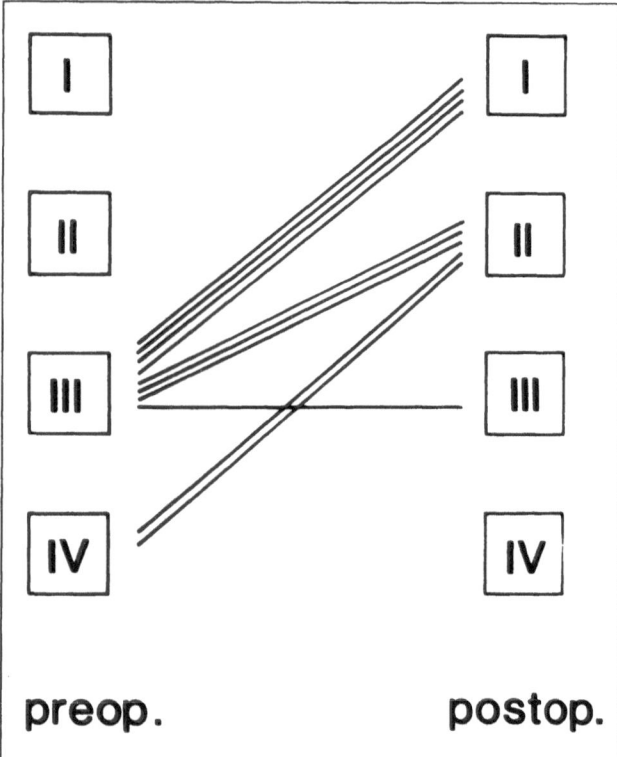

preop.   **postop.**

Figure 17.2 Pre- and postoperative New York Heart Association classification of ten patients who received aortic valve replacement using Starr–Edwards ball valves 14.9 ± 2.4 years ago.

Table 17.2 Rapid filling rate (RFR), mean pulmonary transit time (PTT) and systolic ejection rate (SER) 14.9 ± 2.4 years after aortic valve replacement using Starr–Edwards ball valves

	Rest	Exercise	Statistics
RFR (ml/s)	285 ± 123	460 ± 324	NS
PTT (s)	5.8 ± 0.7	3.9 ± 0.9	$p < 0.05$
SER (ml/s)	233 ± 80	459 ± 232	$p < 0.05$

Table 17.1 Postoperative left ventricular volumes assessed by scintigraphic technique

	Rest	Exercise	Statistics
HR (min⁻¹)	80 ± 15	110 ± 30	$p < 0.05$
EDV (ml)	171 ± 39	178 ± 46	NS
ESV (ml)	78 ± 29	70 ± 30	NS
SV (ml)	93 ± 26	108 ± 48	NS
CO (l/min)	7.9 ± 1.9	10.9 ± 3.1	$p < 0.05$
CI (l/min per m²)	3.9 ± 1.2	5.9 ± 1.5	$p < 0.05$
EF (%)	57 ± 10	60 ± 13	NS

HR = heart rate; EDV = end-diastolic volume; ESV = end-systolic volume; SV = stroke volume; CO = cardiac output; CI = cardiac index; EF = ejection fraction.

Of special interest for the assessment of an aortic prosthesis is the mean systolic ejection rate. This parameter describes the contractility of the left ventricle in regard to the prosthetic valve function in aortic position. Normally, ejection rate must increase considerably. This is not the case if any haemodynamically significant obstruction within the left ventricular outlet exists. After implantation of a Starr–Edwards caged ball valve the blood is forced around the silicon ball, disturbing physiologic laminar blood flow. This causes a pressure gradient present at rest to increase with exercise, ranging from 15 to 20 mmHg, as several investigators reported (Briston and Kremkan, 1975; Glancy *et al.*, 1969; Kloster *et al.*, 1969; Rodriguez, 1970).

Yet, in our patients, the mean systolic ejection rate increased from 233 ± 80 to 459 ± 232 ml/s ($p < 0.02$; Figure 17.3). Therefore, 14.9 ± 2.4 years postoperatively the Starr–Edwards valves in aortic position do not obstruct the outflow tract significantly.

That fact is mirrored by excellent clinical long term results as reported by McManus from the Starr group (McManus *et al.*, 1980): 67% of their patients are still alive after 10 postoperative years, 64% after 15 years. Yet one must bear in mind that the left ventricular function is not all normal. Our patients showed higher end-diastolic volumes and end-systolic volumes at rest than volunteers without Starr–Edwards prostheses. Furthermore, there was an abnormal response to maximum exercise since end-diastolic and end-systolic volumes did not change and the increase of cardiac output depended on heart rate. This might be partially explained by pre-existing myocardial damage, partially by higher pressure gradients of the ball valves especially during peak exercise.

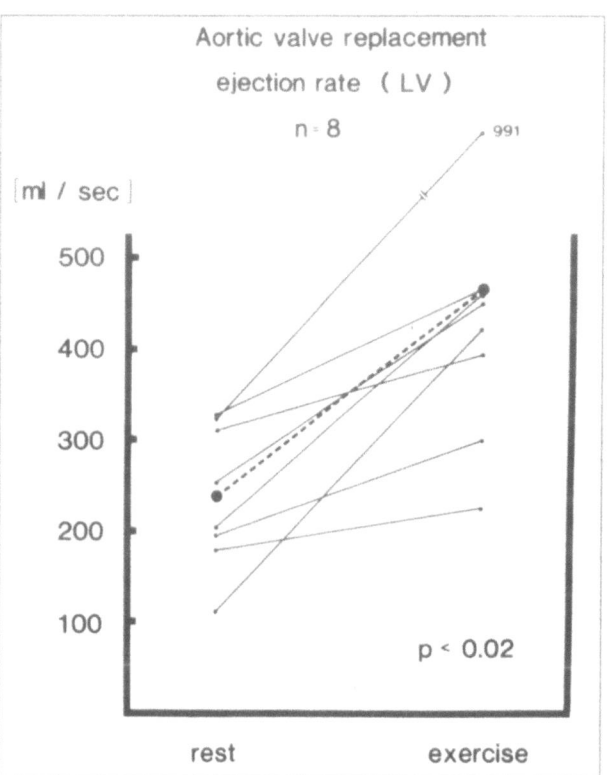

Figure 17.3 Mean systolic ejection rate of eight patients with Starr–Edwards ball valves; the mean values (dashed line) increased from 233 ± 80 to 459 ± 232 ml/s ($p = 0.02$)

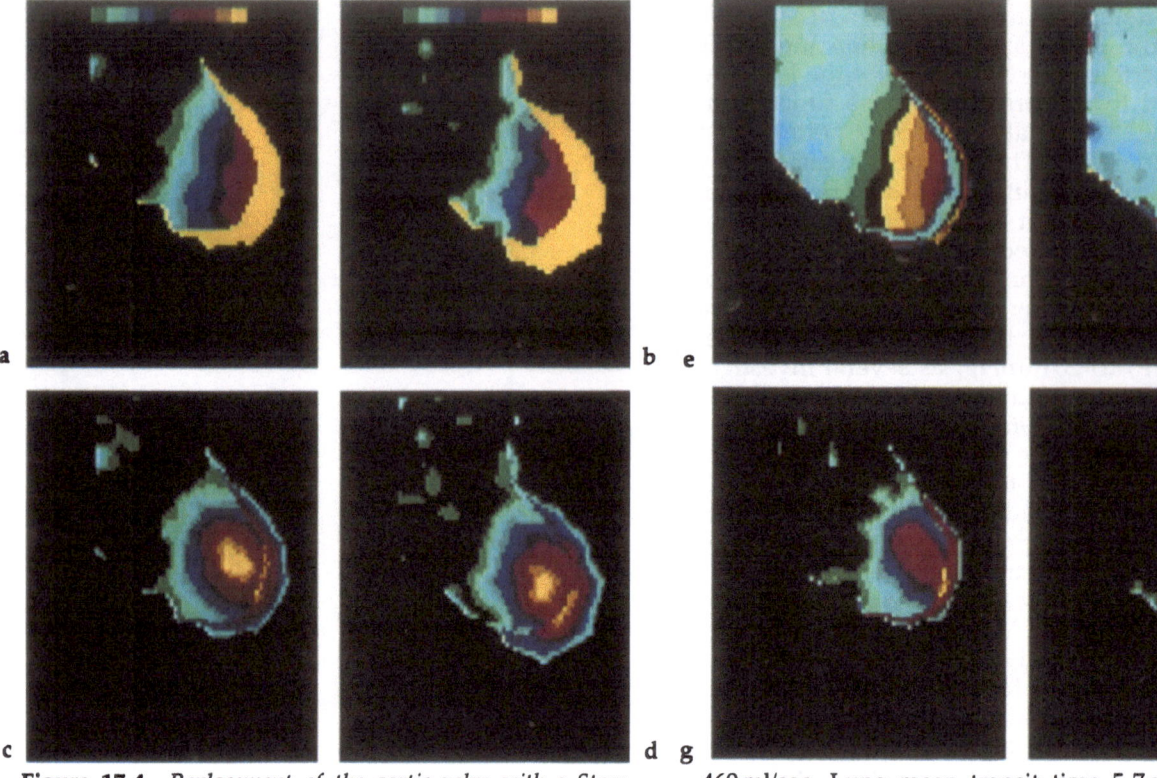

Figure 17.4 *Replacement of the aortic valve with a Starr–Edwards ball prosthesis. Long term follow-up after 18 years. NYHA: pre op III, post op I*

a,b,c,d, Significant improvement of function from rest (left) to exercise (right) along the anterior wall and at the apex, dysfunction of posterior wall on REFI (**a,b**) and REjR (**c,d**). Global ejection rate at rest 200 ml/sec, under stress

460 ml/sec. Lung mean transit time 5.7 s at rest, under stress 2.6 sec.

e,f,g,h, As normally, short mean times along the anterior wall and apex. Prolonged mean times posteriorly at rest (**e**) and exercise (**f**). High rapid filling rates slightly anteriorly displaced, defect posteriorly at rest (**g**) and exercise (**h**).

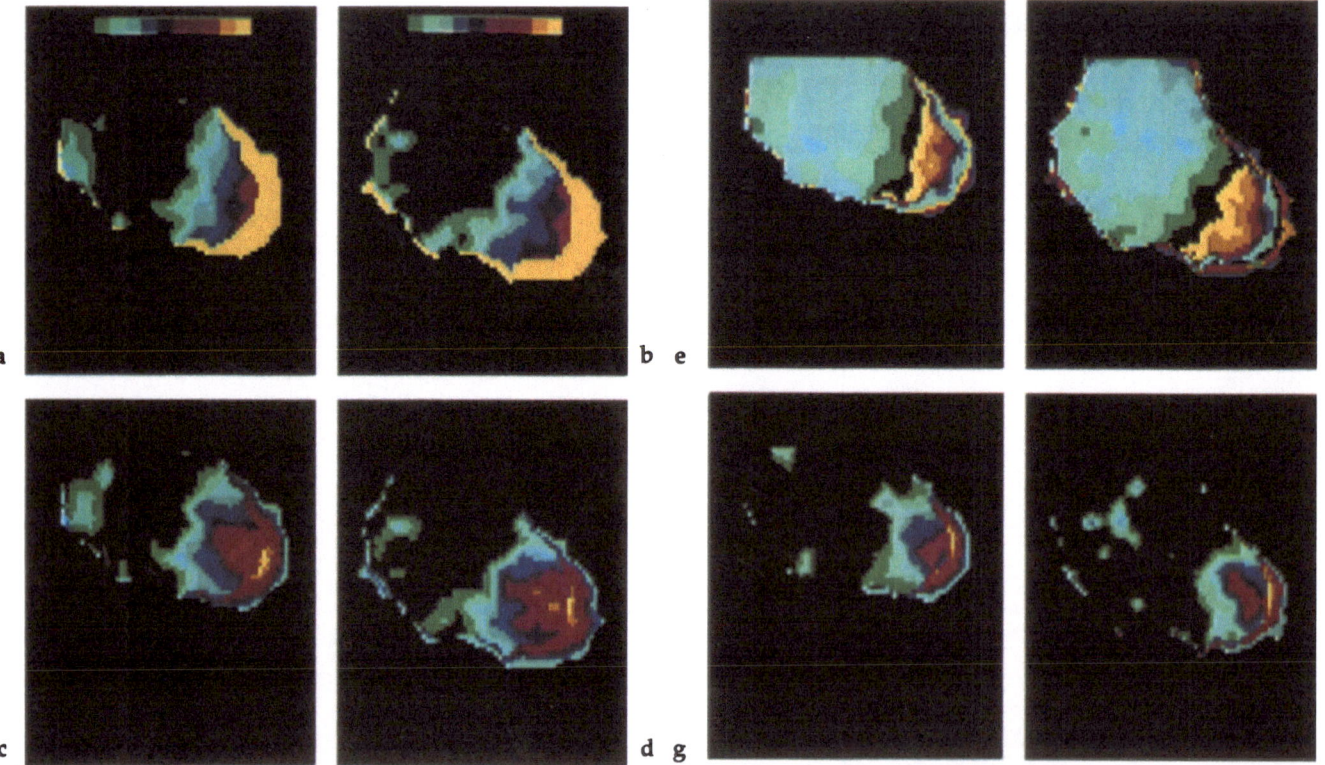

Figure 17.5 *Replacement of the aortic valve with a Starr–Edwards ball prosthesis. Long term follow-up after 14 years. NYHA: pre op IV, post op II*

a,b,c,d, Improvement of function from rest (left) to exercise (right) on REFI (**a,b**) and REjR images (**c,d**). Posterior dysfunction. Global ejection rate at rest 173 ml/sec, under stress 222 ml/sec. Lung mean transit time 5.1 sec at rest and under stress.

e,f,g,h, Short parietal mean times at the anterior and apical wall, prolonged times posteriorly at rest (**e**) and exercise (**f**). Rapid filling rates somewhat anteriorly displaced with posterior defect at rest (**g**) and exercise (**h**).

138

18

Functional Imaging in Patients with Cardiac Pacing, Atrial Fibrillation and Ventricular Rhythm and Conduction Disorders

E. J. ANDREWS JR. AND J. W. FLEMING

Cardiac pacing, atrial fibrillation and ventricular rhythm-conduction disorders do have an affect on regional and global left ventricular (LV) function. The effect upon functional images has been difficult to determine since most patients with these conditions also have other cardiac abnormalities which in themselves may produce wall motion changes. In addition, coronary blood flow can be affected by arrhythmias and cardiac pacing (Benchimol et al., 1972). Limited experience has been gained in patients when rhythm disorders, conduction delays or cardiac pacing were intermittent and correlated with multiple radionuclide ventriculograms (RNV). This chapter will illustrate representative RNV findings correlated with cardiac pacing and ventricular rhythm or conduction disorders.

CARDIAC PACING

Of the three subjects listed in this chapter, cardiac pacing most severely affects left ventricular wall motion (Boucher et al., 1983). An inferior wall motion abnormality (WMA) characteristically is associated with cardiac pacing (see Case 1). This WMA may extend to the LV apex and is usually holosystolic. Similar abnormalities occur with inferior ischaemia or infarction and misinterpretation can be avoided if a simultaneous rhythm strip has been recorded and the interpreter is aware of the presence of a cardiac pacemaker. This abnormality disappears when the pacemaker is not functioning and usually disappears with exercise when the patient is able to achieve a higher intrinsic heart rate overriding the pacemaker.

Case 1 (Figures 18.1 and 18.2) is an example of severe inferior wall motion changes associated with right ventricular (RV) pacing. These changes are not seen in a second study performed on the same day without pacing. The significant difference in the appearance of the inferior wall between these two studies is typical of findings which have been found consistently in a series of other patients studied by RNV during cardiac pacing. Abnormalities of the anterolateral wall usually are not seen in association with RV pacing alone and when present these usually represent significant unrelated findings such as ischaemia or cardiomyopathy.

ATRIAL FIBRILLATION

It is well known that atrial fibrillation (AF) does affect the global LV function on a beat to beat basis. Schneider et al. (1983) and Bacharach et al. (1981) described marked variation in EF in different beats in patients with AF. The effect upon wall motion is more difficult to evaluate because AF is commonly associated with other cardiac abnormalities such as aortic and mitral valve disease, coronary artery disease (CAD), myocarditis, cardiomyopathy, and shunt lesions. These abnormalities in themselves produce WMA which affect the functional image. Limited experience has been gained in patients who have undergone closely successive RNV studies with and without AF.

Case 2 (Figures 18.3 and 18.4) illustrates a patient with CAD with intermittent AF and mild generalized WMA. He had triple vessel coronary disease at cardiac catheterization. Successive RNV studies show no significant changes in WMA between the study obtained in normal sinus rhythm (NSR) and two additional studies obtained during AF on the same day.

Case 3 (Figures 18.5 and 18.6) illustrates that a relatively normal wall motion image can be obtained in a patient with AF. This is representative of other cases in our experience. We feel that AF is not a contraindication to RNV study by the first pass method if careful attention is paid to acquisition, processing technique and interpretation. RNV can be quite helpful in many patients with AF although RNV ejection fractions (EF) are variable and may underestimate true LV performance at rest (Schneider et al., 1983). If there are abnormal WMA in patients with AF, this usually can be attributed to an underlying abnormality or myocardial disease.

PREMATURE VENTRICULAR CONTRACTIONS AND INTRAVENTRICULAR CONDUCTION DELAYS

Multiple premature ventricular contractions (PVC) and intraventricular conduction delays (IVCD) can produce significant changes in global ventricular function. Premature ventricular contractions occur commonly with contrast ventriculography, and it is often a challenge to calculate stroke volume from a single 'normal contraction' occurring within a series of PVCs. Although global function also is affected by the PVC in RNV studies, functional images may remain relatively constant in those cases where careful processing allows these contractions to be excluded from the data. An occasional PVC or other extrasystole can be excluded during data processing resulting in a more reliable evaluation of global and regional LV function.

Left bundle branch block (LBBB) does produce a delay in activation of LV contraction, but it is not always clear whether WMA is due to the conduction delay or diseased myocardium in some of these patients (Swiryn et al., 1981). Since patients with LBBB commonly have an associated underlying myocardial disorder, separation of the two influences is difficult. Functional RNV images in patients with LBBB are usually abnormal but findings in Case 5 with a transient IVCD suggests that IVCD per se may play a relatively minor role in WMA seen in patients with ischaemia. The underlying myocardial abnormality appears to be the most significant contributor to the overall wall motion abnormality.

Case 4 (Figures 18.7 and 18.8) is a 54 year old male with previous history of myocardial infarction and coronary bypass surgery for triple vessel disease. The study shows bigeminy PVCs with exercise. Two exercise studies performed on the same day in this patient with and without bigeminy show very similar wall motion patterns with a typical antero-lateral WMA of ischaemia. Bigeminy does not significantly affect the diagnostic quality of the images in this case. Kaliff et al. (1982) report a similar experience in a series of ten patients.

Case 5 (Figures 18.9 and 18.10) illustrates a patient with CAD who has intermittent IVCD but typical WMA of ischaemia. When this patient exercised to a heart rate of 115 beats per minute, he developed IVCD and ST elevation. With a second exercise effort to a heart rate of 100 beats/min, he developed ST depression but no IVCD. These two studies illustrate that the WMA attributed to ischaemia did not appear to be significantly changed by the presence of an IVCD.

SUMMARY

Functional imaging with RNV in patients with AF, PVCs and IVCD should be interpreted with some caution. This is particularly true in evaluation of inferior WMA in patients who are studied during cardiac pacing. An e.c.g. rhythm strip recording at the time of the radionuclide injection is an important part of the procedure and should be obtained at the precise time that the RN bolus appears in the left ventricle. With experience, careful acquisition and processing of data, and correlation with simultaneous e.c.g. recordings, RNV functional imaging can be useful in evaluating patients with AF, PVCs and IVCD.

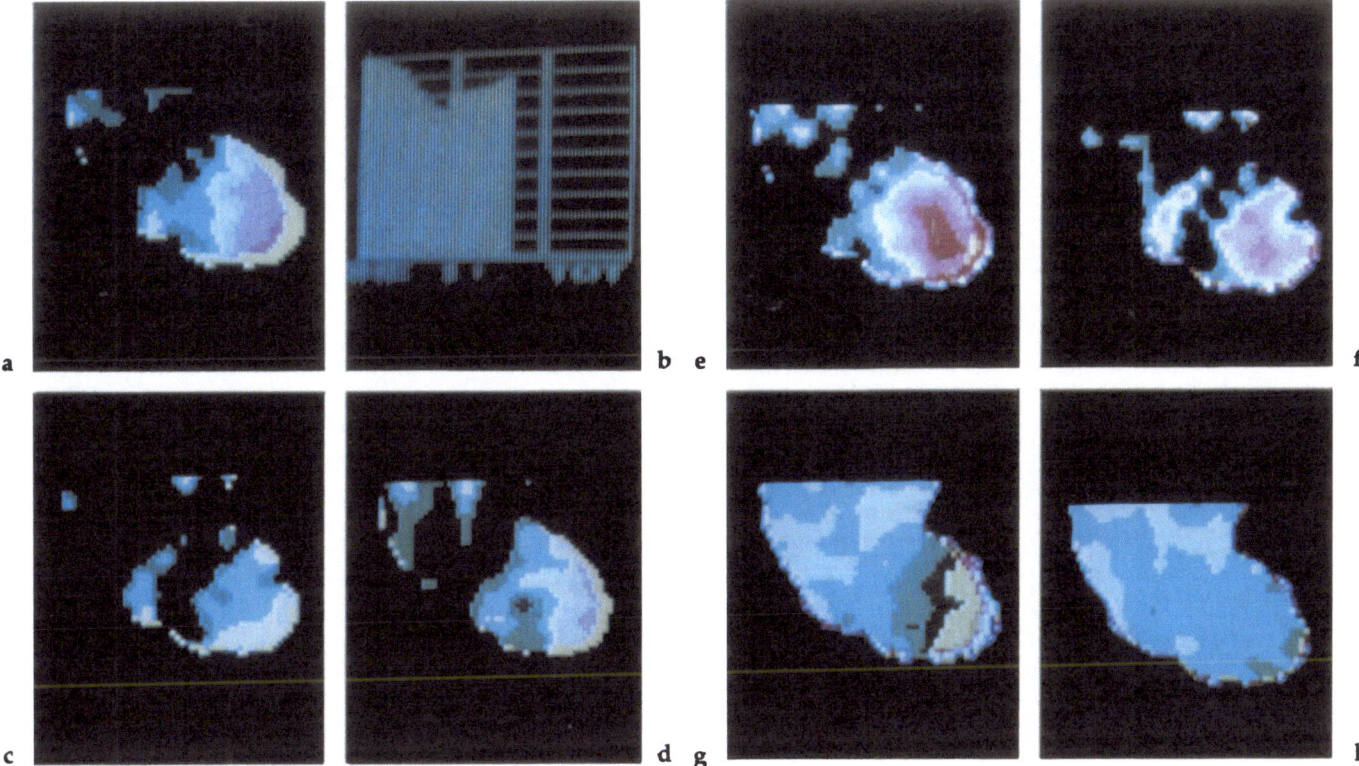

Figure 18.1 *Case 1. Sinus rhythm*, bradycardia, minimal coronary arteriosclerosis, anterior, rest, LVEF 46%. Images obtained during sinus rhythm show only mild wall motion abnormalities inferiorly and in the high lateral wall related to minimal focal ischaemia. **a**, REFI; **b**, volume curve; **c**, first half REFI; **d**, second half REFI; **e**, ejection rate; **f**, first half ER; **g**, transit; **h**, first half transit.

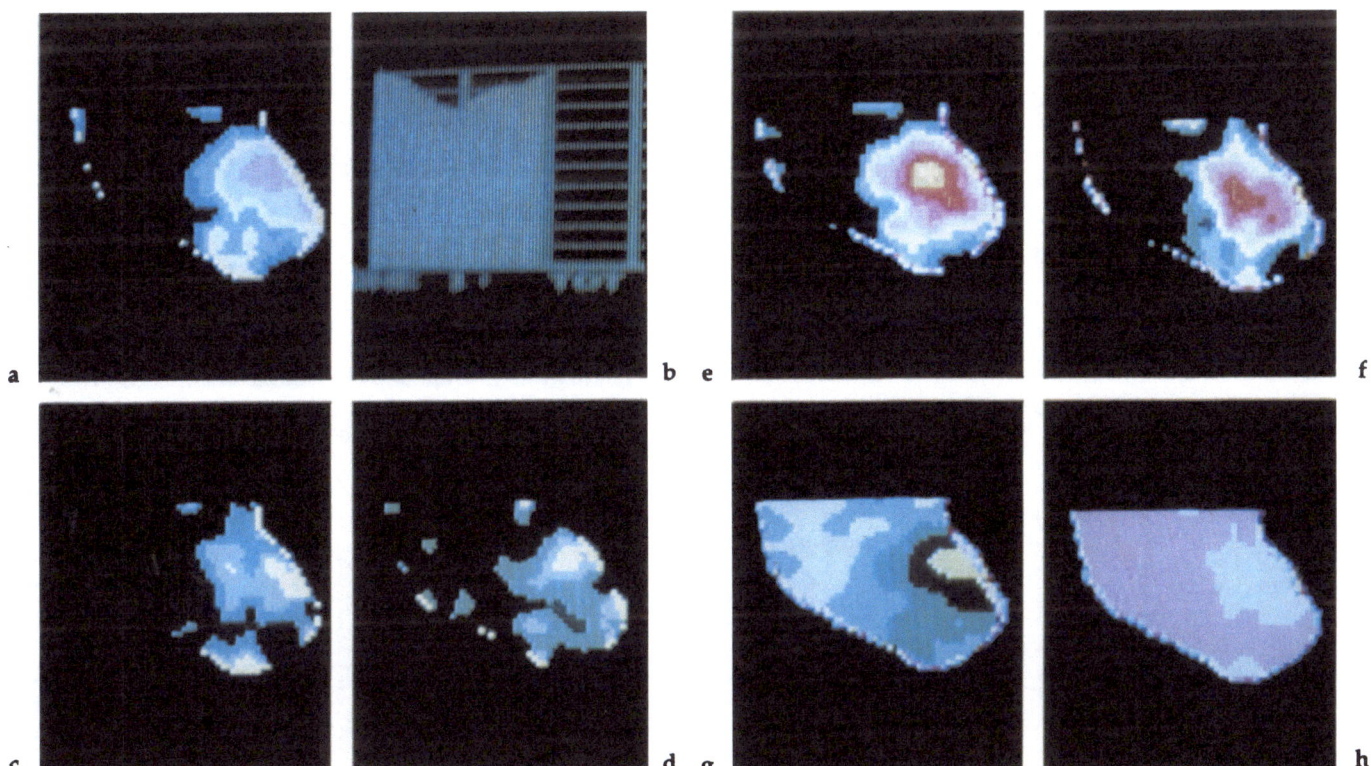

Figure 18.2 *Case 1. Cardiac pacing*, rest, anterior, LVEF 30%.) With cardiac pacing global function decreases slightly and a severe inferior wall motion abnormality does develop occurring early as well as late in systole, as seen in the first and second half REFI images. The REFI image becomes abnormal inferiorly as do the rate and transient time images. **a**, REFI; **b**, volume curve; **c**, first half REFI; **d**, second half REFI; **e**, ejection rate; **f**, first half ER; **g**, transit; **h**, first half transit.

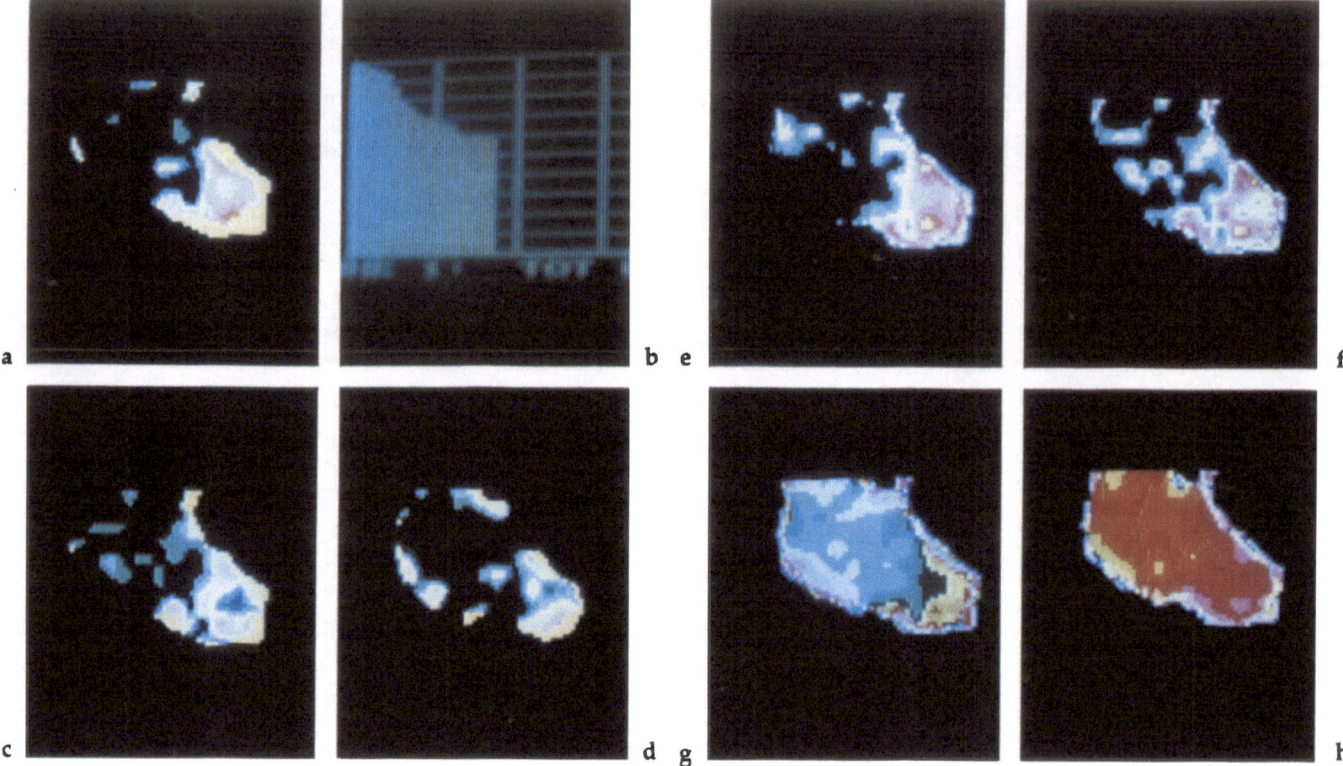

Figure 18.3 *Case 2. Sinus rhythm*, CAD, recent myocardial infarction, rest, anterior. Images show mild wall motion changes most pronounced anterolaterally consistent with ischaemia. **a**, REFI; **b**, volume curve; **c**, first half REFI; **d**, second half REFI; **e**, ejection rate; **f**, first half ER; **g**, transit; **h**, first half transit.

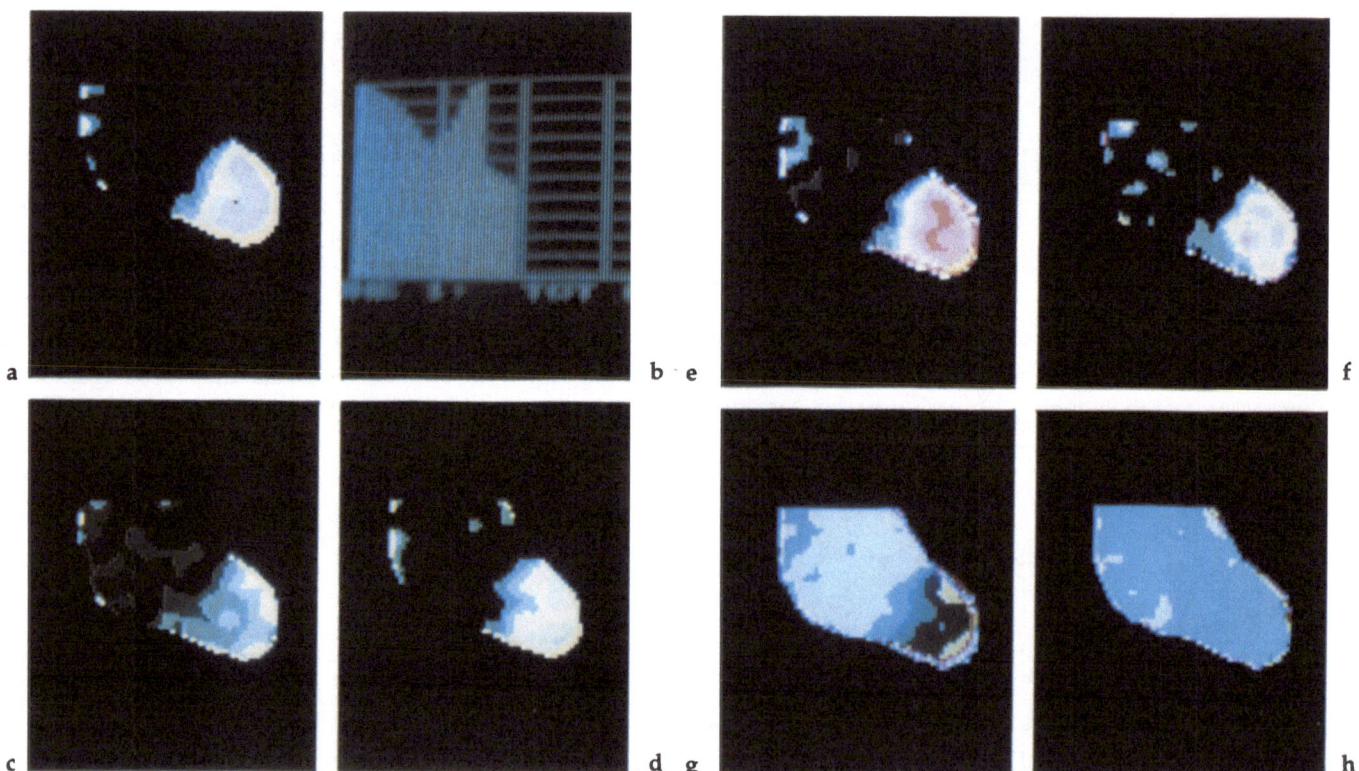

Figure 18.4 *Case 2. Atrial fibrillation*, rest, anterior. Images obtained the same day during atrial fibrillation show essentially the same wall motion abnormality as seen during sinus rhythm. Global function also remains the same. In this example atrial fibrillation did not appreciably change the diagnostic quality of the images. **a**, REFI; **b**, volume curve; **c**, first half REFI; **d**, second half REFI; **e**, ejection rate; **f**, first half ER; **g**, transit; **h**, first half transit.

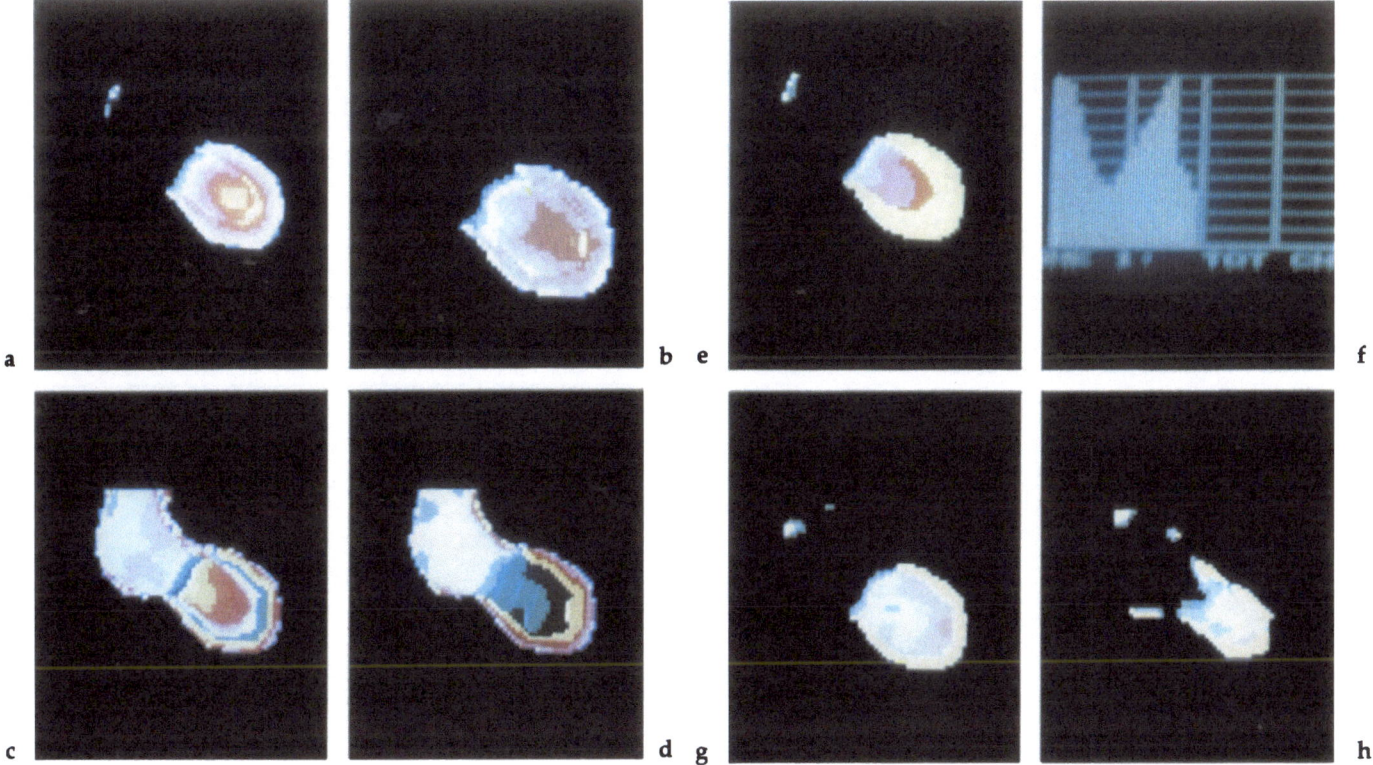

Figure 18.5 *Case 3. Atrial fibrillation*, normal coronary arteries, mitral valve prolapse, rest, anterior, LVEF 60%. Images show essentially normal wall motion in this patient with atrial fibrillation. **a**, REFI; **b**, volume curve; **c**, first half REFI; **d**, second half REFI; **e**, ejection rate; **f**, first half ER; **g**, transit; **h**, first half transit.

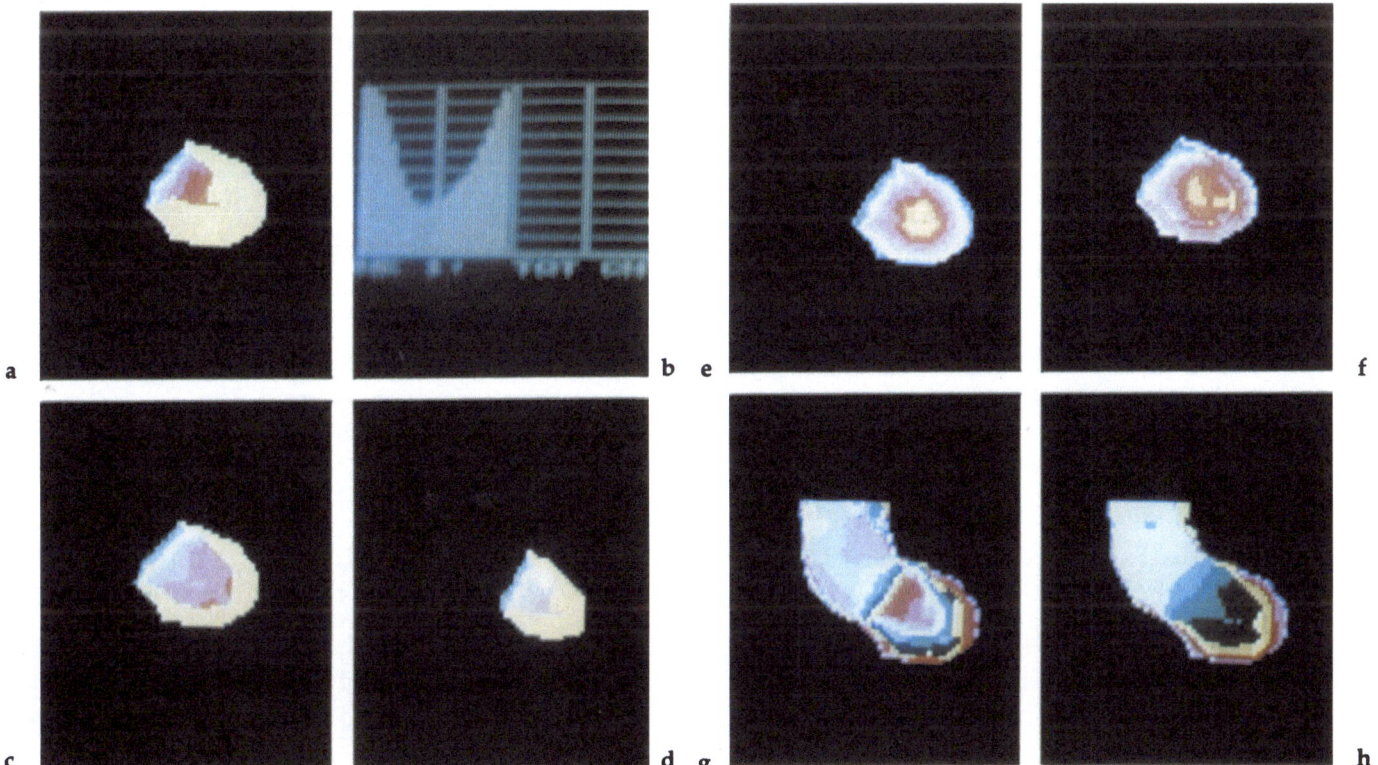

Figure 18.6 *Case 3. Atrial fibrillation*, anterior, exercise, LVEF 65%. With exercise images remain normal in this patient with atrial fibrillation. **a**, REFI; **b**, volume curve; **c**, first half REFI; **d**, second half REFI; **e**, ejection rate; **f**, first half ER; **g**, transit; **h**, first half transit.

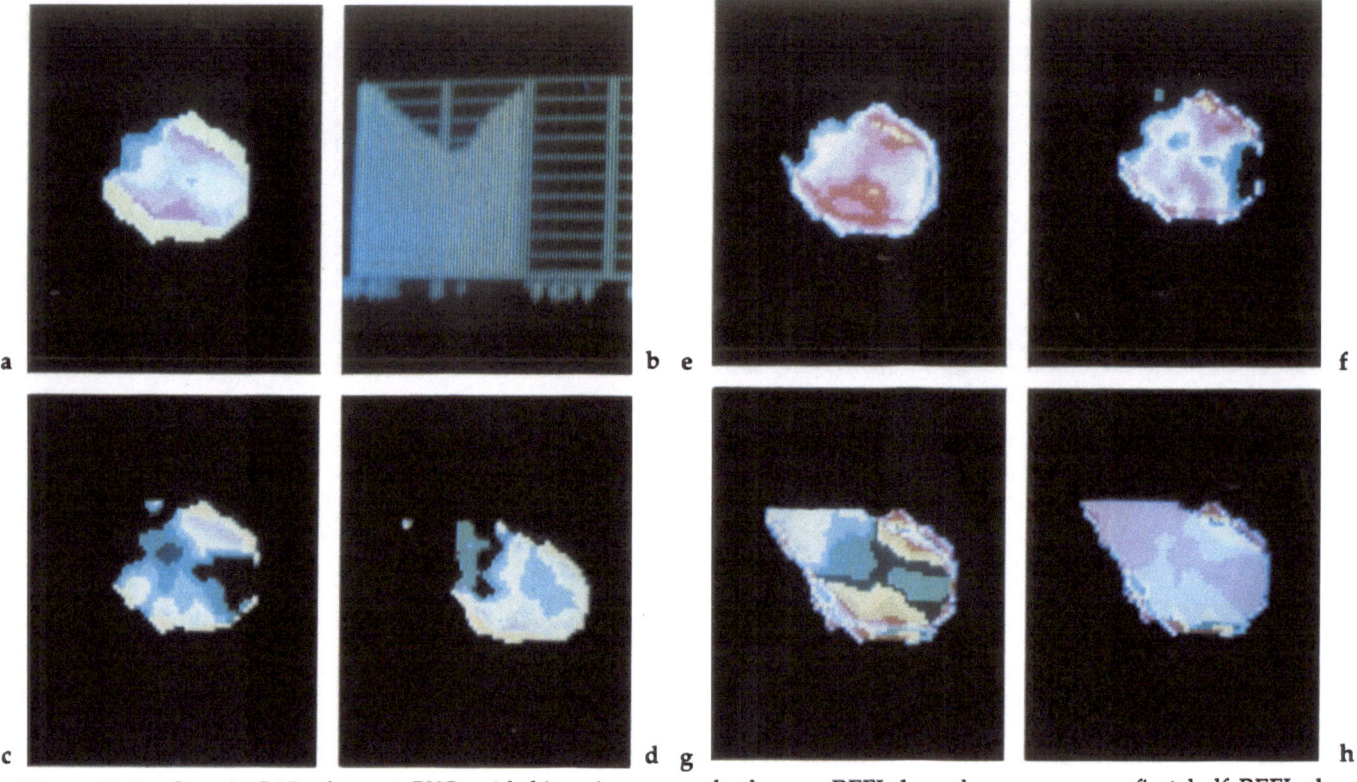

Figure 18.7 *Case 4. CAD, frequent PVCs* with bigeminy, anterior, exercise LVEF 46%. Images show diffuse wall motion changes most pronounced at the apex consistent with ischaemia. This study was obtained during sinus rhythm. **a,** REFI; **b,** volume curve; **c,** first half REFI; **d,** second half REFI; **e,** ejection rate; **f,** first half ER; **g,** transit; **h,** first half transit.

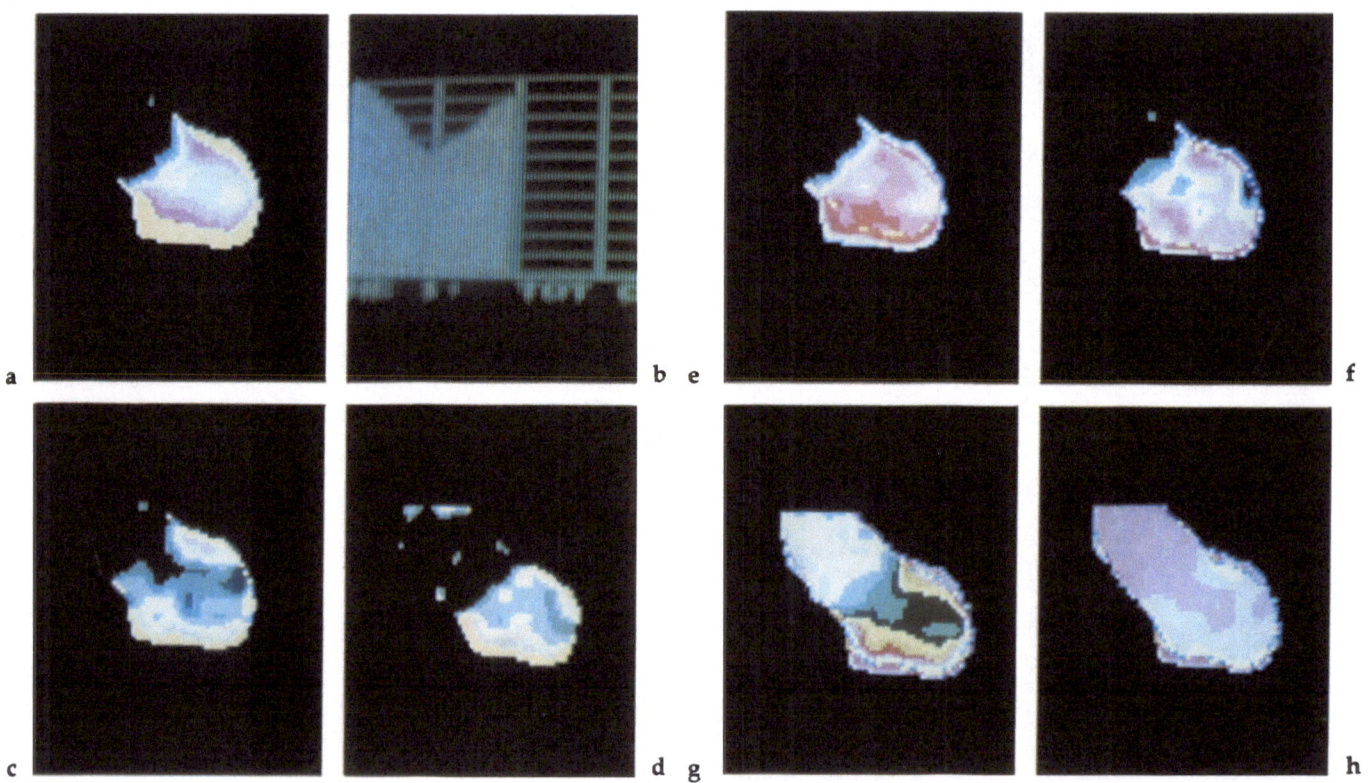

Figure 18.8 *Case 4. Bigeminy PVCs,* exercise, repeat study LVEF 36%. Repeat study during episode of bigeminy shows little change in global function or appearance of images. Anterolateral wall motion changes are again seen in all images consistent with ischaemia. **a,** REFI; **b,** volume curve; **c,** first half REFI; **d,** second half REFI; **e,** ejection rate; **f,** first half ER; **g,** transit; **h,** first half transit.

144

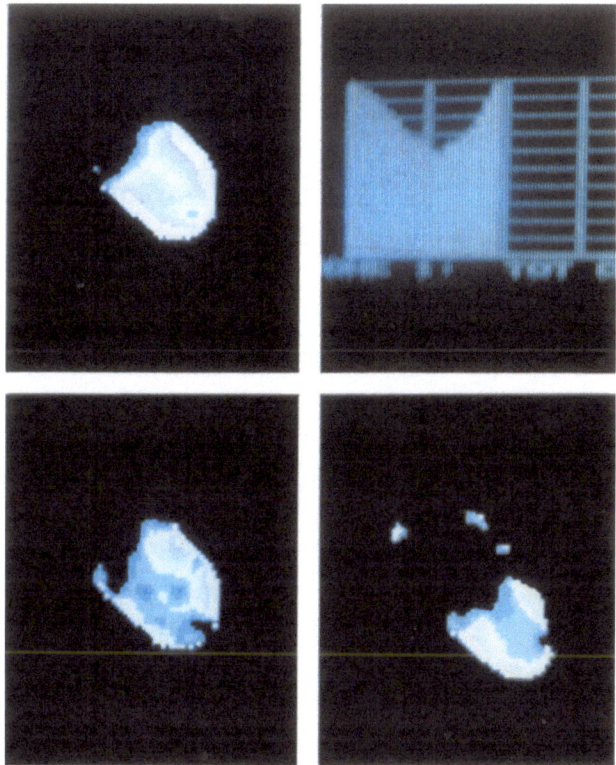

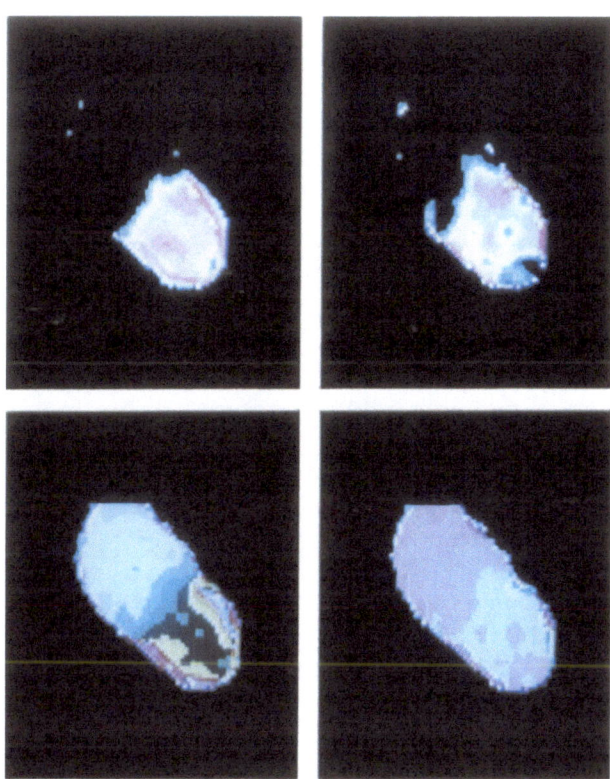

Figure 18.9 *Case 5. Intraventricular conduction delay,* CAD, exercise, anterior LVEF 40%. Images show typical wall motion changes of ischaemia extending to the cardiac apex mostly pronounced on the early systolic images. This

study was obtained during a time of *normal* conduction. **a**, REFI; **b**, volume curve; **c**, first half REFI; **d**, second half REFI; **e**, ejection rate; **f**, first half ER; **g**, transit; **h**, first half transit.

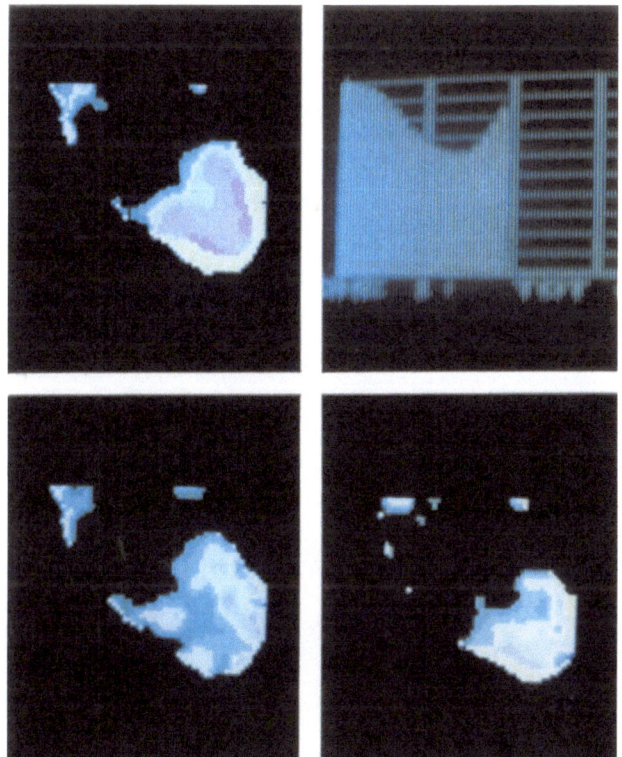

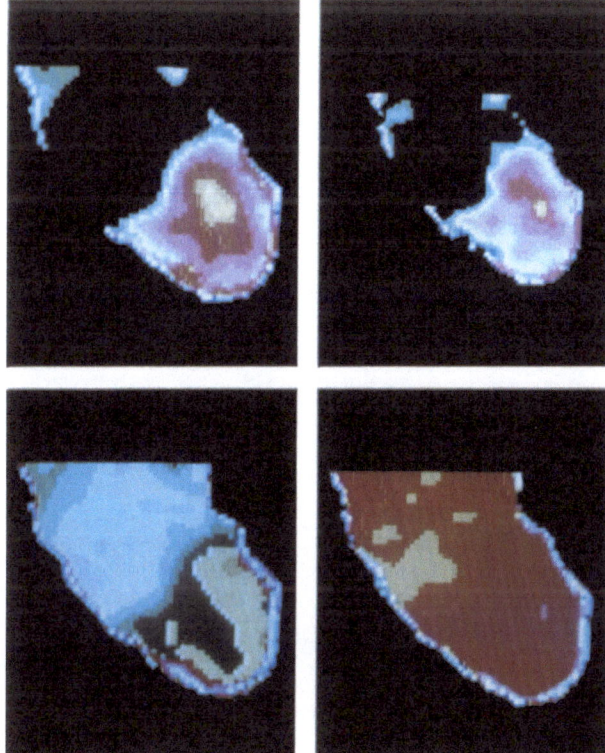

Figure 18.10 *Case 5. Intraventricular conduction delay,* anterior, exercise. With heart rate above 115, this patient develops an intraventricular conduction delay. Repeat exercise heart rate 120 done on the same day during an episode of intraventricular conduction delay confirmed by

e.c.g. Wall motion remains essentially the same, still showing ischaemic change extending into the cardiac apex. **a**, REFI; **b**, volume curve; **c**, first half REFI; **d**, second half REFI; **e**, ejection rate; **f**, first half ER; **g**, transit; **h**, first half transit.

19

Functional Imaging of the Right Heart in Various Clinical Conditions Including Left to Right Shunts

E. J. ANDREWS JR. AND J. W. FLEMING

Although most of the interest in radionuclide ventriculography (RNV) evaluation of the heart has centred around the left ventricle (LV), Schad and Nickel (1979) and Berger *et al.* (1979a) described the usefulness of first pass radionuclide assessment of the right ventricle (RV). In routine first pass RNV studies, data are available for right heart evaluation as the bolus passes through the RV, but most laboratories process only the LV information. However, RV evaluation can be useful and should be performed more often in cases where the clinical picture is confusing and where LV analysis does not satisfactorily explain the diagnosis. The same type of functional images described in Chapter 2 applies to RV studies. In addition to ejection fraction (EF), RV volumes, and pulmonary transit times can be calculated. The cases discussed in this chapter are only a few examples of potential applications of information available through right heart evaluation. Function of the RV can be significantly affected by a number of clinical conditions. Some of these will be discussed briefly.

SEVERE ACUTE PULMONARY HYPERTENSION

Global RV function (EF) is a sensitive indicator of pulmonary hypertension (Korr *et al.*, 1982). More recently, Friedman (1982) described the use of RVEF during the second half of systole (a number) as a predictor of pulmonary arterial systolic pressure.

Case 1 (Figures 19.1 and 19.2) is an example of early use of RV evaluation when LV information did not explain the clinical picture. This 60-year-old male was transferred from an outside hospital for cardiac evaluation with a diagnosis of severe congestive heart failure unresponsive to therapy. Resting RNV revealed an LVEF of 65% with no evidence of significant LV ischaemia on functional images. RVEF on the other hand was 23% and pulmonary transit time was 19 seconds. RV images showed diffuse wall motion abnormality and diagnosis of severe pulmonary hypertension was made. The patient had significant bradycardia with a 2:1 AV block and cardiac catheterization confirmed suspected pulmonary hypertension. Systemic pressures were found in the RV and there was

normal global left ventricular function but findings suggested IHSS. After insertion of a cardiac pacemaker and medical therapy, symptoms improved dramatically with pulmonary artery pressures returning to normal per flotation catheter study. Repeat RNV evaluation showed improvement in RVEF (52%) and wall motion. Pulmonary transit time decreased to 6 seconds. Since patients with IHSS do not appear to tolerate bradycardia well, a permanent pacemaker was recommended. The patient remains well 3 years after the intial episode of RV failure. This case is somewhat unusual but illustrates the value of right heart evaluation in an acute situation.

PULMONARY VENOUS HYPERTENSION

Elliott (1976) described the use of the plain chest X-ray in the diagnosis of pulmonary venous hypertension. In addition, he clearly categorized the conditions which lead to this diagnosis indicating the site of increased resistance at the mitral valve or distal to the mitral valve. Each of these two categories has a distinctly different effect upon the cardiac configuration in the chest X-ray, but the physiological effect of pulmonary venous hypertension upon the right heart is similar. The conditions which are associated with the increased resistance distal to the mitral valve are categorized as 'left ventricular stress' and include LV ischaemia, aortic stenosis, coarctation and systemic hypertension. The second category is designated 'mitral' and includes mitral valve disease and left atrial myxoma.

Ischaemia

While myocardial ischaemia more commonly affects the left ventricle, the right ventricle can also be affected, and RV infarction presents as a different clinical picture. Case 2 (Figure 19.3) presented with a history of angina of several months' duration with nocturnal angina as well as dyspnoea. There was a probable myocardial infarction (LV) several months earlier. RNV showed severe biventricular dysfunction with LVEF of 30% and RVEF of 35%. Images revealed diffuse wall motion abnormalities typical of RV ischaemia, most pronounced during early systole. Cardiac catheterization revealed total occlusion of the left anterior descending coronary artery and 95% narrowing of the proximal right coronary artery. Right heart pressures were normal. Case 3 (Figure 19.4) a 48-year-old male with congestive failure, was found to have a total occlusion of the left main coronary artery with collateral filling via the RCA. LVEF was 17%.

Valvular disease

Although aortic stenosis and mitral stenosis have a distinctly different effect upon the cardiac contour as seen by the plain chest X-ray, both lead to the same findings of pulmonary venous hypertension and effect upon the right heart. The effect upon the left ventricle has been previously discussed in Chapter 13. The effect upon the right heart is related to the amount of resistance created by the lesion. In general, stenotic lesions lead to high pressures in the pulmonary vascular bed and consequently have a greater effect upon RV function. However, long-standing valvular insufficiency can also produce severe RV dysfunction. Cases 4 and 5 contrast mitral stenosis and mitral regurgitation. In Case 4 (Figure 19.5) very severe mitral stenosis was diagnosed at cardiac catheterization with a calculated mitral valve area of $0.7 \, cm^2$; the main pulmonary artery systolic pressure was 80 mmHg with a mean wedge pressure of 35 mmHg. In contrast, Case 5 (Figure 19.6) illustrates RV function in a patient with severe mitral regurgitation graded at 4+. There is also left ventricular dysfunction with LVEF of 38%. However, pulmonary pressures were found to be normal with main pulmonary artery systolic pressure 27 mmHg with a mean wedge pressure of 10 mmHg. There is a striking difference in the appearance of the RV functional images in these two patients as would be expected from the standpoint of the different vascular resistance. However, Winzelberg et al. (1981) found no correlation between RVEF and right atrial pressure in a series of 56 patients with valvular heart disease. Cases 6 (Figure 19.7) and 7 (Figure 19.8) contrast aortic valve disease. Here wall motion and global function are more severely affected in Case 6 (AS), who had elevated pulmonary artery and wedge pressures.

PULMONARY ARTERIAL HYPERTENSION

Right heart function is also affected by conditions compromising the pulmonary capillary bed which produce increased pulmonary artery pressure and right ventricular dysfunction. These conditions include pulmonary embolism and chronic obstructive pulmonary disease (COPD).

Pulmonary embolism

Case 8 (Figures 19.9 and 19.10) is a 70-year-old male with pleural effusion and congestive failure. RNV study shows RV dysfunction with RVEF 38%, tricuspid insufficiency, and pulmonary transit time of 10 seconds. There was no evidence for LV ischaemia and the RNV picture was compatible with pulmonary hypertension. Cardiac catheterization 5 days later revealed normal coronary arteries with pulmonary artery pressure of 55 mmHg and pulmonary wedge pressure 15 mmHg. Pulmonary angiogram was consistent with multiple pulmonary emboli.

Chronic obstructive pulmonary disease

Berger et al. (1979a) describe the use of RVEF in the evaluation of patients with COPD and suggest that RNV studies are a simple reproducible means of following such patients and assessing pharmacological intervention. RVEF was consistently lower in patients with cor pulmonale. There was no apparent relation of RV to LV function.

Case 9 (Figure 19.11) illustrates mildly decreased RV function in a patient with severe COPD. There is relative preservation of wall motion in the functional images, but there is an overall depression of global function (RVEF 30%), mild tricuspid insufficiency, and prolonged pulmonary transit time of 7.5 seconds. Function however does not improve with exercise. RV function is more severely affected in Case 10 (Figure 19.12) with bullous emphysema. Pulmonary transit time was 10 seconds.

TRICUSPID INSUFFICIENCY

Tricuspid insufficiency (TI) is difficult to evaluate by RNV studies and is usually related to an underlying condition which produces increased RV volume and pressure. Tu'meh et al. (1982) described a method whereby TI can be assessed by RNV studies using hepatic activity as a region of interest. Hepatic counts are significantly increased with significant TI. However, two-dimensional echocardiography with contrast enhancement is the more commonly accepted method of evaluation (Meltzer et al., 1983; DePace et al., 1983). Echocardiography, however, is less helpful in evaluating associated RV function and pulmonary transit time. Angiographic evaluation is also difficult because of the necessary presence of the catheter across the tricuspid valve. First pass RNV studies with functional imaging can detect TI as well as provide additional information regarding RV function, pulmonary transit time, and LV function.

Case 11 (Figure 19.13), a 44-year-old female with intermittent tachycardia, presented with the clinical findings of tricuspid insufficiency confirmed by two-dimensional echocardiography. LVEF was 37% and EDV was 194 ml. LV wall motion was consistent with cardiomyopathy. RVEF was 40% with EDV 212 ml. Pulmonary transit time was relatively normal at 6.2 seconds. Because of persistence of activity in the right atrium, shunt evaluation by a standard computer was falsely positive. Functional imaging can help make the important differentiation between left and right shunt versus tricuspid insufficiency. In the latter instance, right heart evaluation shows increased activity in the region of the right atrium in the systolic portion of the rate image.

LEFT TO RIGHT SHUNTS

Three important questions are raised in the evaluation of patients with left to right shunts: (1) is a shunt present? (2) what is the location of the defect (atrial, ventricular, or aortic)? and (3) what are the effects upon the RV? Evaluation of the RV by RNV with functional imaging can address all three of these questions and provide valuable information regarding right heart function. Of particular importance is the evaluation for the presence of associated pulmonary hypertension due to the effect of volume overload upon the pulmonary vascular bed.

A shunt program is available which generates a gamma variate fit (Parker and Treves, 1977) of the lung transit curve. Early recirculation due to a shunt produces a 'hump' on the downslope of the curve which can be quantitated (Jones, 1979). Functional imaging, on the other hand, enables one to visualize the shunt and thereby determine its location. However, imaging is dependent upon processing those frames of data obtained when flow through the defect is maximum. For example, in an atrial septal defect (ASD) maximum flow occurs during late systole and early diastole. Data processed from this portion of the cardiac cycle shows changing counts in the area of the defect, often producing a definite abnormality in the rate and transit time images.

Atrial septal defect

The ASD may be a significant clinical problem in the adult population and is often misdiagnosed as mitral valve disease. RNV studies can be helpful in differentiation as well as assessing RV function. RVEF is often increased in patients with ASD when compared to the normal population but may fall significantly following surgical repair of the defect (Konstam et al., 1983). Liberthson et al. (1981) found a close correlation between RV function and the clinical course in 20 patients undergoing ASD repair. This study concludes that nuclear imaging appears to be helpful in assessing the older symptomatic adult. Figure 19.14 shows excellent RV function in a 44-year-old female with an ASD (Case 12). Cardiac catheterization revealed a left to right shunt of 2.25:1 with a systolic pulmonary artery pressure of 44 mmHg and a mean wedge pressure of 7 mmHg.

Ventricular septal defect

The ventricular septal defect is less common in the adult population but can be evaluated by RNV.

Figure 19.15 is an example of a VSD in a 20-year-old female (Case 13). The shunt itself is visualized in the upper portion of the interventricular septum and is seen in the rate and mean transit time images of the RV. Superimposition of the right and left ventricles can be made with black and white transparencies as illustrated in this case. Normal right heart pressures were found at cardiac catheterization. There is evidence that lifelong volume overload may be detrimental to myocardial function (Jablonsky et al., 1983), and radionuclide evaluation of the right heart may be helpful in evaluating these patients.

MASS LESIONS

In addition to intrinsic and functional abnormalities of the RV, intrinsic and extrinsic masses can distort the contour of the RV and affect function. Case 14 (Figure 19.16), a 50-year-old male transferred from an outside hospital with intermittent chest pain and dyspnoea, was felt to have LV failure secondary to CAD. RNV shows LVEF of 42% and RVEF of 29%. A filling defect in the RV cavity is seen as an area where counts do not change in the REFI, second half REFI and rate images. A similar finding was seen with two-dimensional echocardiography. Cardiac catheterization showed a completely occluded RCA, subtotal occlusion of the circumflex branch of the LCA, and a mass in the RV cavity with the same contour as the defect seen by RNV. This was confirmed at cardiac catheterization to be a large thrombus and the source of multiple pulmonary emboli.

Case 15 (Figure 19.17), in contrast, shows a large contour defect of the inferior wall of the RV. Presenting symptoms were peripheral oedema, fatigue and dyspnoea with mild exertion. There was a previous history of rheumatic pericarditis. Contrast enhanced two-dimensional echocardiography showed narrowing of the RV inflow. The same finding was found at cardiac catheterization, and at surgery, an old organized pericardial thrombus was successfully removed. Indentation of the floor of the RV is seen in the RNV functional images with relative preservation of wall motion and global function (RVEF = 60%).

SUMMARY

The above cases represent only a small sample of interesting applications of right heart evaluation by first pass RNV. There is a great deal of physiology which can be learned from these non-invasive studies which may prove helpful in patient management. Hopefully, automation and more rapid data processing will make right heart evaluation a part of the routine examination in the future.

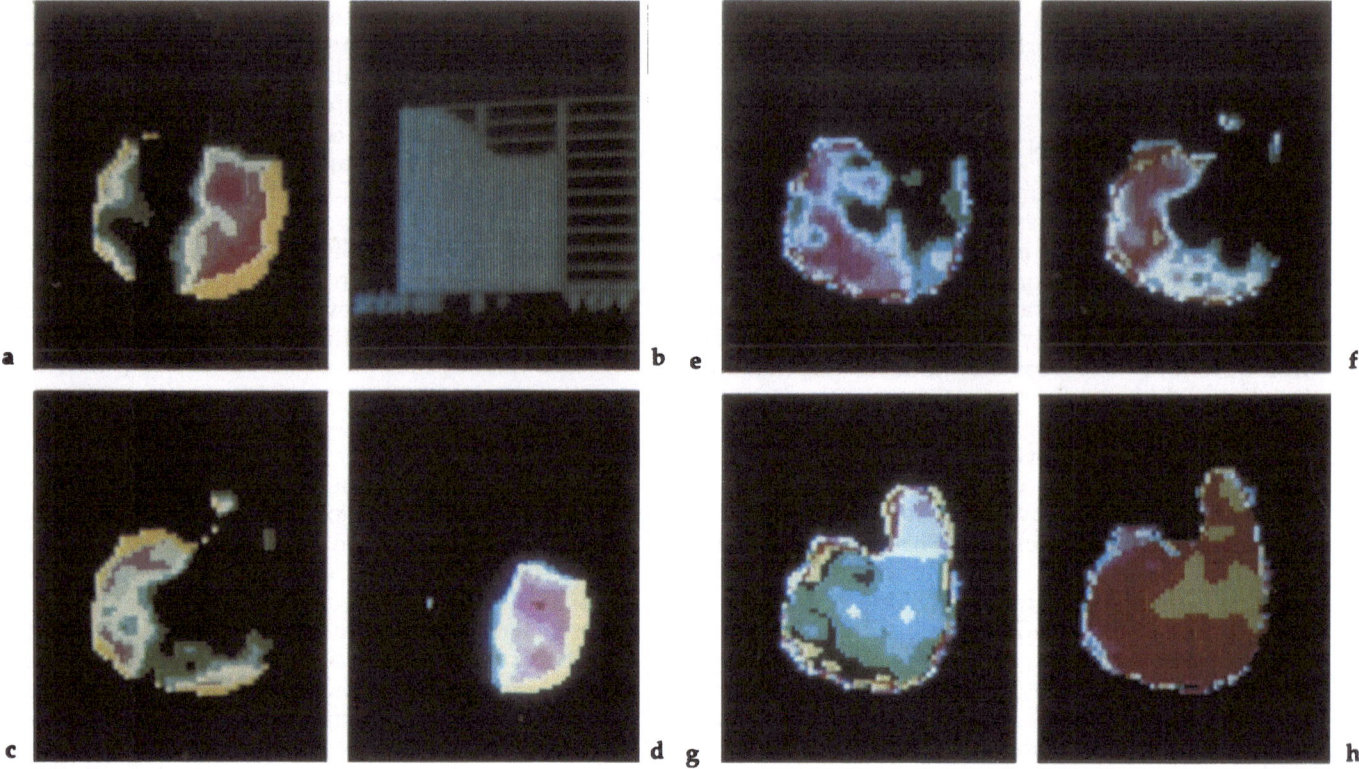

Figure 19.1 *Case 1. Acute pulmonary hypertension.* Symptoms of severe congestive heart failure unresponsive to therapy. Cardiac catheterization revealed severe pulmonary hypertension, IHSS, and normal coronary arteries. Electrocardiogram: 2:1 AV block. Rest anterior RVEF 26%. Images showed diffuse wall motion changes with all images abnormal. Pulmonary transit time was 19 s. **a**, REFI; **b**, volume curve; **c**, first half REFI; **d**, second half REFI; **e**, rejection rate; **f**, first half ER; **g**, transit; **h**, first half transit.

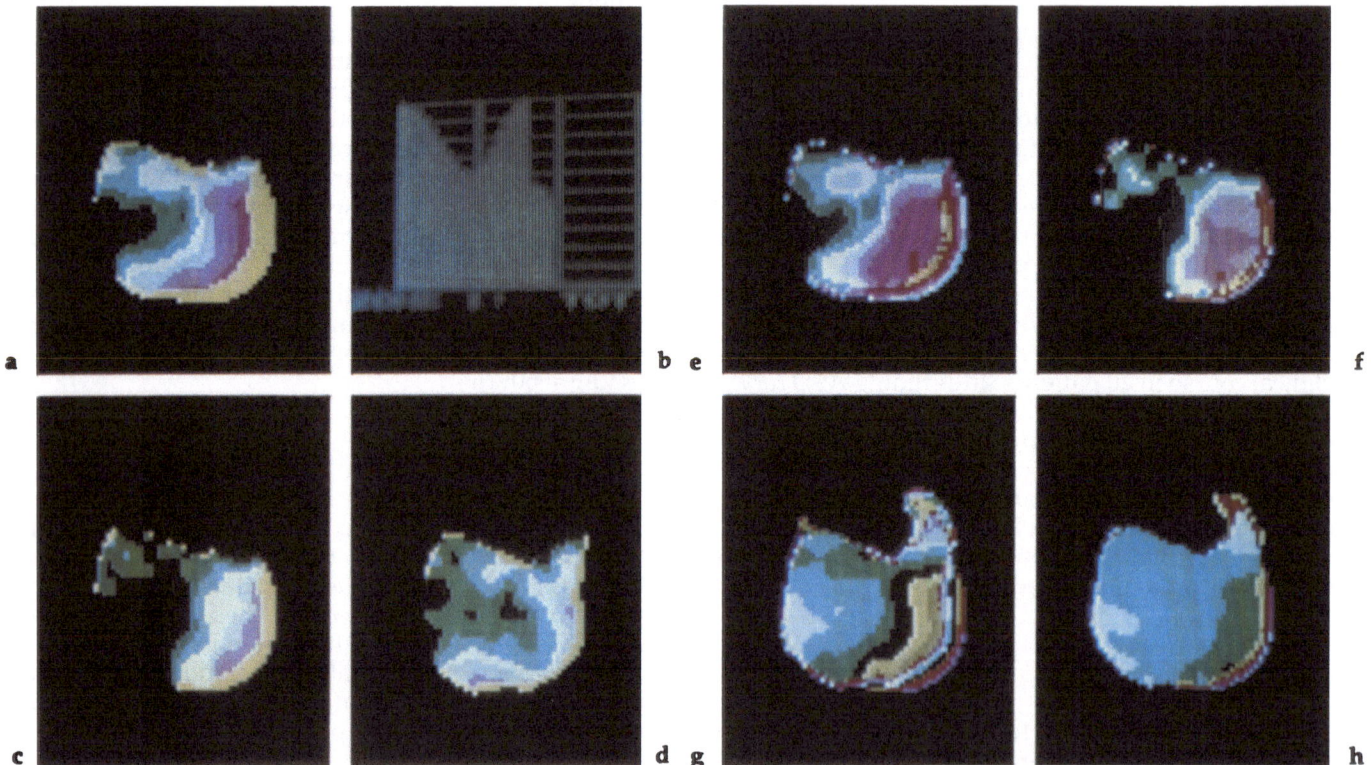

Figure 19.2 *Case 1.* Rest, anterior, RVEF 45%. Follow-up study after medical management and cardiac pacing. Images show marked improvement in wall motion. Pulmonary transit time decreased to 6 seconds. Pulmonary artery pressures have returned to normal. **a**, REFI; **b**, volume curve; **c**, first half REFI; **d**, second half REFI; **e**, rejection rate; **f**, first half ER; **g**, transit; **h**, first half transit.

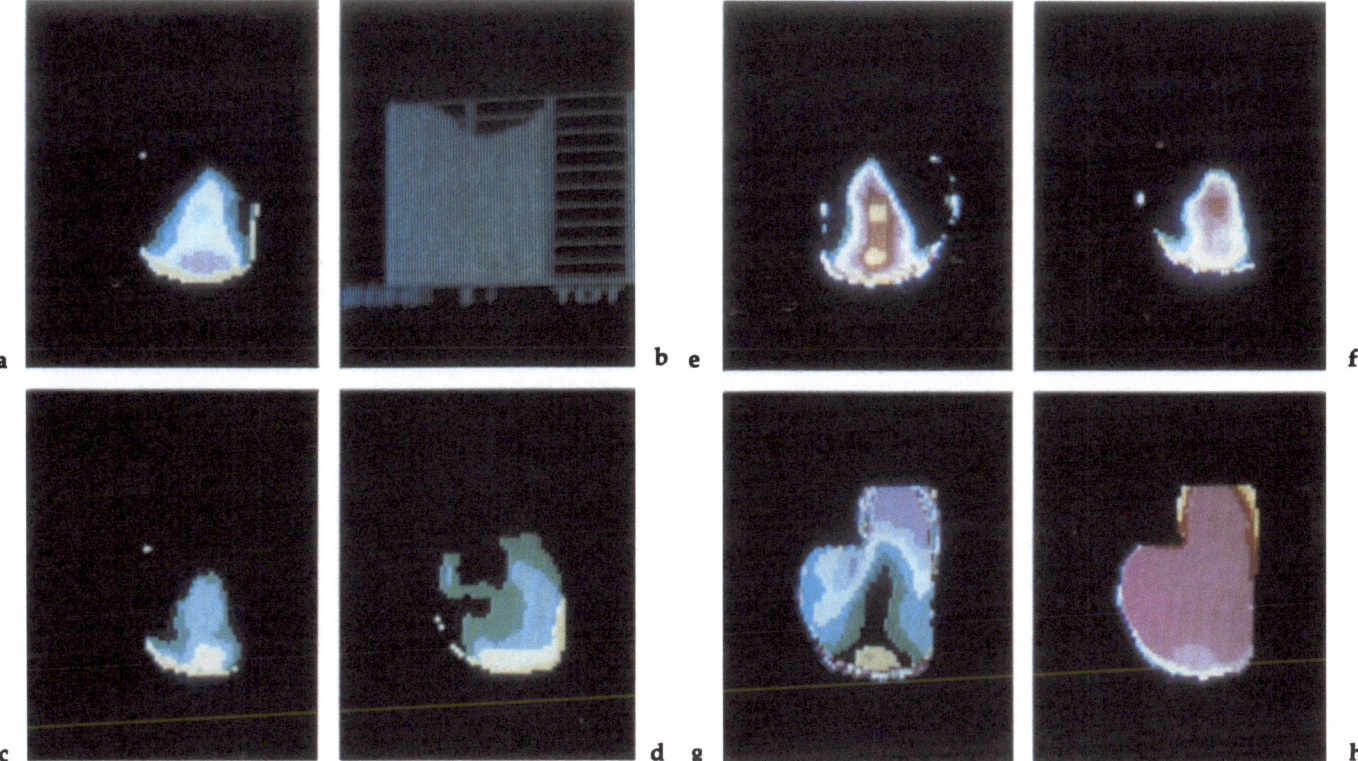

Figure 19.3 *Case 2.* *Ischaemia* (total LAD, 95% RCA) angina and dyspnoea with recent myocardial infarction. Rest, anterior, LVEF 30%, RVEF 35%. Images show diffuse abnormality but most pronounced during early systole. This is consistent with right ventricular ischaemia. **a,** REFI; **b,** volume curve; **c,** first half REFI; **d,** second half REFI; **e,** rejection rate; **f,** first half ER; **g,** transit; **h,** first half transit.

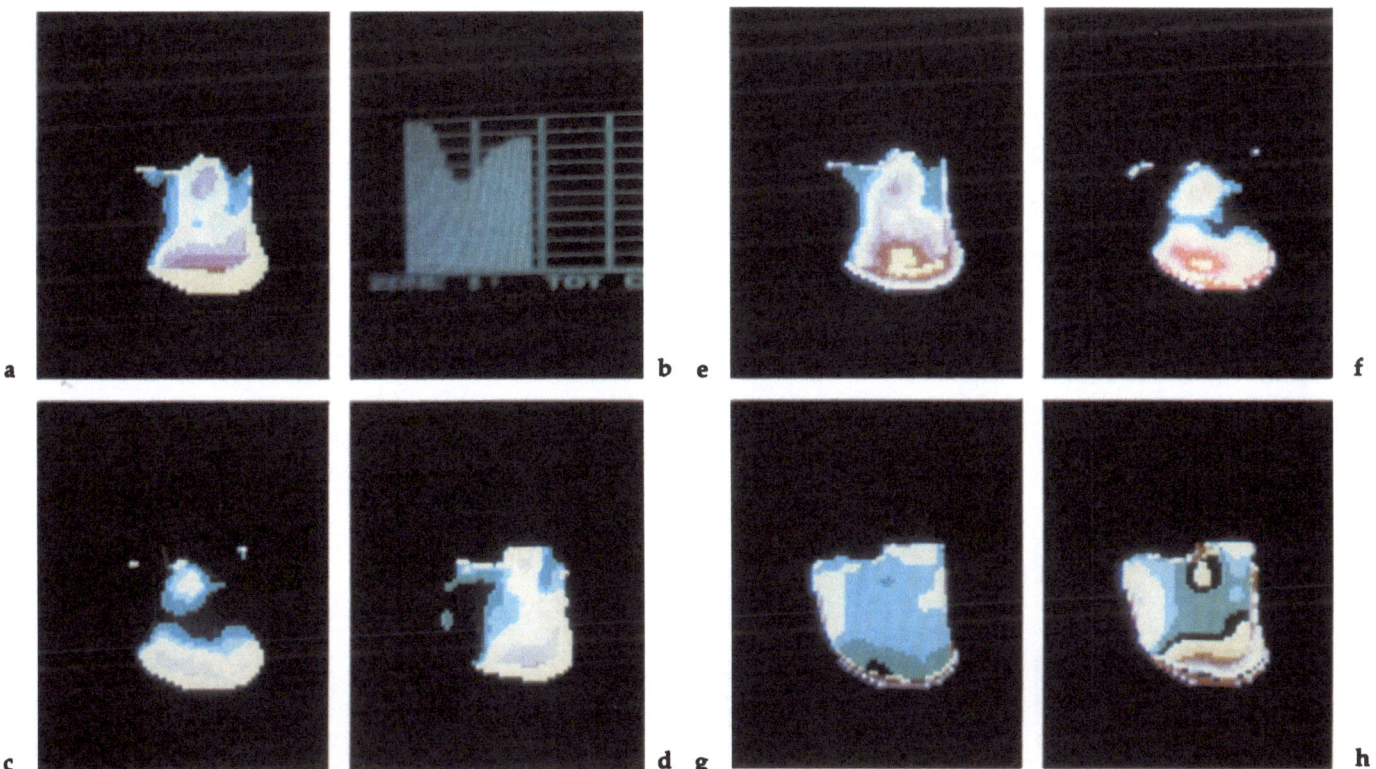

Figure 19.4 *Case 3.* *Ischaemia* (total left main coronary). Congestive failure and probable recent myocardial infarction. Cardiac catheterization revealed total occlusion of the left main coronary artery and 50% narrowing of the RCA. LVEF 17%, RVEF 45%. Global function as well as wall motion is relatively well preserved with images more indicative of pulmonary hypertension than ischaemia in contrast to Figure 19.3. **a,** REFI; **b,** volume curve; **c,** first half REFI; **d,** second half REFI; **e,** rejection rate; **f,** first half ER; **g,** transit; **h,** first half transit.

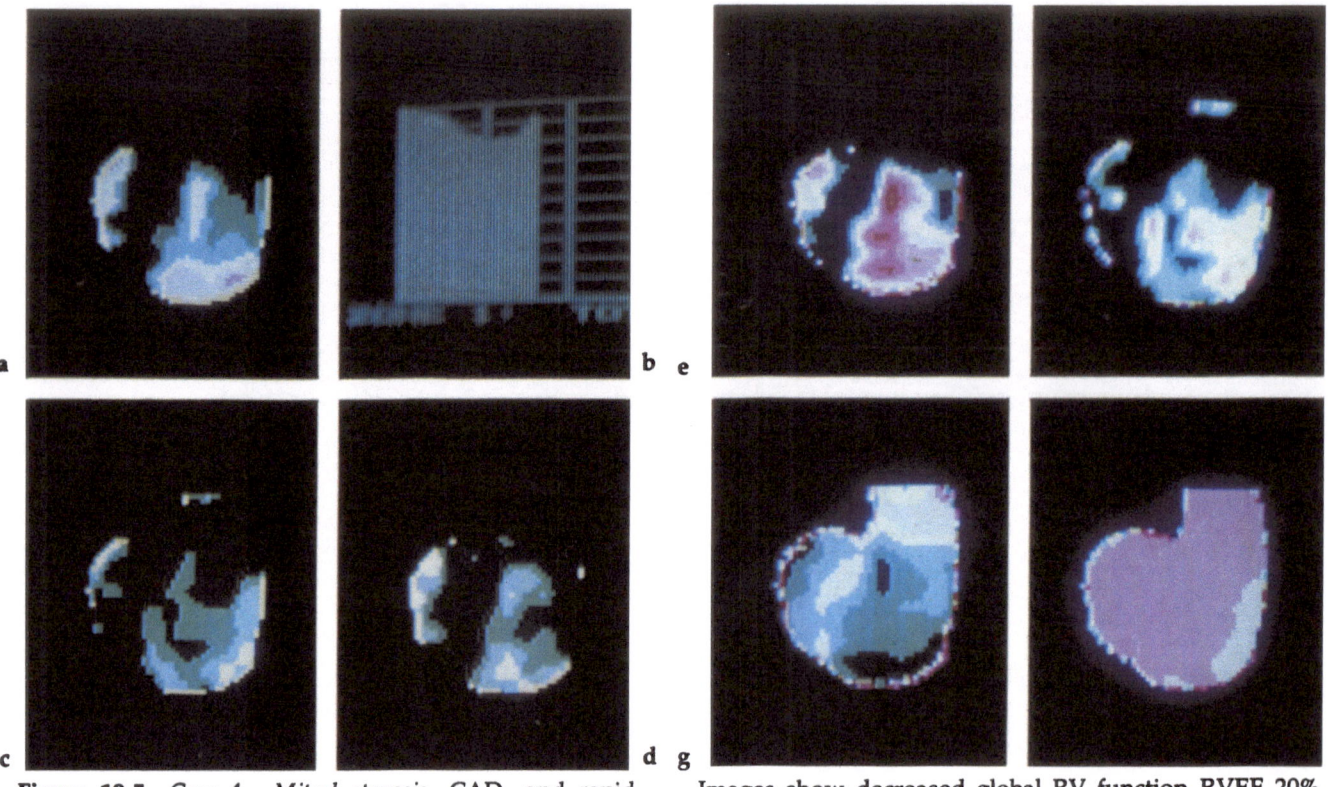

Figure 19.5 *Case 4.* *Mitral stenosis*, CAD, and rapid atrial fibrillation with pulmonary oedema. Cardiac catheterization revealed mitral valve areas 0.7 cm². Main pulmonary artery pressure 80 mmHg with a mean wedge pressure of 35 mmHg and 75% narrowing of the mid LAD.

Images show decreased global RV function RVEF 20%, LVEF 48%. RV is enlarged with diffuse wall motion changes consistent with pulmonary hypertension. **a**, REFI; **b**, volume curve; **c**, first half REFI; **d**, second half REFI; **e**, rejection rate; **f**, first half ER; **g**, transit; **h**, first half transit.

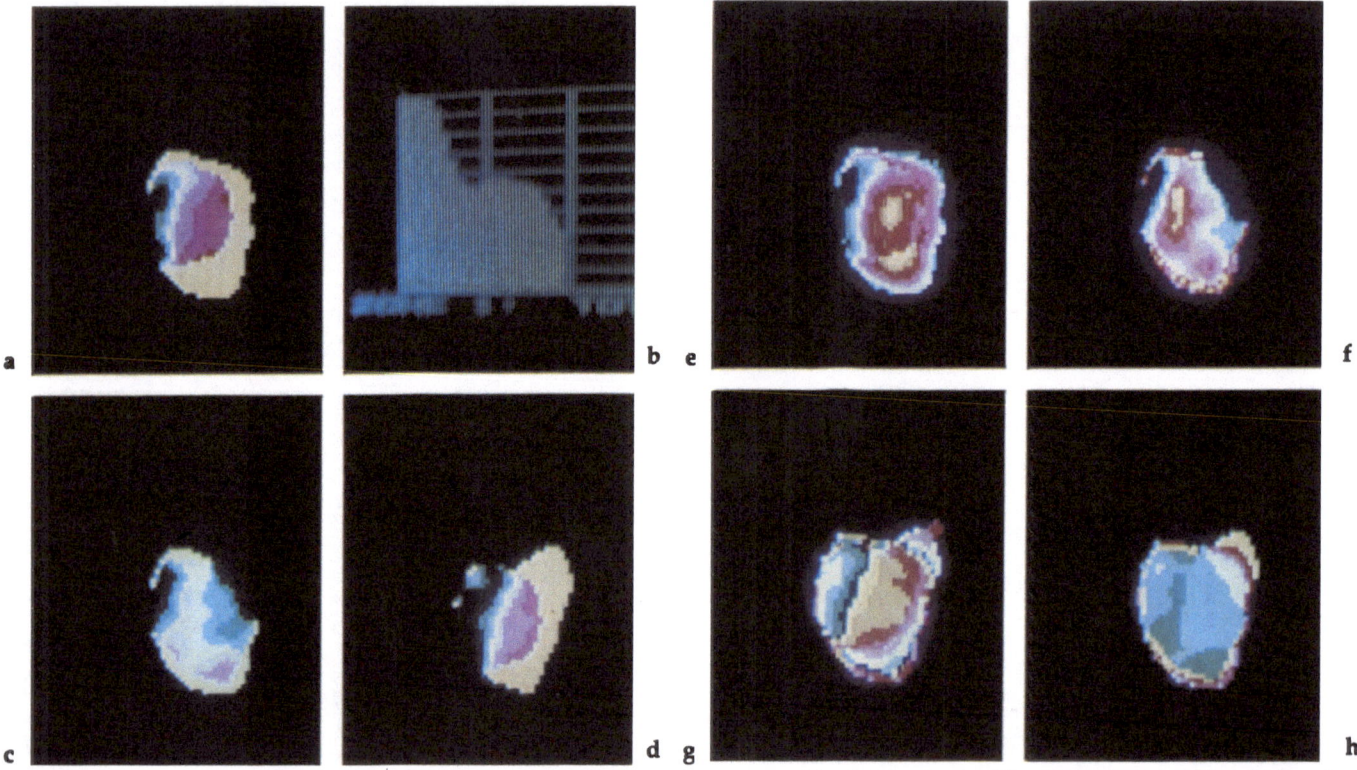

Figure 19.6 *Case 5.* *Mitral regurgitation*, symptomatic. Cardiac catheterization reveals 4+ mitral regurgitation with a left atrial dilatation and main pulmonary artery pressure 27 mmHg with wedge pressure 10 mmHg. Global function as well as wall motion is relatively well

preserved in this patient with relatively normal right heart pressures in spite of severe MR. **a**, REFI; **b**, volume curve; **c**, first half REFI; **d**, second half REFI; **e**, rejection rate; **f**, first half ER; **g**, transit; **h**, first half transit.

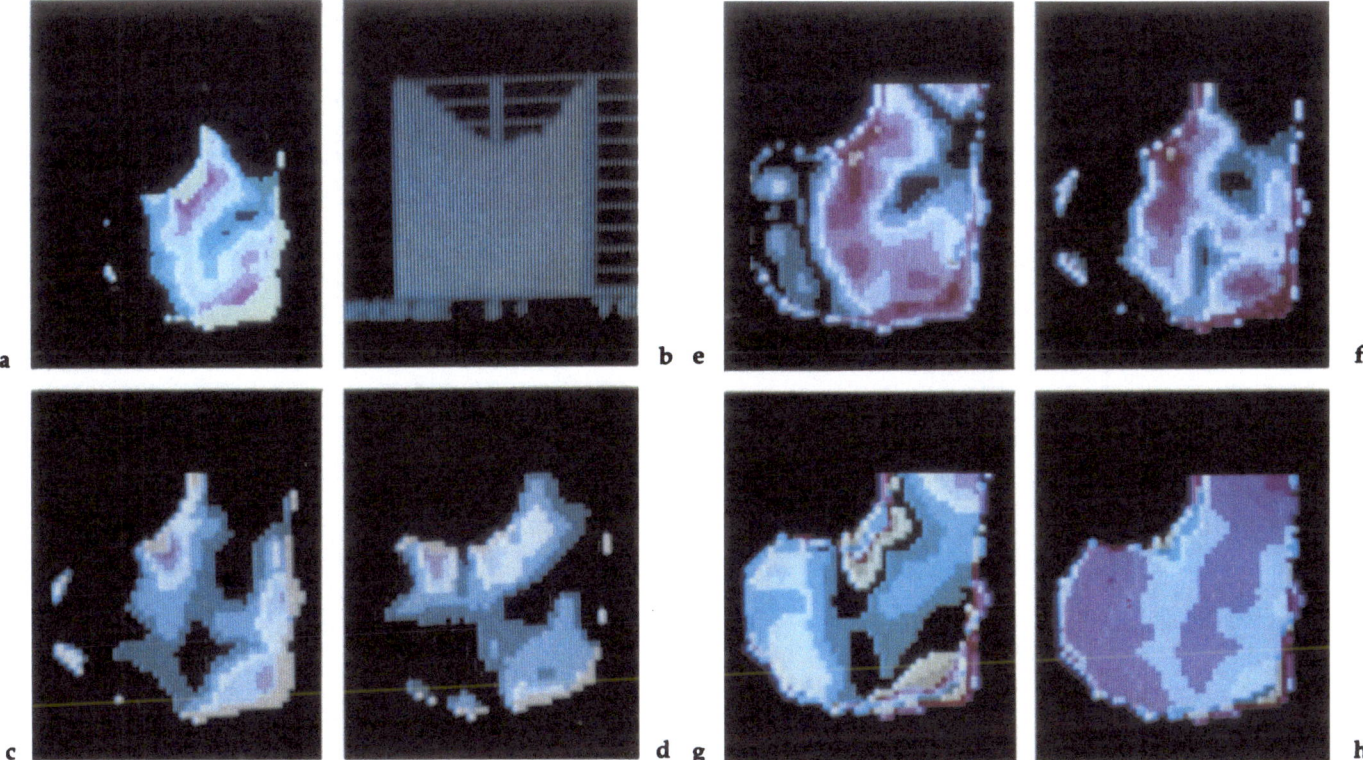

Figure 19.7 *Case 6. Aortic stenosis.* Normal coronary arteries with previous aortic valve replacement known to be malfunctioning. Rest, anterior, LVEF 32%, RVEF 30%, main pulmonary systolic pressure 65 mmHg. Mean wedge pressure 25 mmHg, 35 gradient 65 mmHg. Images show decreased global and regional right ventricular function related to pulmonary hypertension. **a**, REFI; **b**, volume curve; **c**, first half REFI; **d**, second half REFI; **e**, rejection rate; **f**, first half ER; **g**, transit; **h**, first half transit.

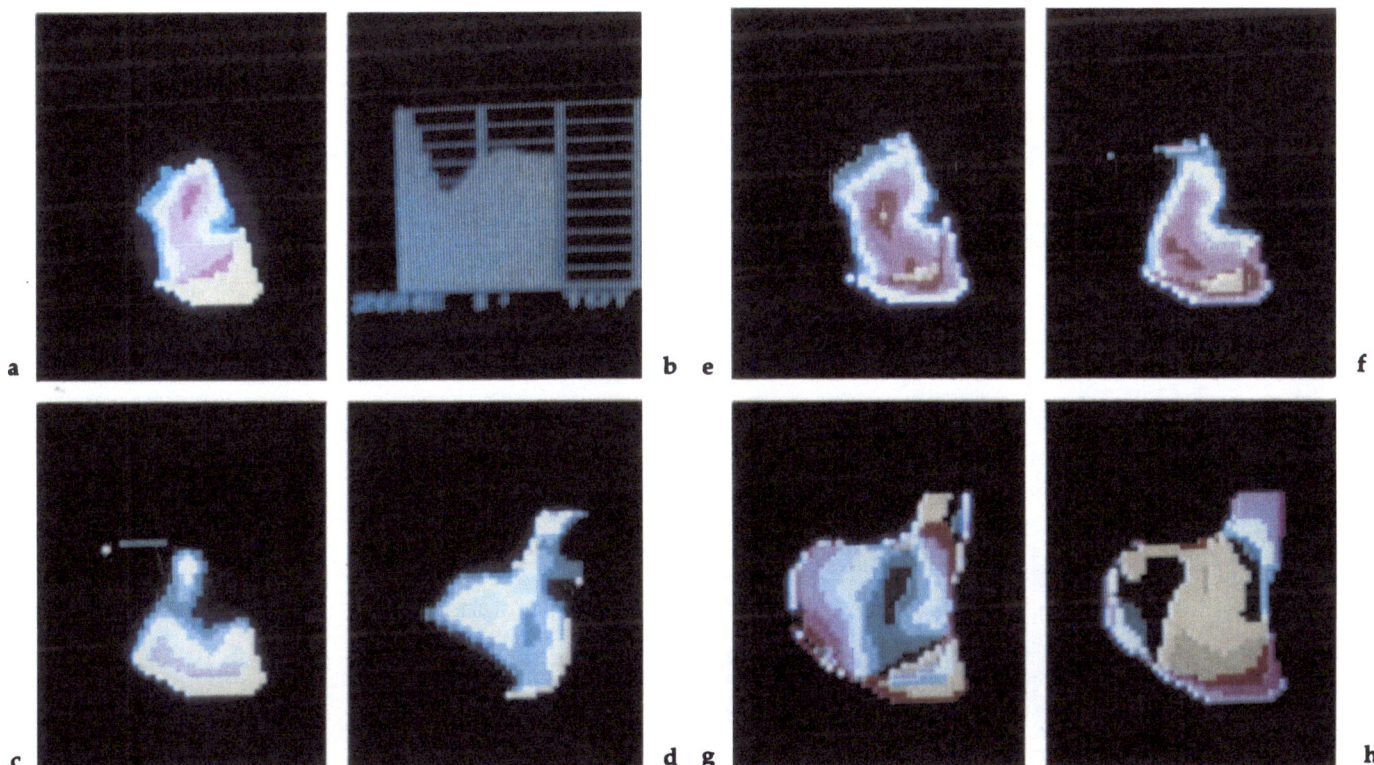

Figure 19.8 *Case 7. Aortic regurgitation.* Mild CAD (40% RCA). Dyspnoea on exertion 4+ aortic insufficiency, pulmonary artery systolic pressure 25 mmHg, mean wedge pressure 8 mmHg. Rest, anterior, LVEF 49%, RVEF 40%. Images show relative preservation of global and regional function in this patient with relatively normal pulmonary pressures in contrast to the previous case. **a**, REFI; **b**, volume curve; **c**, first half REFI; **d**, second half REFI; **e**, rejection rate; **f**, first half ER; **g**, transit; **h**, first half transit.

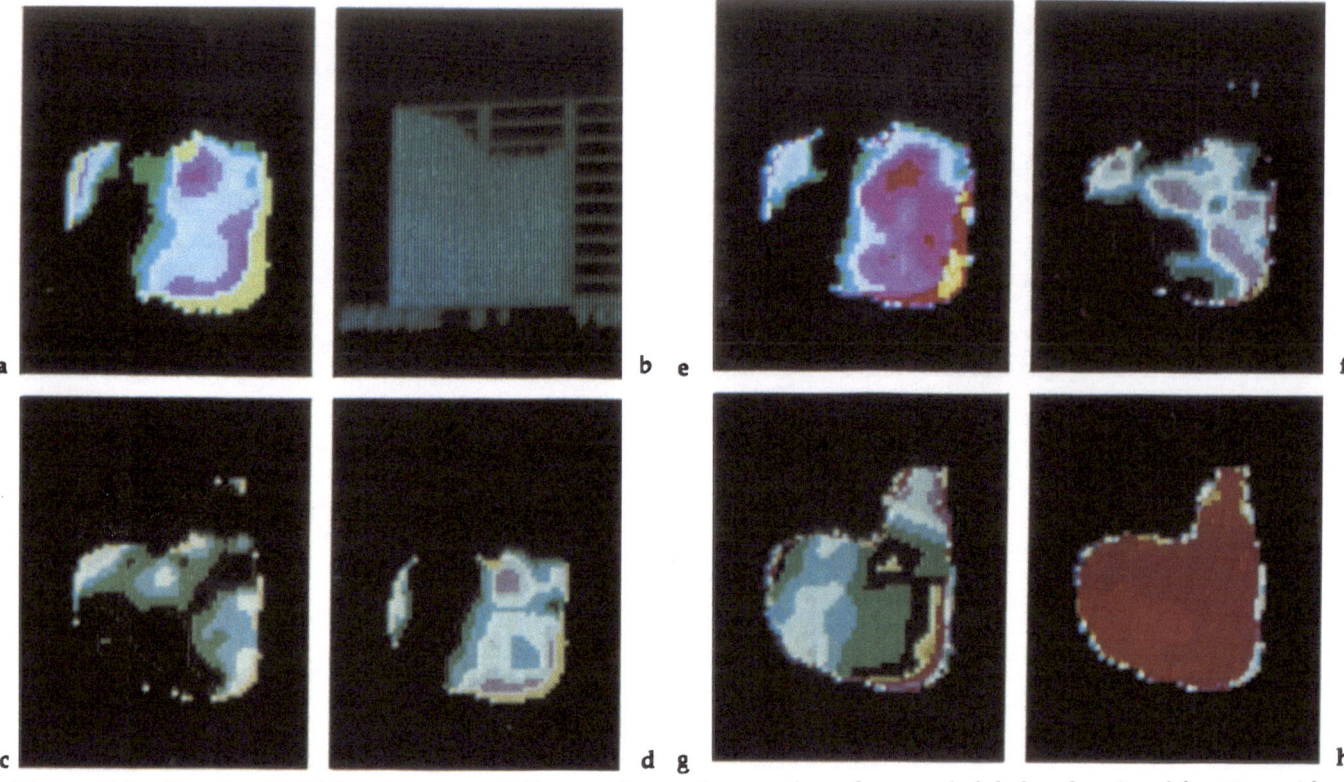

Figure 19.9 *Case 8.* *Multiple pulmonary emboli,* normal coronary arteries, symptoms of congestive heart failure. Catheterization revealed normal coronary arteries and pulmonary artery pressure 55 mmHg, wedge pressure 16 mmHg. Pulmonary angiogram revealed multiple pulmonary emboli. Rest, anterior, LVEF 61%, RVEF 30%.

Images show decreased global and regional function with tricuspid regurgitation consistent with pulmonary hypertension. **a,** REFI; **b,** volume curve; **c,** first half REFI; **d,** second half REFI; **e,** rejection rate; **f,** first half ER; **g,** transit; **h,** first half transit.

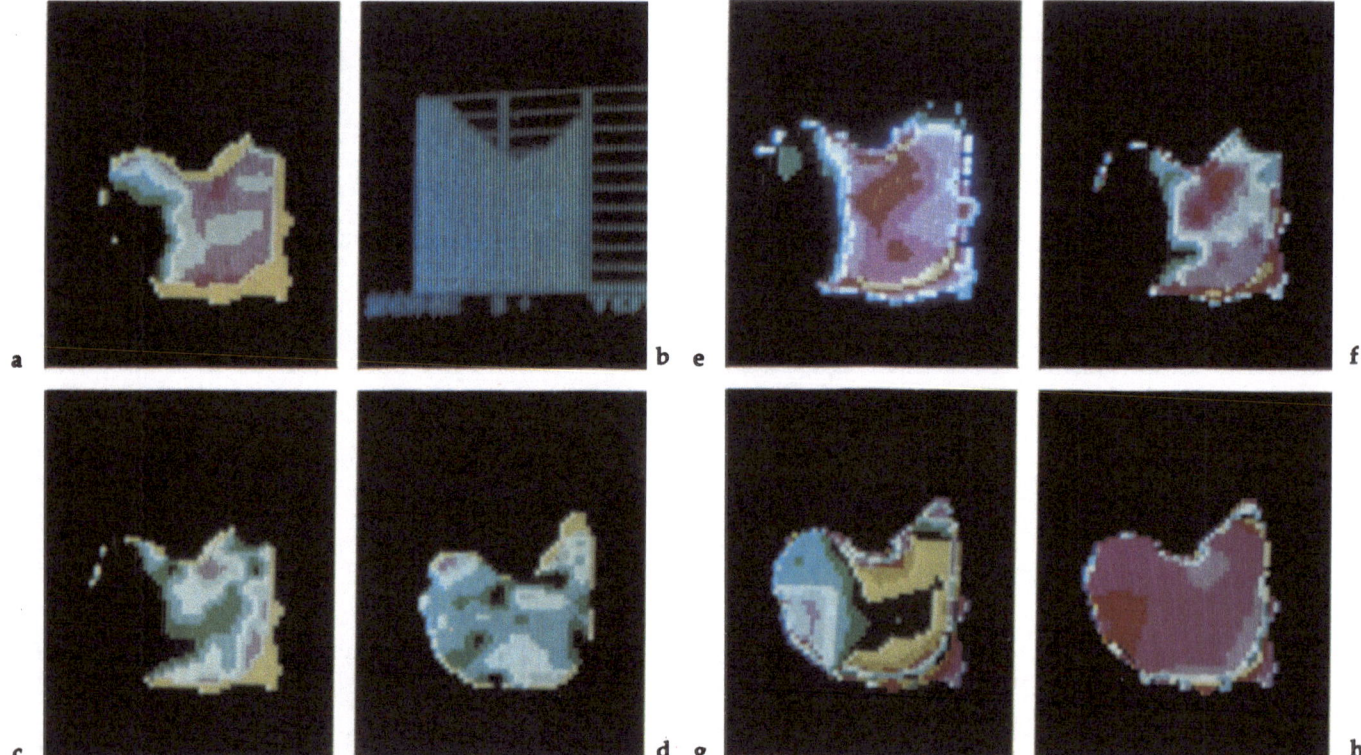

Figure 19.10 *Case 8.* *Multiple pulmonary emboli,* exercise, anterior, LVEF 63%, RVEF 35%. Function does improve slightly with exercise but images reflect pulmonary hypertension secondary to multiple pulmonary emboli. **a,**

REFI; **b,** volume curve; **c,** first half REFI; **d,** second half REFI; **e,** rejection rate; **f,** first half ER; **g,** transit; **h,** first half transit.

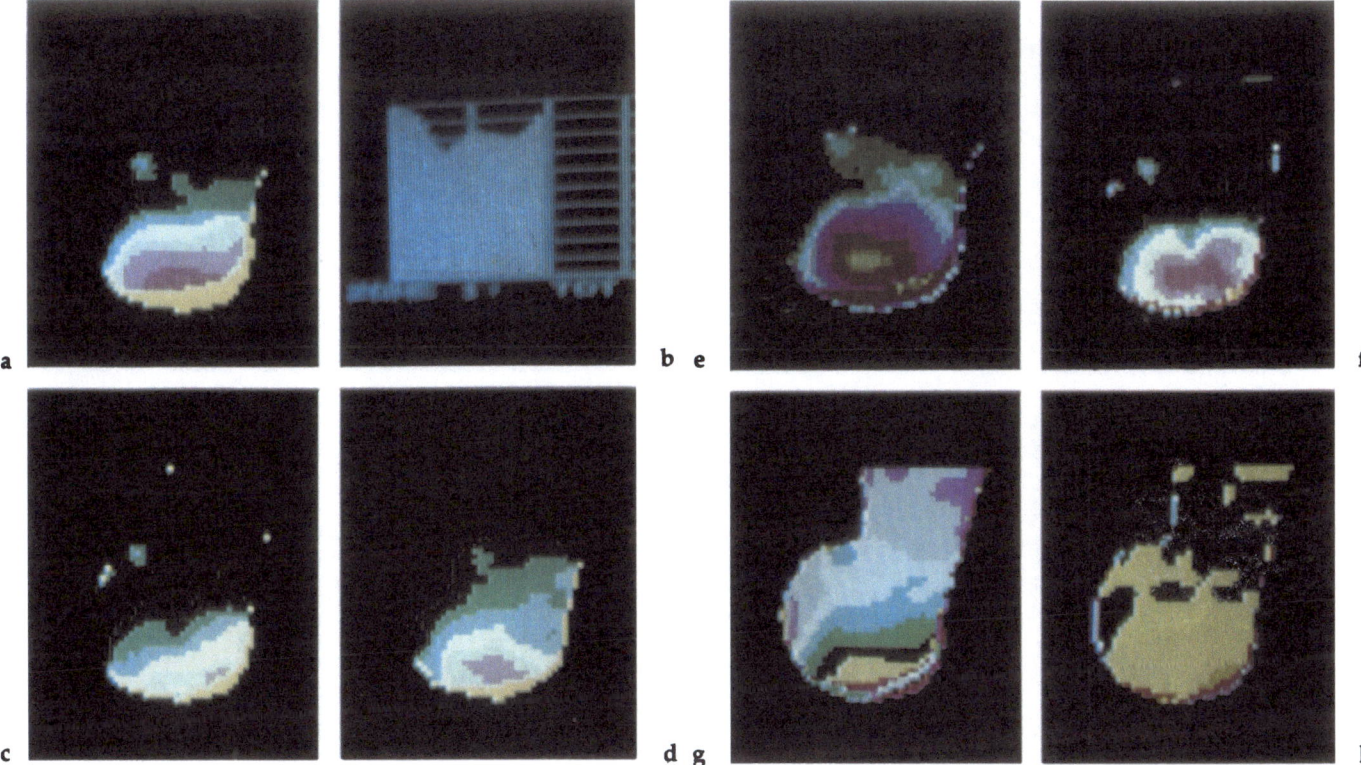

Figure 19.11 *Case 9. COPD,* chest pain with left pneumothorax. Rest, anterior, LVEF 30%, RVEF 16%. Pulmonary transit time 7.5 seconds. Images show only mild diffuse wall motion changes in spite of severely decreased global function. **a,** REFI; **b,** volume curve; **c,** first half REFI; **d,** second half REFI; **e,** rejection rate; **f,** first half ER; **g,** transit; **h,** first half transit.

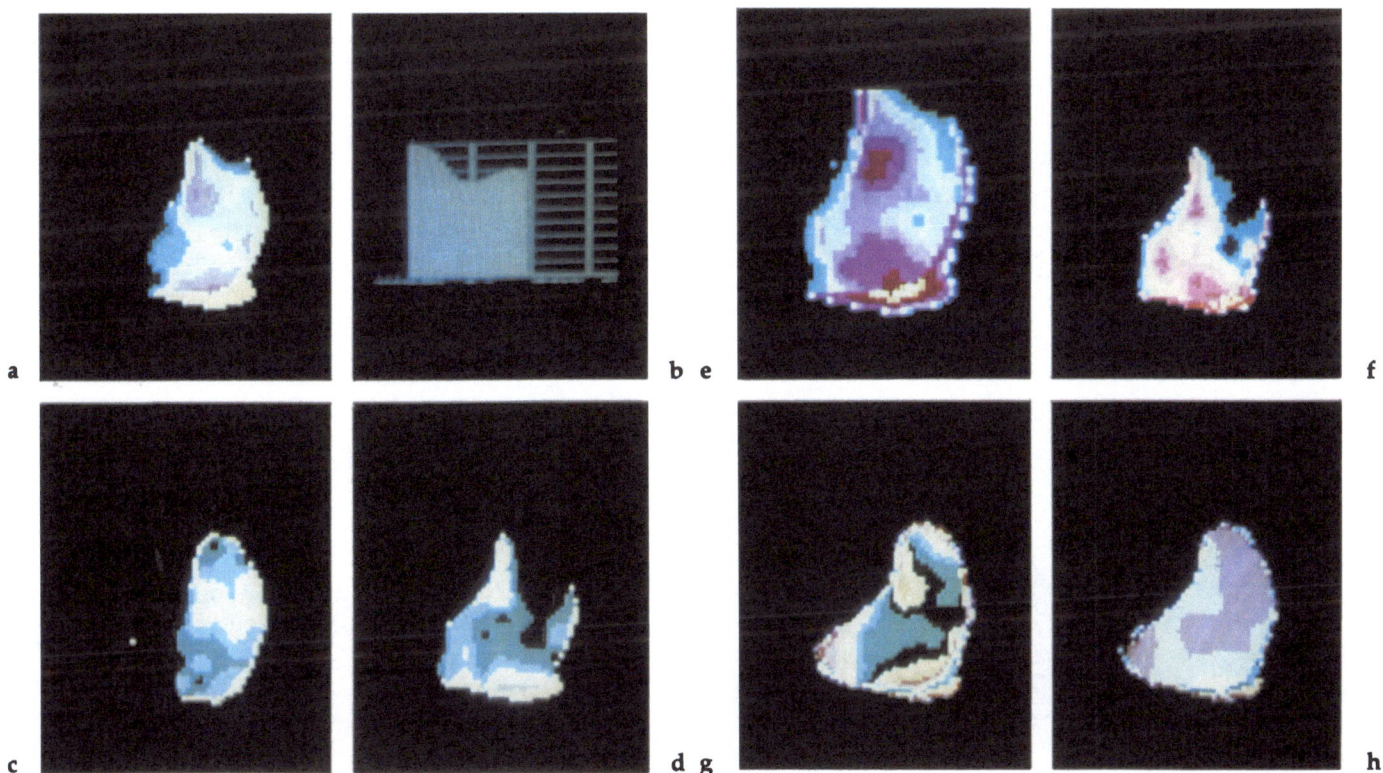

Figure 19.12 *Case 10. Bullous emphysema,* symptoms of congestive failure and COPD. Rest, anterior, LVEF 61%, RVEF 36%. There are diffuse wall motion changes which are relatively mild but compatible with pulmonary venous hypertension. **a,** REFI; **b,** volume curve; **c,** first half REFI; **d,** second half REFI; **e,** rejection rate; **f,** first half ER; **g,** transit; **h,** first half transit.

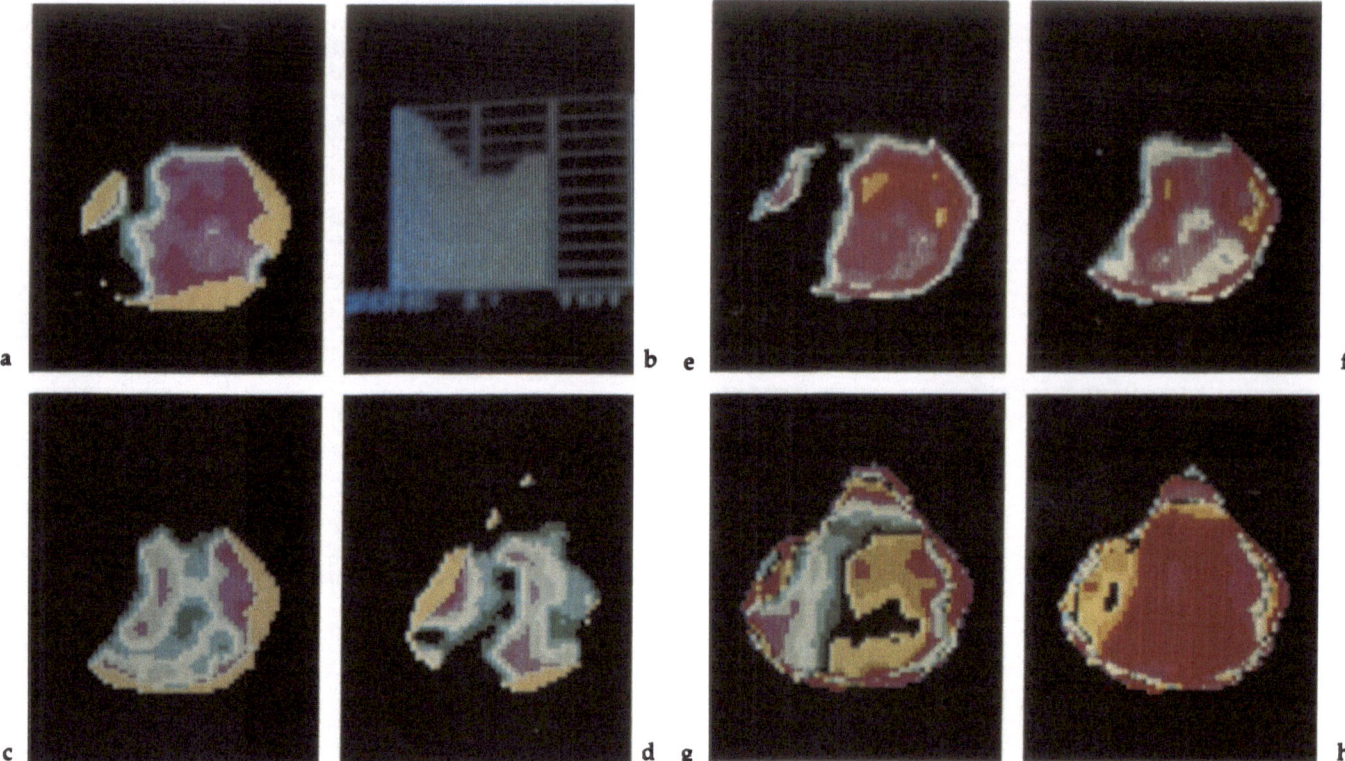

Figure 19.13 *Case 11. Tricuspid insufficiency*, intermittent tachycardia, but otherwise asymptomatic, rest, anterior, RVEF 37%, LVEF 38%. Images show enlarged right ventricle with diffuse wall motion changes and tri-

cuspid insufficiency. **a,** REFI; **b,** volume curve; **c,** first half REFI; **d,** second half REFI; **e,** rejection rate; **f,** first half ER; **g,** transit; **h,** first half transit.

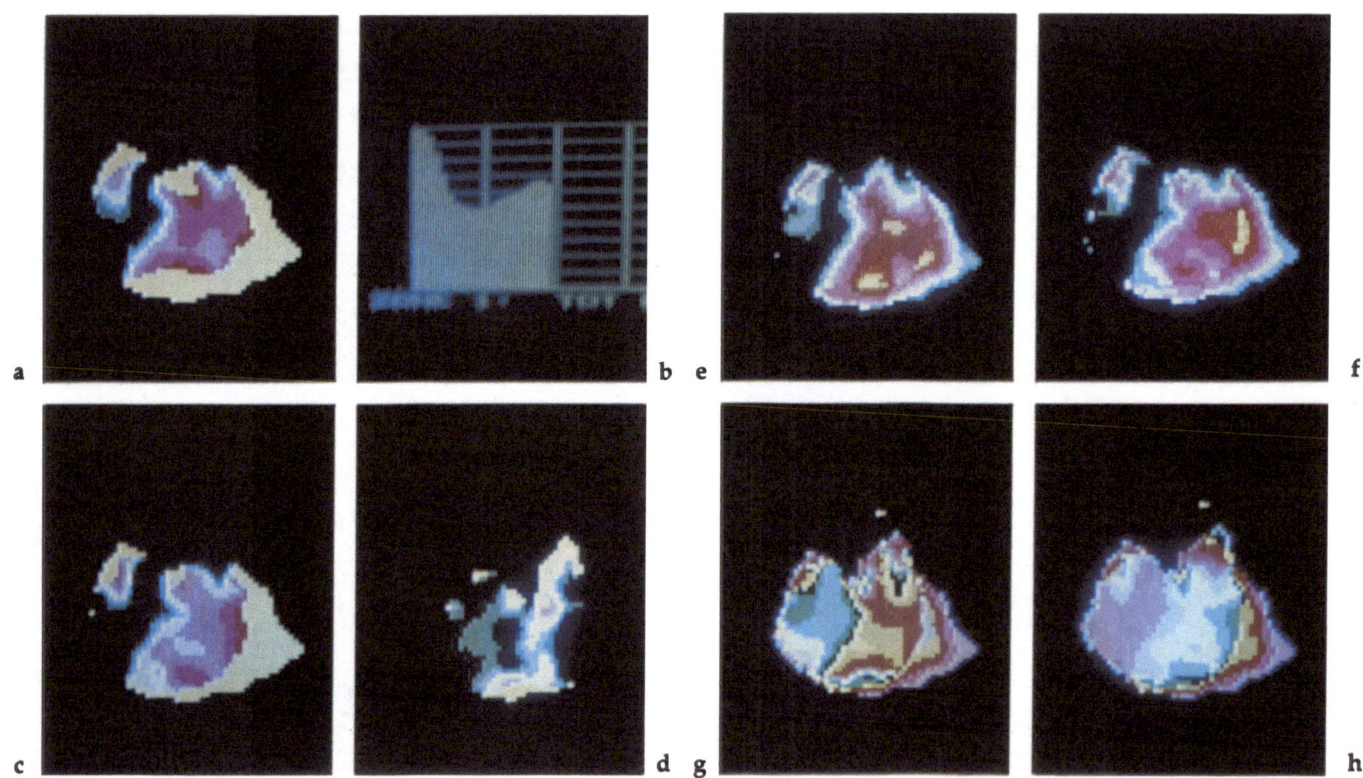

Figure 19.14 *Case 12. Atrial septal defect*, normal coronary arteries. Left to right shunt 2.25:1 with main pulmonary artery systolic pressure 42 mmHg with mean pressure 25 mmHg and wedge pressure 7 mmHg. Rest, anterior, LVEF 34%, RVEF 50%. Images reflect pulmonary

hypertension but with relative preservation of global function LV was more severely affected by volume overload in this patient. **a,** REFI; **b,** volume curve; **c,** first half REFI; **d,** second half REFI; **e,** rejection rate; **f,** first half ER; **g,** transit; **h,** first half transit.

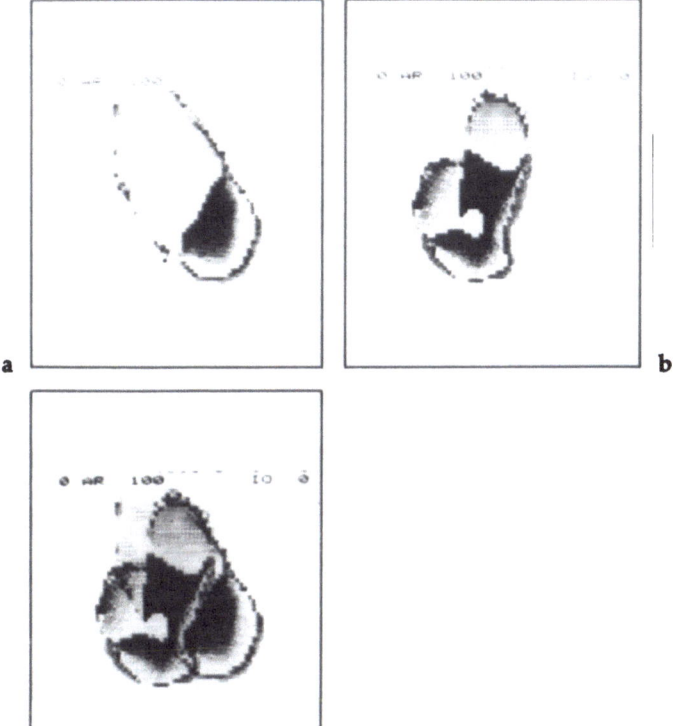

Figure 19.15 *Case 13.* *VSD* without associated aortic regurgitation. Exercise LV and RV are shown as well as superimposition of RV and LV using transparent overlays. The last image is the mean transit image showing small central area in the region of the septum where there was no count change. This correlated well with surgical location of the VSD. Global function is preserved. LVEF 63%, RVEF 58%. **a,** left ventricle; **b,** right ventricle; **c,** superimposed RV and LV.

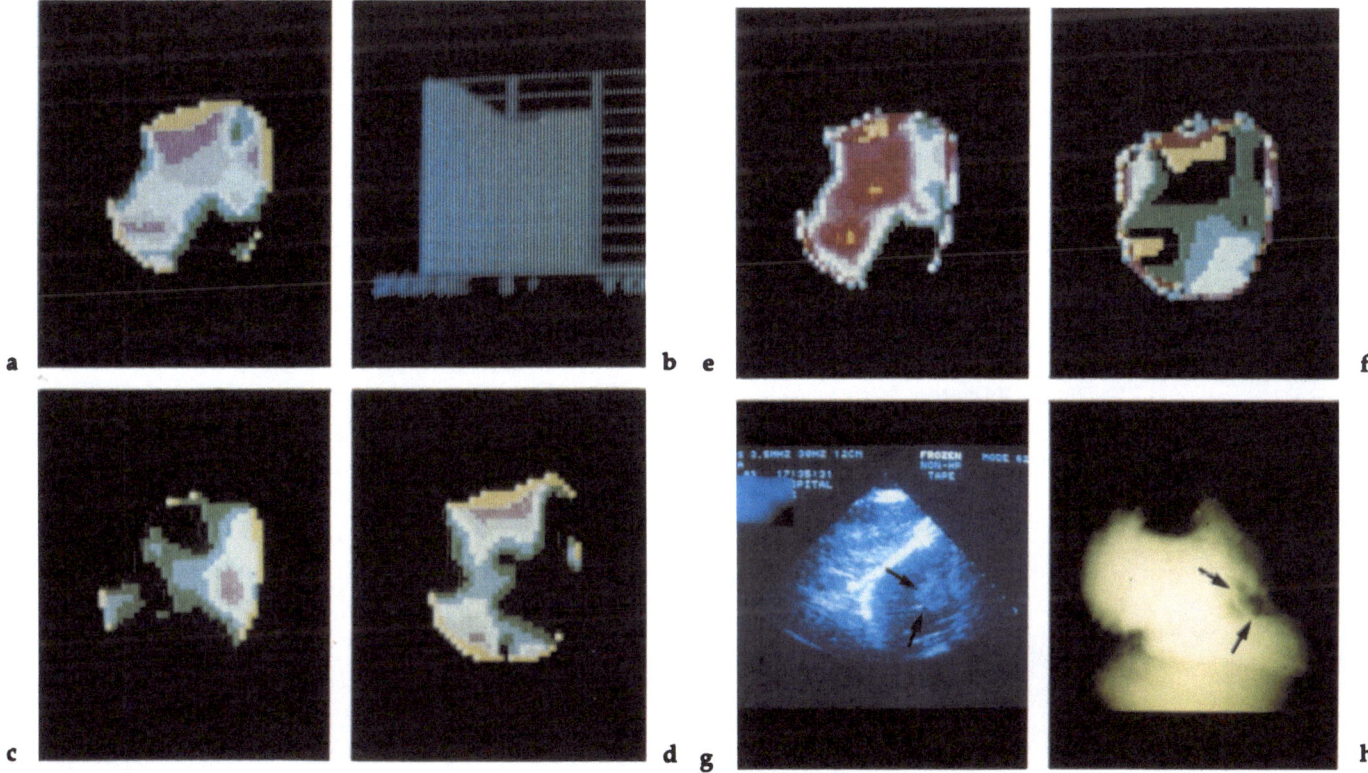

Figure 19.16 *Case 14.* RV thrombus. Symptoms of chest pain and shortness of breath. Cardiac catheterization revealed large filling defect in the RV. There was complete occlusion of the RCA and total occlusion of the circumflex with normal LAD. Rest anterior LVEF 42%, RVEF 20%. REFI, first and second half REFI and rate images showing an abnormality in the inferior aspect of the RV. Echocardiographic findings and angiographic findings correlate well. **a,** REFI; **b,** volume curve; **c,** first half REFI; **d,** second half REFI; **e,** ejection rate; **f,** transit; **g,** echocardiogram; **h,** RV angiogram.

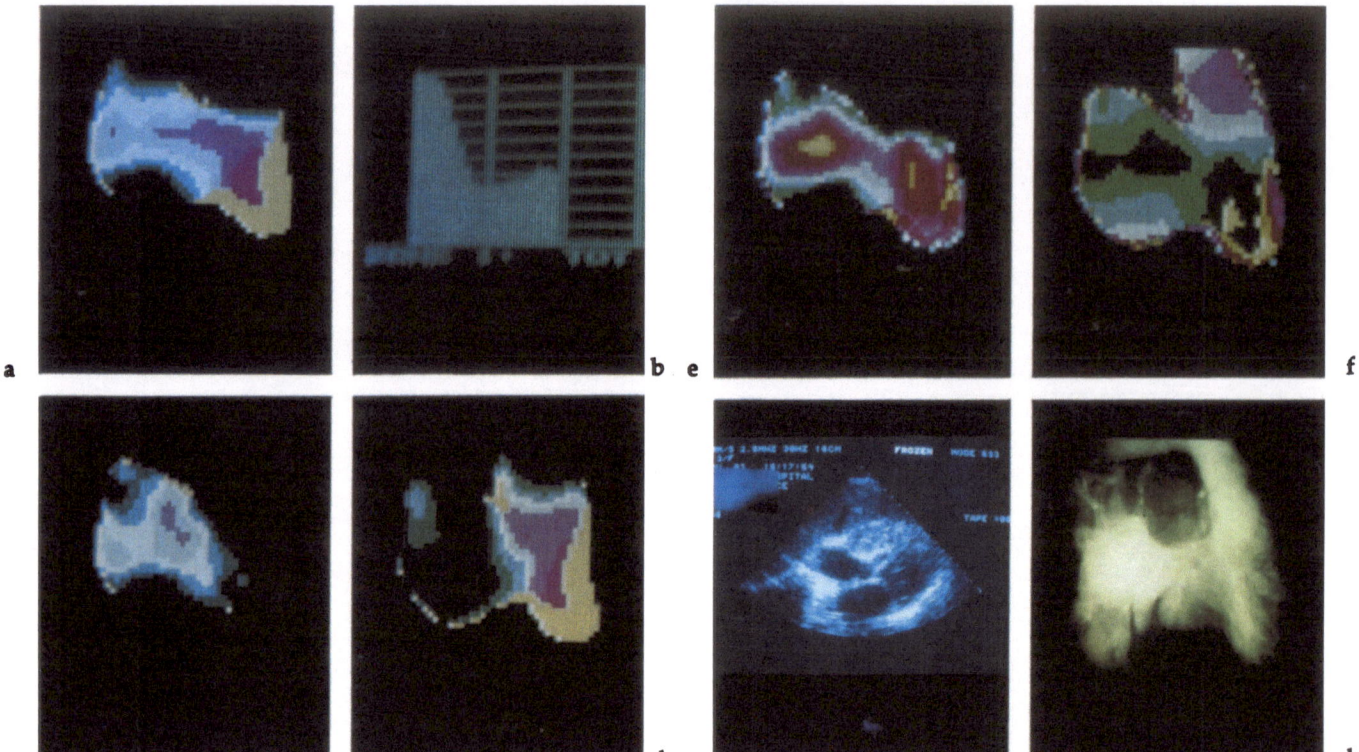

a   b   e   f

c   d   g   h

Figure 19.17 *Case 15. Extrinsic mass*, normal coronary arteries, shortness of breath, anterior, LVEF 46%, RVEF 40%. Images show a large extrinsic contour defect on the inferior aspect of the right atrium in the region of the RV inflow. Though distorted, RV wall motion remains good. Echocardiographic and angiographic findings show similar changes. **a**, ejection rate right atrium and RV; **b**, transit RA and RV; **c**, echocardiogram; **d**, angiogram.

20

Functional Imaging after Cardiac Transplantation

B. REICHART, N. SCHAD, B. REBLE, B. M. KEMKES, E. KREUZER AND R. HATZ

In the past 3 years cardiac transplantation has made remarkable advances and is now on its way to become a clinically accepted surgical procedure. Soon after the first human heart had been transplanted in 1967, a wave of enthusiasm broke out throughout the medical world. But it was not long before many researchers recognized that numerous problems still had to be solved before acceptable long term results could be achieved. Therefore, many abandoned the method in the following years. However, others like N. E. Shumway and his team at Stanford University in Palo Alto, California continued clinical heart transplantation. They made important contributions concerning the question of donor and recipient selection and developed new methods to recognize early acute rejection, such as endomyocardial biopsy and accurate immunological monitoring of immunosuppressive therapy with corticosteroids, azathioprine and anti-thymocyte-globulin. They also showed that retransplantation is possible.

The discovery of cyclosporin A by Borel *et al.* (1977) and its introduction to clinical use by Sandoz/ Basel in the early 1980s led to a new era in cardiac transplantation. In December 1980 Stanford was the first to use the new immunosuppressive drug in heart transplant cases; cyclosporin A impressively improved short term results.

At present, recipients selected for transplantation are usually in the final stage of cardiac disease. Every other type of conservative medical therapy and conventional surgery such as revascularization procedures and resection of ventricular aneurysms should have been utilized before patients are considered for transplantation.

Most of the transplant candidates suffer from cardiomyopathy. While waiting for transplantation these patients show constant changes in cardiac function and clinical status. There are periods when they are in stable condition and feel fine, whereas at any time they may decompensate. This constant alternation between stable and unstable conditions is a characteristic of this disease. In order to determine the appropriate time for surgery, radionuclide cardiography can be used repeatedly during the preoperative period because it is non-invasive and practically without risk to the patient.

The implantation of the donor's heart usually takes 3–4 hours. The recipient's heart is exposed by a median sternotomy and the arterial cannula of the heart–lung machine is inserted into the ascending aorta. Two cannulae placed into the inferior and superior vena cava provide venous return. During cardiopulmonary bypass the aorta is cross-clamped, and the heart is exercised in a caudo-cranial direction. The lateral right and left atrial walls are incised just ventral to the vena cava and pulmonary veins. The atrial septum is then divided, the pulmonary artery is transected distal to the valvular commissures, and the aorta is transected distal to the coronary ostia. A running suture of the atrial cuffs to the donor heart – which is totally excised – is started at the lateral portion of the left atrial wall and continued through the atrial septum. The anastomosis of the right atrium is performed in the same fashion. Then the great vessel anastomoses are completed.

As mentioned earlier, the introduction of cyclosporin A to clinical immunosuppressive therapy after cardiac transplantation has improved short and long term results impressively. One-year survival rates increased from 65% under conventional immunosuppression to 81% under cyclosporin A medication. In the years following transplantation, however, there may be rapid progression of arteriosclerosis in the transplanted heart's coronary system, especially in the presence of hyperlipidaemia. The precise cause is unknown, but it may be an immunological problem. The rate of progression of this coronary artery disease is alarming: 35% of all transplant recipients are affected seven years postoperatively. Because these patients are without heart innervation, they have no angina pectoris. This is why our patients are controlled on a yearly basis using technetium 99m pertechnetate scintigraphy (Schad, 1978a; Reichart *et al.*, 1982). It gives valuable information in helping to decide if retransplantation has to be performed, and when it should take place.

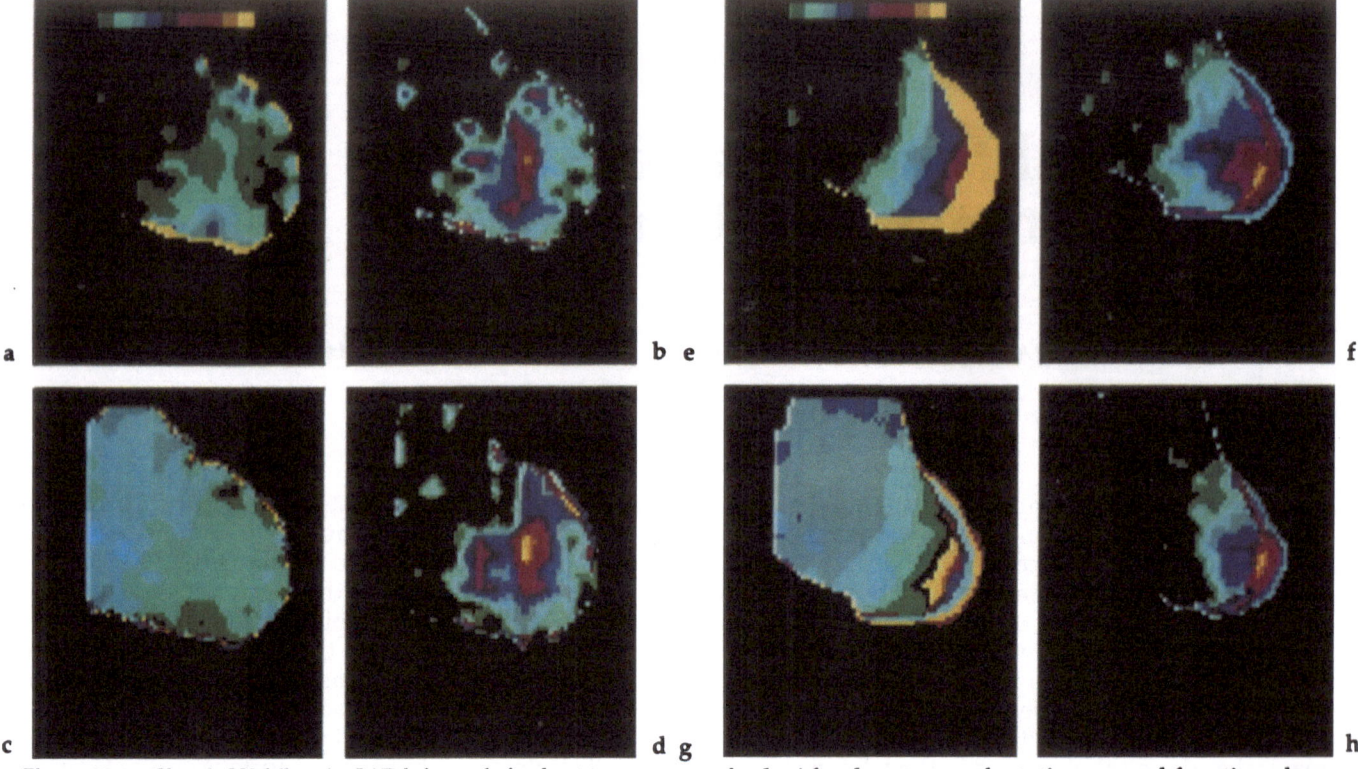

Figure 20.1 *Chronic LV failure in CAD before and after heart transplantation. One year after heart transplantation.*
a,b,c,d, Before transplantation dilated LV with diffusely reduced function, with a minimum along the anterior wall seen on REFI (**a**) and REjR (**b**) images. Very long parietal mean times extending over the entire ventricular cavity (**c**). Rapid filling rates (**d**) reduced along the anterior and inferior wall.

e,f,g,h, After heart transplantation normal function along the anterior wall, dysfunction posteriorly on the REFI (**e**) and REjR (**f**) images as well as on the MTT image (**g**). Rapid filling rates directed to the apex with defect posteriorly (**h**).

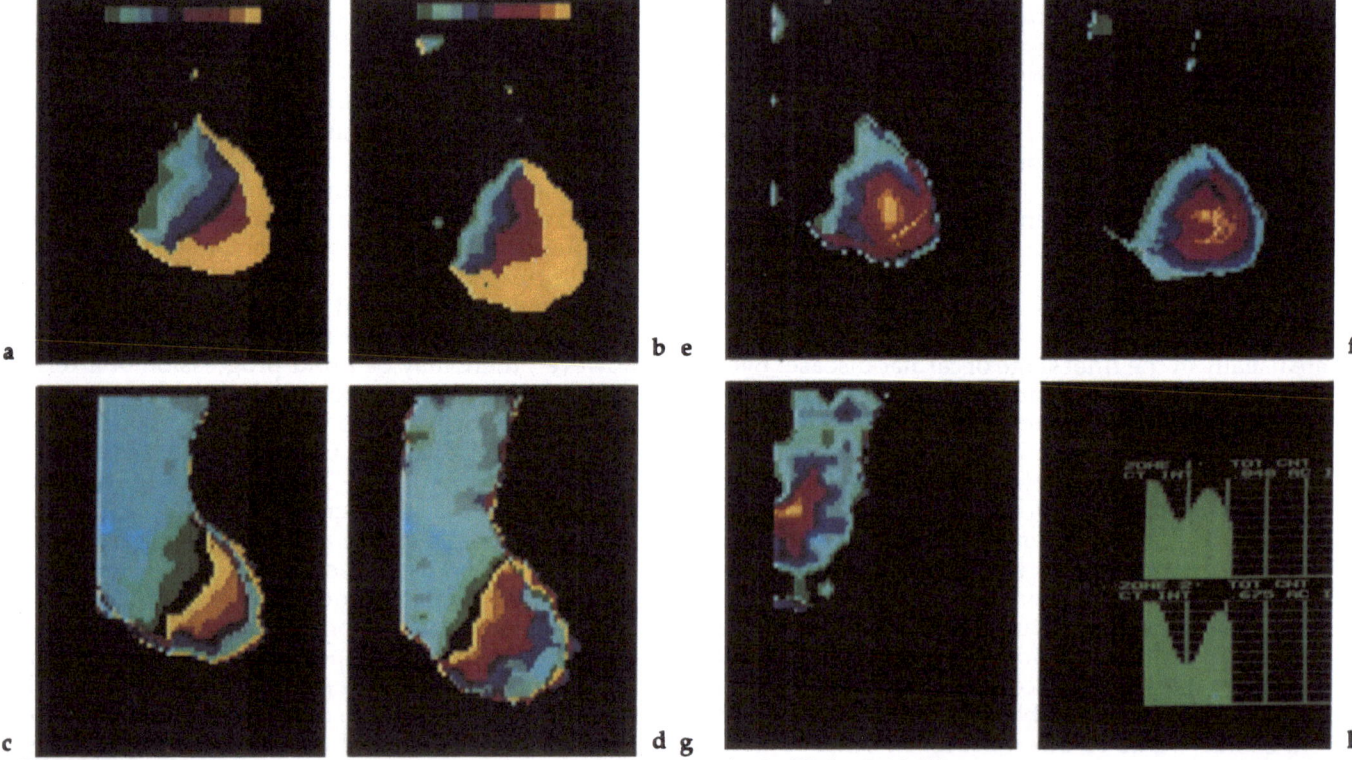

Figure 20.2 *Transplanted heart at rest and exercise. One year after heart transplantation.*
a,b,c,d, Significant improvement of function from rest (left) to exercise (right) of REFI (**a,b**) and MTT (**c,d**) images.

e,f,g,h, High rapid filling rates as normally directed to the apex. No defects at rest (**e**) and exercise (**f**). No paradoxical inward motion at rest (**g**) and exercise. Significant increase of global EF with exercise (**h**).

21

Functional Imaging of Coronary Flow with Intracoronary Injections

N. SCHAD AND F. BRUZZONE

Non-invasive first pass radionuclide angiography performed with an intravenous injection of a small radionuclide bolus of technetium 99m pertechnetate or gold Au 195m allows screening for coronary artery disease with a high degree of accuracy if regional functional imaging of left ventricular systolic and diastolic events is adopted (*see* Chapters 4 and 5). Information about the degree of regional dysfunction can also be obtained, and by examination before and after administration of nitrates (*see* Chapters 6 and 11) myocardial reserve in infarcted and ischaemic segments can be non-invasively assessed.

In clinical evaluation of patients with coronary angiography one can also inject a small radionuclide bolus directly into a coronary artery and record the first pass through the coronary circulation. Thus far, the techniques most adopted for assessment of flow distribution in the coronary vascular tree are the injection of labelled microspheres and the measurement of xenon clearance. With the advent of short-lived radionuclides, the question arises if the coronary-inflow distribution pattern can be visualized by bolus injection of gold 195m. The short half-life of gold 195m – 30.5 seconds only – would allow repeated bolus injections into the left and right coronary artery in different projections provided the injected substance causes no adverse effects on the myocardium.

The biological-pharmacological properties of gold-195m injections as well as the physical characteristics of the gold generator and its use for first pass examinations have been described extensively (Garcia *et al.*, 1981; Panek *et al.*, 1982; Mena *et al.*, 1982, 1983; Wackers *et al.*, 1982; Dymond *et al.*, 1982a). 1596 intravenous injections of gold 195m performed in our laboratory in 792 patients have been well tolerated without any significant complications (Schad *et al.*, 1984a). In a preliminary study of 14 intracoronary gold 195m injections in nine patients no significant pressure or e.c.g. changes during and after injections or subsequent rise of enzymes were observed (Schad *et al.*, 1984a).

The patient is positioned in the right anterior oblique (RAO) or left anterior oblique (LAO) projection under the multicrystal gamma-camera after introduction of the catheter into the coronary artery. Three to five minutes after flushing the generator, the intracoronary injection is initiated at onset of

ventricular diastole. The gold 195m bolus is flushed into the coronary artery by 7 ml of 5% glucose solution at an injection rate of 5 ml/s. Injection is performed with a conventional contrast injector and timer. Recording starts simultaneously with the flush at a frame rate of 25 per second (40 ms accumulation interval). Before and during injection and recording of frames, the electrocardiogram is continuously acquired. Before and immediately after injection, the intracoronary arterial pressure is also measured.

The intracoronary injection is started with the ventricular diastole since maximum coronary flow takes place during the diastolic phase. The flushing volume of 7 ml results from the capacity of the connecting tubing (50 cm) and catheter. Two millilitres are displaced at the moment of elution and the filling of the connecting tubing with the activity. During injection possibly the total of 7 ml volume should be injected, so that the eluate enters the coronary and the catheter is emptied. This facilitates later imaging of the heart because a remaining high count density over the catheter by the process of image normalization during display would suppress the lower densities over the heart and the coronary vessels. Some reduction of injection volume, however, is possible by using a shorter connecting tubing. With the use of 5% glucose solution for flushing, no or only minimal and very short-lasting repolarization changes were noticed. These changes usually subsided at the end of recording. No significant pressure changes or rise of enzymes were observed.

The rate of generation of gold 195m is rapid; within 3 minutes more than 98% of the theoretical maximum amount has been formed. The fast decay of Au 195m enables repeated injections after 3–5 minutes without any need of background subtraction of residual activity. Thus, after repositioning the patient in the LAO view or after introduction of a catheter into the other coronary artery, a second injection can be performed. Two to four hours after examination, an e.c.g. is repeated, and the next day serum enzymes are obtained.

Signals of each frame are recorded along with the electrocardiogram so that exact synchronization of the frames with the cardiac phases can be obtained. For evaluation of coronary inflow, the frames of two early cycles are selected; for coronary inflow–outflow the frames of three to four cycles are taken.

The injection time is kept short and as a rule should not exceed two heart cycles. This reduces interference of injection with the time period of imaging, which usually begins at the first systole or second diastole after the start of injection. Since only two cycles are then taken for inflow evaluation, a high framing rate is necessary to sample information as frequently as possible. To be able to select the precise cycles is mandatory. To visualize the venous phase, one can extend the imaging to three or four cycles or image only the second or third cycle.

Functional images of inflow and outflow were processed by the use of the computer programs that demonstrate regional rates of increase and decrease during a preselected time-interval (see Chapter 3). Because of the least squares fit through the data points, some smoothing occurs so that the resulting regions of rates of increase or decrease are clearly delineated. The other two images are the result of an algorithm that determines for each pixel the time of the centre of gravity (mean transit time) of the curve through the data points. One image shows only a few levels (e.g. shades of colours); the second image, by subdividing each level into eight sublevels, provides better regional discrimination. The inflow and outflow patterns observed are as follows.

As long as only *two initial consecutive cycles* are processed, the rate of decrease or outflow image normally visualizes the injection site and the initial portion of the coronaries. During the same time interval, the rate of increase or inflow image shows the distribution of peripheral filling with a central maximum (RAO view) or two maxima (left coronary, LAO view). For the same time period, the mean-transit-time images present short times at the base of the heart and increasingly longer times toward parietal periphery indicating a longer persistence of activity in the peripheral myocardium than at the base. Some lengthening of the bolus as it passes through the arterial circulation may also account for this phenomenon.

If only the *first cycle* is selected for processing, a shorter initial part of the coronaries and a more central or basal maximum of increase rates is visualized in the rate of decrease image or increase image, respectively, than if two cycles are employed for processing. Accordingly, the maximum of persistence of activity on the regional mean transit time images will not yet have reached the area of the coronary venous sinus. Selection of the *second cycle* only changes the appearance of the functional images fundamentally. With LAD injections the rate of decrease image may now show the more peripheral part of the arteries and the central tissue that already washes out, whereas the increase image illustrates the coronary veins and sinus flow. The mean transit time image may present the coronary arteries and veins simultaneously and an increasing persistence of activity in the direction of the coronary venous sinus.

Pathological cases showed reduced inflow rates in the LAD territory with a ventricular aneurysm, particularly if only the first cycle was processed, and in the LAO projection (Figure 21.1). An almost totally occluded right coronary artery could be seen on a rate of increase image with only one cycle processed since no tissue perfusion had yet occurred (Figure 21.2). On the increase images processed somewhat later, a slight peripheral filling and a small area of tissue perfusion could be visualized corresponding, on the coronary angiogram, to the region of collateral flow from the LAD and therefore probably not infarcted. The infarcted area, however, did not show any tissue perfusion. In the latter and another case, retrograde filling of the posterior descending artery from the LAD could be demonstrated with LAD injections on the mean transit time image and/or rate of increase images with processing of one or two cycles.

SUMMARY

It is possible to visualize inflow and outflow distributions by intracoronary injections of the short-lived radionuclide gold Au 195m and utilization of first pass functional imaging. The interesting fact is that central arteries and veins become visible on functional images because, in comparison to the tissue, they present higher flow rates and therefore more rapid changes in activity concentration as long as short bolus input and transit are guaranteed. As expected on the original images, however, they are not visible. To obtain the inflow pattern phasic overlap has to be avoided, i.e. it is necessary to process only two early cycles, as well as each heart cycle, independently. Demonstration of regional flow distribution may become useful in evaluation of patients with prior myocardial infarction or with territories partially supplied by collateral flow. Extent and relative degree of inflow and outflow can be established by functional imaging (Figures 21.1 and 21.2).

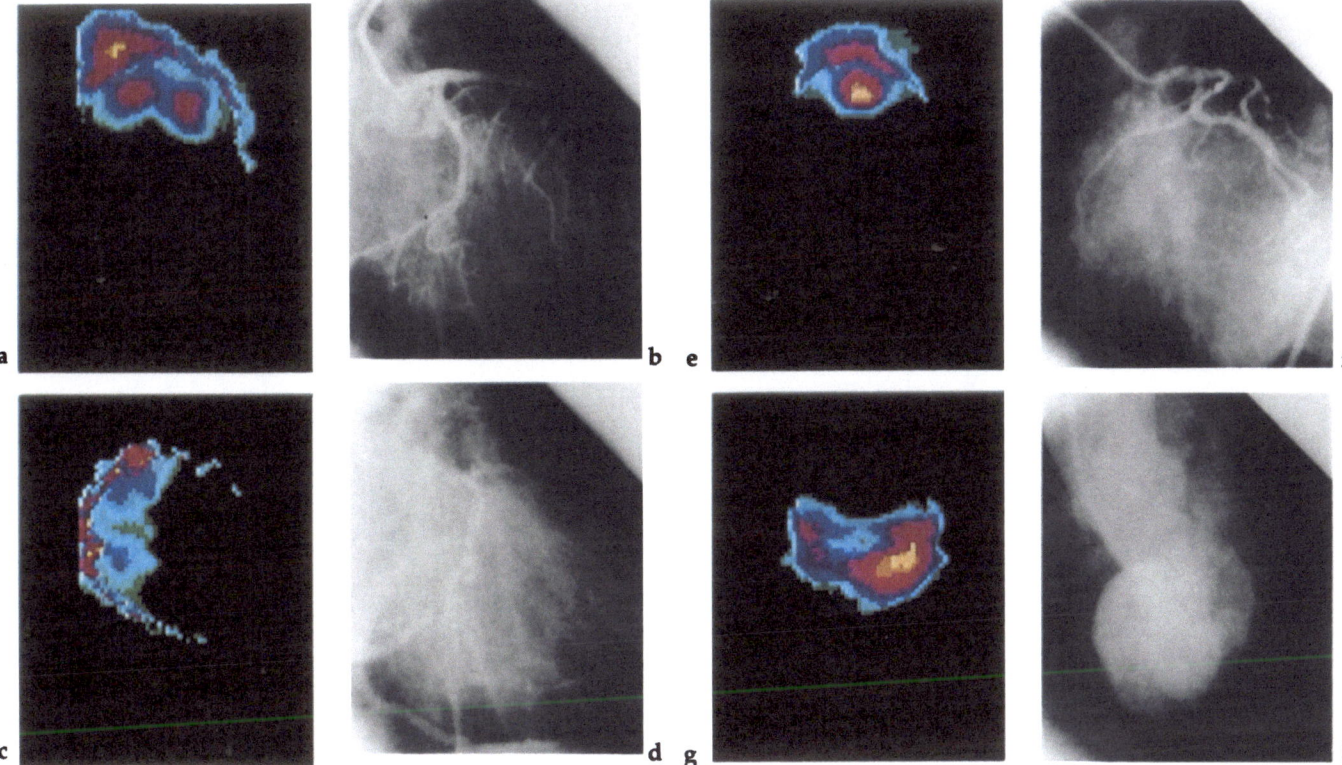

Figure 21.1 *Intra-coronary injection of Au 195m. Septal LV aneurysm.*
a,b,c,d, RAO-view outflow rates from LAD and from the territories of upper branches during the first two cycles after diastolic injection (**a**) show the initial part of the LAD, compare with (**b**). Inflow rates during the second cycle already demonstrate the coronary veins emptying into the coronary sinus, compare with (**d**).

e,f,g,h, LAO view: Outflow rates from LAD, CX and the territories of the upper branches during the first two cycles after diastolic injection (**e**) show the initial part of the LAD and CX, compare with (**f**).

Inflow rates during the first two cycles demonstrate the coronary inflow into the peripheral LAD and CX territories, significant reduced inflow into the LAD territory (**g**). The LV-angiogram shows the septal aneurysm (**h**).

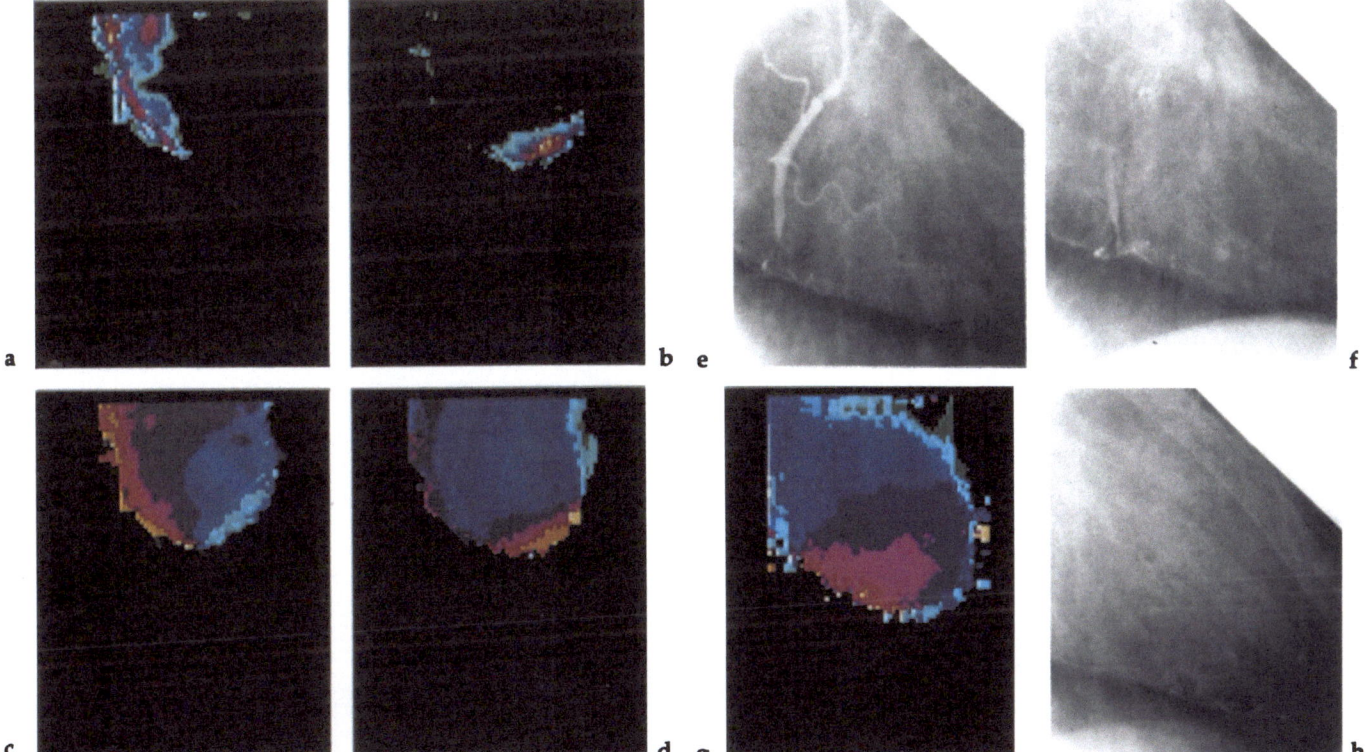

Figure 21.2 *Intra-coronary injection of Au 195m. Subtotal occlusion of the RC. RAO view.*
a,b,c,d,e,f,g,h, Inflow rates during the first cycle after diastolic injection into the obstructed RC show the vessel and some tissue-inflow proximal to the obstruction (**a**), compare with (**e**). 200 ms later delayed inflow into the peripheral RC territory sparing the posterior infarcted one,

compare with (**f**). Mean transit times corresponding to (**a**) show long persistence of blood within the proximal RC (**c**) and later in the distal perfused territory (**d**). Left coronary injection shows long persistence at the inferior zone (**g**) corresponding to the collateral flow from the LAD to the posterior descending artery (**h**).

163

References

Adam, W. E., Tarkowska, A., Bitter, F. and Stauch, M. (1979). Equilibrium (gated) radionuclide ventriculography. *Cardiovasc. Radiol.*, **2**, 161–73

Ahmad, M., Sullivan, T., Haibach, H., Sandock, K., Logan, K. and Holmes, R. (1979). Exercise induced changes in left ventricular function in patients with mitral valve prolapse. (Abstr.) *J. Nucl. Med.*, **20**, 640

Ahmed, S. S., Levinson, G. E., Fiore, J. J. and Regan, T. J. (1980). Spectrum of heart muscle abnormalities related to alcoholism. *Clin. Cardiol.*, **3**, 335–41

Anderson, P. A. W., Rerych, S. K., Moore, T. E. and Jones, R. H. (1981). Accuracy of left ventricular end-diastolic dimension determinations obtained by radionuclide angiocardiography. *J. Nucl. Med.*, **22**, 500–505

Andrews, E. J., Fleming, J. W., Schad, N., Nickel, O. and Mello, M. (1981). New computer programs for radionuclide evaluation of ventricular wall motion in ischemic heart disease. Presented at *28th Annual Meeting*, RSNA, 1981 (Abstr.)

Appelbaum, A., Kouchoukos, N. T., Blackstone, E. H. and Kirklin, J. W. (1976). Early risks of open heart surgery for mitral valve disease. *Am. J. Cardiol.*, **37**, 201

Ashburn, W. L., Schlebert, H. R. and Verba, J. W. (1978). Left ventricular ejection fraction: A review of several radionuclide angiographic approaches using the scintillation camera. In Holman, B. L., Sonnenblick, E. H. and Lesch, M. (eds.) *Principles of Cardiovascular Nuclear Medicine*, pp. 171–88. (New York: Grune & Stratton)

Attarian, D. E., Jones, R. N., Currie, W. D., Hill, R. C., Sink, J. D., Olsen, C. O., Chitwood, W. R. and Wechsler, A. S. (1981). Characteristics of chronic left ventricular hypertrophy induced by subcoronary valvular aortic stenosis. I. Myocardial blood flow and metabolism. *J. Thorac. Cardiovasc. Surg.*, **81**, 382–8

Bacharach, S. L., Green, M. V., Bonow, R. O., Findley, S. L., Ostrow, H. G. and Johnston, G. S. (1981). Measurement of ventricular function by ECG gating during atrial fibrillation. *J. Nucl. Med.*, **22**, 226–31

Bache, R. J. and Vrobel, T. R. (1979). Effects of exercise on blood flow in hypertrophied heart. *Am. J. Cardiol.*, **44**, 1029–33

Backet, T., Bical, O., Goudot, B., Menu, P., Richard, T., Barbagelatta, M. and Guilmet, D. (1979). Early structural failure of porcine xenografts in young patients. In Sebening, F. (ed.) *Bioprosthetic Valves*, pp. 341–9. (Munich: Deutsches Herzzentrum)

Barlow, J. B., Bosman, C. K., Pocock, W. A. *et al.* (1968). Late systolic murmurs and non-ejection ('mid-late') systolic clicks. An analysis of 90 patients. *Br. Heart J.*, **30**, 203–18

Barlow, J. B. and Pocock, W. A. (1979). Mitral valve prolapse, the specific billowing mitral leaflet syndrome,

or an insignificant non-ejection systolic click. *Am. Heart J.*, **97**, 277–85

Barnett, H. J. M., Boughner, D. R., Taylor, D. W. *et al.* (1980). Further evidence relating mitral-valve prolapse to cerebral ischemic events. *N. Engl. J. Med.*, **302**, 139

Barnhorst, D. A., Oxman, H. A., Connolly, D. C., Pluth, J. R., Danielson, G. K., Wallace, R. B. and McGoon, D. C. (1976). Isolated replacement of the mitral valve with the Starr–Edwards-prosthesis; an eleven year review. *J. Thorac. Cardiovasc. Surg.*, **71**, 230

Benchimol, A., Matsuo, S., Wang, T. F. and Gartlan, J. L. (1972). Phasic coronary arterial flow velocity during arrhythmias in man. *Am. J. Cardiol.*, **29**, 604–10

Berger, H. J., Matthay, R. A., Pytlik, L. M., Gottschalk, A. and Zaret, B. L. (1979). First-pass radionuclide assessment of right and left ventricular performance in patients with cardiac and pulmonary disease. *Sem. Nucl. Med.*, **9**, 275–95

Berger, H. J., Reduto, L. A., Johnstone, D. E. *et al.* (1979b). Global and regional left ventricular response to bicycle exercise in coronary artery disease. Assessment by quantitative radionuclide angiocardiography. *Am. J. Med.*, **66**, 13–21

Berger, H. J., Milton, J. S., Davies, R. A. *et al.* (1981). Exercise left ventricular performance in patients with chest pain, ischemic-appearing exercise electrocardiograms, and angiographically normal coronary arteries. *Ann. Intern. Med.*, **94**, 186–91

Berman, D. S., Salel, A. F., De Nardo, G. L., Bogren, G. and Mason, D. T. (1974). Clinical assessment of left ventricular regional contraction patterns and ejection fraction by high resolution gated scintigraphy. *J. Nucl. Med.*, **16**, 865

Bishop, V. S., Stone, H. L. and Guyton. A. C. (1964). Cardiac function curves in conscious dogs. *Am. J. Physiol.*, **207/3**, 677

Block, P. C., Myler, R. and Stertzer, S. (1981). Morphology after transluminal angioplasty in human beings. *N. Engl. J. Med.*, **305**, 382–5

Block, P. C., Cowley, M. and Kaltenbach, M. (1984). Percutaneous angioplasty of stenoses of bypass grafts or of bypass graft anastomotic sites. *Am. J. Cardiol.*, **53**, 666–8

Bodenheimer, M. M., Banka, V. S., Fooshee, C. M. *et al.* (1978). Quantitative radionuclide angiography in the right anterior oblique view: comparison with contrast ventriculography. *Am. J. Cardiol.*, **41**, 718–25

Bolen, J. L. and Alderman, E. L. (1977). Ventriculographic and hemodynamic features of mitral regurgitation of cardiomyopathic, rheumatic and nonrheumatic etiology. *Am. J. Cardiol.*, **39**, 177–83

Bonow, R. D., Bacharach, S. L., Green, M. C., Kent, K. M., Rosing, D. R., Lipson, L. C., Leon, M. B. and Epstein, S. E. (1981). Impaired left ventricular diastolic filling in patients with coronary artery disease: assessment with radionuclide angiography. *Circulation*, **64**, 315

Borel, J. F., Feurer, C., Maquee, C. and Stähelin, H. (1977). Effects of the antilymphotic peptide Cyclosporin A in animals. *Immunology*, **32**, 1017–52

Borer, J. S., Bacharach, S. L., Green, M. V., Kent, K. A., Epstein, S. E. and Johnston, G. S. (1977). Real-time radionuclide cineangiography in the noninvasive evaluation of global and regional left ventricular function at rest and during exercise in patients with coronary-artery disease. *N. Engl. J.*, **296**, 839–44

Borer, J. S., Bacharach, S. L., Green, M. V., Kent, K. M., Henry, W. L., Rosing, D. R., Seldes, S. F., Johnston, G. S. and Epstein, S. E. (1978). Exercise-induced left ventricular dysfunction in symptomatic and asymptomatic patients with aortic regurgitation: assessment with radionuclide cineangiography. *Am. J. Cardiol.*, **42**, 351–7

Borer, J. S., Kent, K. M., Bacharach, S. L. *et al.* (1979). Sensitivity, specificity and predictive accuracy of radionuclide cineangiography during exercise in patients with coronary artery disease. Comparison with exercise electrocardiography. *Circulation*, **60**, 572–80

Borer, J. S., Philipps, P., Moses, J. W., Goldberg, H. L. and Fisher, J. (1982). Determination of prognosis in patients with coronary artery disease by noninvasive radionuclide-based methods applied during exercise. *Adv. Cardiol.*, **31**, 23–7

Boucher, C. A., Bingham, J. B., Osbakken, M. D., Okada, R. D., Strauss, H. W., Block, P. C., Levine, F. H., Phillips, H. R. and Pohost, G. M. (1981). Early changes in left ventricular size and function after correction of left ventricular volume overload. *Am. J. Cardiol.*, **47**, 991–1004

Boucher, C. A., Kanarek, D. J., Okada, R. D., Hutter, A. M., Straus, H. W. and Pohost, G. M. (1983a). Exercise testing in aortic regurgitation: comparison of radionuclide left ventricular ejection fraction with exercise performance at the anaerobic threshold and peak exercise. *Am. J. Cardiol.*, **2**, 801–8

Boucher, C. A., Pohost, G. M., Okada, R. D., Levine, F. H., Strauss, H. W. and Harthorne, J. W. (1983b). Effect of ventricular function assessed by radionuclide angiography. *Am. Heart J.*, **106**, 1105–11

Bourassa, M. G., Lesperance, J., Campeau, L. and Saltiel, J. (1972). Fate of left ventricular contraction following aortocoronary venous graft. *Circulation*, **47**, 724

Boyer, K. W., Konstantinow, G., Rerych, S. K. and Jones, R. H. (1978). Nuclear cardiology: selected computer aspects. *Symposium proceedings*. Atlanta, GA, January 22–23, 1978. Sponsored by the Computer Council of the Society of Nuclear Medicine. New York, Society of Nuclear Medicine.

Braunwald, E. (1969). Mitral regurgitation: Physiologic, clinical and surgical considerations. *N. Engl. J. Med.*, **281**, 425

Braunwald, E. (1980). Valvular disease. In Braunwald, E. (ed.) *Heart Disease. A Textbook of Cardiovascular Medicine*, pp. 1119 ff. (Philadelphia, Toronto, London: W. B. Saunders)

Braunwald, E. and Kloner, R. A. (1982). The stunned myocardium: prolonged, post-ischemic ventricular dysfunction. *Circulation*, **66**, 1146–1149

Briston, J. D. and Kremkan, E. L. (1975). Hemodynamic changes after valve replacement with Starr–Edwards prostheses. *Am. J. Cardiol.*, **35**, 716

Brower, R. W., Serrys, P. W., Bos, E. and Nauta, J. (1979). Regional myocardial shortening in relation to graft-reactive hyperemia and flow after coronary bypass surgery. *J. Thorac. Cardiovasc. Surg.*, **77**, 92

Burton, N. A., Stinson, E. B., Oyer, P. E. and Shumway, N. E. (1979). Left ventricular aneurysm: preoperative risk factors and long-term postoperative results. *J. Thorac., Cardiovasc. Surg.*, **77**, 65

Bussmann, W. D., Mager, V. and Kaltenbach, M. (1979). Ventricular function at rest, during raising and physical exercise before and after aortocoronary bypass surgery. *Am. J. Cardiol.*, **43**, 486

Carpentier, A. (1969). Le valvuloplastie reconstructive. Une nouvelle technique de valve plastie mitrale. *Presse Med.*, **77**, 251

Carpentier, A., Gueninson, J., Deloche, A., Fabiani, J. N. and Relland, J. (1976). Pathology of the mitral valve. In Kalmanson, D. and Anold, E. (eds.) *The Mitral Valve. A Pluridisciplinary Approach*, p. 65.

Carpentier, A., Chauvaud, S., Fabiani, J. N., Deloche, A., Relland, J., Lessana, A., d'Allaines, Ch., Blondeau, Ph., Piwnica, A. and Dubost, Ch. (1980). Reconstruction surgery of mitral valve incompetence. Ten year appraisal. *J. Thorac. Cardiovasc. Surg.*, **79**, 338

Carpentier, A. (1983). Cardiac valve surgery – the 'French correction'. *J. Thorac. Cardiovasc. Surg.*, **86**, 323

Casarotto, D., Bortolotti, U., Thiene, G., Gallucci, V. and Cévese, P. G. (1979). Long-term results (from 5 to 7 years) with the Hancock S-G-P bioprosthesis. *J. Cardiovasc. Surg.*, **20**, 399–406

Chazov, E. I., Matveeva, L. S., Mazaev, A. V. and Ruda, M. Ya. (1976). Intracoronary introduction of fibrolysin at myocardial infarction. *VII Eur. Congr. Cardiol.*, Abstract I

Chesebro, J. H., Ritman, E. I., Fryre, R. I., Smith, H. C., Conolly, D. C., Rutherford, B. D., Davis, G. D. *et al.* (1976). Videometric analysis of regional left ventricular function before and after aortocoronary bypass surgery. *J. Clin. Invest.*, **58**, 1339

Chesler, E., King, R. A. and Edwards, J. E. (1983). The myxomatous mitral valve and sudden death. *Circulation*, **67**, 632

Cipriano, P. R., Gutman, S. I., Kline, S. A., Alonso, D. R. and Baltaxe, H. A. (1975). Left ventricular myocardial function and structure in patients with mitral valve prolapse. (Abstr.) *Circulation*, 51–2, Suppl II:69

Cobbs, B. W. Jr. (1974). Clinical recognition and medical management of rheumatic heart disease and other acquired valvular disease. In Hurst, J. W. (ed.) *The Heart: Arteries and Veins*. 3rd Edn. pp. 874–5, 881–9 (New York: McGraw-Hill)

Cobbs, B. W. Jr. and King, S. B. (1977). Ventricular buckling: a factor in the abnormal ventriculogram and peculiar hemodynamics associated with mitral valve prolapse. *Am. Heart J.*, **93**, 741–58

Cohen, M. V., Shah, P. K. and Spindola-Franco, H. (1979). Angiographic-echocardiographic correlation in mitral valve prolapse. *Am. Heart J.*, **97**, 43–52

Cohn, L. H., Mudge, G. H., Pratter, F. and Collins, J. J. (1981). Five to eight-year follow-up of patients undergoing porcine heart-valve replacement. *N. Engl. J. Med.*, **304**, 258–62

Curry, G. C., Elliott, L. P. and Ramsey, H. W. (1972). Quantitative left ventricular angiocardiographic findings in mitral stenosis. Detailed analysis of the anterolateral wall of the left ventricle. *Am. J. Cardiol.*, **29**, 621–7

Deeg, P., Schad, N., Haubitz, I., v.d. Emde, E. and Schneider, K. W. (1980). Nichtinvasive und invasive Erfolgskontrolle nach ACVB-Operation. (Bad Nauheim: Verh. Dtsch. Ges. Herz-u. Kreisl.-Forsch.)

DeMaria, A. N., Neumann, A., Lee, G. *et al.* (1977). Echocardiographic identification of the mitral valve prolapse syndrome. *Am. J. Med.*, **62**, 819–29

DePace, N. L., Ren, J. F., Kotler, M. N., Mintz, G. S., Kimbiris, D. and Kalman, P. (1983). Two-dimensional echocardiographic determination of right atrial emptying volume: A noninvasive index in quantifying the degree of tricuspid regurgitation. *Am. J. Cardiol.*, **52**, 525–9

Devereux, R. B., Perloff, J. K., Reichek, N. *et al.* (1976). Mitral valve prolapse. *Circulation*, **54**, 3–14

Dotter, C. T. and Judkins, M. P. (1964). Transluminal treatment of arterosclerotic obstruction: description of a new technique and a preliminary report of its application. *Circulation*, **30**, 654–70

Dotter, C. T., Rösch, J. and Seaman, A. J. (1974). Selective clot lysis with low-dose streptokinase. *Radiology*, **111**, 31

Dymond, D. S., Elliot, A. T. and Flatman, W. (1982a). First pass radionuclide angiography in man using Gold-195 m (T1/2 30.5 sec.). *J. Nucl. Med.*, **23**, 71

Dymond, D. S., Elliott, A., Stone, D. *et al.* (1982b). Factors that affect the reproducibility of measurements of left ventricular function from first-pass radionuclide ventriculograms. *Circulation*, **65**, 311–22

Dymond, D. S., Grenier, R. P., Carpenter, J. and Schmidt, D. H. (1984). First-pass radionuclide angiography via pulmonary arterial catheters. A critical analysis of background components. *Radiology*, **150**, 819–23

Elliott, L. P. (1976). Decisional tree analysis of the plain chest film in heart disease. Part I. Approach and pulmonary vascularity. *Diagn. Radiol.*, 553–4

Fazio, F., Gerundini, P. and Maseri, A. (1982). First pass radionuclide angiography using Au 195 m. *J. Nucl. Med.*, **23**, 71

Ferrans, V. J., Spray, T. L., Billingham, M. E. and Roberts, W. C. (1978). Structural changes in glutaraldehyde-treated porcine heterografts used as substitute cardiac valves. *Am. J. Cardiol.*, **41**, 1159–84

Fleming, J. W. (1982). Functional imaging of the left ventricle. Presentation before *The Seventh Annual Nuclear Cardiology Symposium*, Milwaukee, WI, 24 Sept. 1982

Fleming, J. W., Andrews, E. J., Arenson, N. *et al.* (1980). First pass radionuclide wall motion abnormalities associated with mitral valve prolapse syndrome. (Abstr.) *Am. J. Cardiol.*, **45**, 409

Foster, C., Anholm, J. D., Hellman, C. K. *et al.* (1981). Left ventricular function during sudden strenuous exercise. *Circulation*, **63**, 592–6

Foster, C., Dymond, D. S., Anholm, J. D. *et al.* (1983). Effect of exercise protocol on the left ventricular response to exercise. *Am. J. Cardiol.*, **51**, 859–64

Friedman, B. J. and Homan, B. L. (1982). Scintigraphic prediction of pulmonary arterial systolic pressure by regional right ventricular ejection fraction during the second half of systole. *Am. J. Cardiol.*, **50**, 1114–19

Gaasch, W. H., Levine, H. J., Quinones, M. A. and Alexander, J. K. (1976). Left ventricular compliance: mechanisms and clinical implications. *Am. J. Cardiol.*, **38**, 645

Gaffney, F. A., Karlsson, E. S., Campbell, W. *et al.* (1979). Autonomic dysfunction in women with mitral valve prolapse syndrome. *Circulation*, **59**, 894

Garcia, E., Mena, I. and de Jong, R. B. J. (1981). Gold Au-195m, short-lived single photon emitter for hemodynamic studies. *J. Nucl. Med.*, **22**, 71

Geha, A. S., Laks, H., Stansel, H. C., Comhill, J. F., Kilman, J. W., Buckley, M. J. and Roberts, W. C. (1979). Late failures of porcine valve heterografts in children. *J. Thorac. Cardiovasc. Surg.*, **78**, 351–64

Gibbons, R. J., Lee, D. L., Cobb, F. and Jones, R. H. (1981). Ejection fraction response to exercise in patients with chest pain and normal coronary arteriograms. *Circulation*, **64**, 952–7

Gibbons, R. J., Lee, K. L., Cobb, F. R., Coleman, R. E. and Jones, R. H. (1982). Ejection fraction response to exercise in patients with chest pain, coronary artery disease and normal resting ventricular function. *Circulation*, **66**, 643–8

Gibson, D. G. and Brown, D. J. (1979). Abnormal left ventricular wall movement in patients with chest pain and normal coronary arteriograms. Relation to inferior T wave changes and mitral prolapse. *Br. Heart J.*, **41**, 385–91

Glancy, D. L., O'Brien, K. P., Reis, R. L. *et al.* (1969). Hemodynamic studies in patients with 2M and 3M Starr–Edwards prostheses: evidence of obstruction to left atrial emptying. *Circulation*, **39–40** (Suppl. I), 113

Gooch, A. S., Ficencia, F., Maranhao, V. and Goldberg, H. (1972). Arrhythmias and left ventricular asynergy in the prolapsing mitral leaflet syndrome. *Am. J. Cardiol.*, **20**, 611–20

Gottdiener, J. S., Borer, J. S., Bacharach, S. L. *et al.* (1979). Left ventricular dysfunction in mitral valve prolapse. (Abstr.) *Am. J. Cardiol.*, **43**, 387

Gravanis, M. B. and Campbell, W. G. Jr. (1982). The syndrome of prolapse of the mitral valve: an etiologic and pathogenic enigma. *Arch. Pathol. Lab. Med.*, **106**, 369–74

Grondin, C. M. (1984). Late results of coronary artery grafting: Is there a flag on the field? *J. Thorac. Cardiovasc. Surg.*, **87**, 161

Grossman, W. and McLaurin, L. P. (1976). Diastolic properties of the left ventricle. *Ann. Intern. Med.*, **84**, 316

Gruntzig, A. (1978). Transluminal dilatation of coronary artery stenosis. *Lancet*, **1**, 263

Gruntzig, A, Senning, A. and Siegerhalter, W. E. (1979). Nonoperative dilatation of coronary artery stenosis: percutaneous transluminal coronary angioplasty. *N. Engl. J. Med.*, **301**, 61–8

Gruntzig, A. R. (1984). Percutaneous transluminal coronary angioplasty: six years experience. *Am. Heart J.*, **107**, 818–19

Hagl, S., Meisner, H., Heimisch, W. and Sebening, F. (1978). Acute effects of aorto coronary bypass surgery on left ventricular function and regional myocardial mechanics: A clinical study. *Ann. Thorac. Surg.*, **26**, 548

Hairston, P., Newmann, W. H. and Daniell, H. B. (1973). Myocardial contractile force as influenced by direct coronary surgery. *Ann. Thorac. Surg.*, **15**, 364

Hancock, W. F. (1984). Valvular heart disease. In *Scientific American Medicine*. Chap. 1, part XI, p. 8. (New York: Scientific American)

Hancock Laboratories (1980). Durability assessment of the Hancock porcine bioprosthesis; a multicenter retrospective analysis of patients operated prior to 1975. *Anaheim*, 1–16

Hartzler, G. O. (1983). Percutaneous transluminal coronary angioplasty in multi-vessel disease. *Cath. and CUD*, **9**, 537–41

Hecht, H. S. and Hopkins, J. M. (1981). Exercise-induced regional wall notion abnormalities on radionuclide angiography. Lack of reliability for detection of coronary artery disease in the presence of valvular heart disease. *Am. J. Cardiol.*, **47**, 861–5

Hecht, H., Taylor, R., Wong, M. and Shah, P. (1981). Comparative evaluation of segmental asynergy in remote myocardial infarction by radionuclide angiography, two-dimensional echocardiography, and contrast ventriculography. *Am. Heart J.*, **101**, 742

Hellman, C. K. (1978). Dynamic evaluation of ventricular function. *Symposium on nuclear cardiology: Principles and applications*. Milwaukee, October 1978

Hetzer, R., Heim, K., Borst, H. G., Amende, J. and Sigwart, U. (1976). Röntgenkinematographische Studien der lokalen Ventrikeldynamik vor und nach aortokoronarem Bypass. *Thoraxchirurgie*, **24**, 296

Hoffman, M. A., Fallon, J. T., Block, P. C. *et al.* (1981). Arterial pathology after percutaneous transluminal angioplasty. *Am. J. Radiol.*, **137**, 147–9

Hollman, J., Garth, A., Gruntzig, A. et al. (1983). Coronary artery spasm at the site of angioplasty in the first four months after successful percutaneous transluminal coronary angioplasty. J. Am. Coll. Cardiol., 2, 1039–45

Holman, B. L. (1979). Cardiac nuclear medicine: An overview. Cardiovasc. Radiol., 2, 141–8

Jablonsky, G., Hilton, J. D., Liu, P. P., Morch, J. E., Druck, M. N., Bar-Shlomo, B. and McLaughlin, P. R. (1983). Rest and exercise ventricular function in adults with congenital ventricular septal defects. Am. J. Cardiol., 51, 293–8

Jenge, J. A., Uszler, J. M., Freeman, R. et al. (1978). Upright exercise stress first pass radionuclide detection of coronary artery disease. 2nd international congress of nuclear medicine and biology, September 1978, p. 95

Jengo, J. A., Mena, I., Blaufuss, A. and Criley, J. M. (1978). Evaluation of left ventricular function (ejection fraction and segmental wall motion) by single pass radioisotope angiography. Circulation, 57, 326

Jeresaty, R. M. (1971). Mitral ballooning – a possible mechanism of mitral insufficiency in diseases associated with reduced endsystolic volume of the left ventricle. (Editorial) Chest, 60, 114–15

Jeresaty, R. M. (1975). Etiology of the mitral valve prolapse-click syndrome. (Editorial) Am. J. Cardiol. 36, 110–13

Jeresaty, R. M. (1978). Mitral valve prolapse-click syndrome: etiology, clinical findings, and therapy. Cardiovasc. Med., 3, 597–613

Johnson. L. L., Ellis, K., Schmidt, D., Weiss, M. B. and Cannon, P. J. (1975). Volume ejected in early systole: A sensitive Index of left ventricular performance in Coronary Artery Disease. Circulation, 52, 378

Johnson, L. L., Powers, E. R., Tzall, W. R., Feder, J., Sciacca, R. R. and Cannon, P. J. (1983). Left ventricular volume and ejection fraction response to exercise in aortic regurgitation. Am. J. Cardiol., 51, 1379–85

Jones, E. L. and King, S. B. (1984). Intraoperative balloon-catheter dilation in the treatment of coronary artery disease. Am. Heart J., 107, 836–7

Jones, R. H., Sabiston, D. C. Jr., Bates, B. B. et al. (1972). Quantitative radionuclide angiocardiography for determination of chamber to chamber cardiac transit times. Am. J. Cardiol., 30, 855

Jones, R. H., Newmann, G. E., Rerych, S. K., Scholz, P. M., Upton, M. T. and Sabiston, D. C. (1978a). Rest and exercise radionuclide angiography in surgical patients. Wld. Fed. Nucl. Med. Biol. 2nd Intern. Congr., Washington 1978, p. 95

Jones, R. H., Rerych, S. K., Newmann, G. E., Scholz, P. M., Howe, W. R., Oldman, H. N., Goodwich, J. K. and Sabiston, D. C. (1978b). Noninvasive radionuclide procedures for diagnosis and management of myocardial ischemia. Wld. J. Surg., 2, 811

Jones, R. H., McEwan, P., Newman, G. E., Port, S. T., Rerych, S. K., Scholz, P. M., Upton, M. T., Peter, C. E., Austin, E. H., Leong, K. H., Gibbons, R. J., Cobb, F. R., Coleman, R. E. and Sabiston, D. (1981). Accuracy of diagnosis of coronary artery disease by radionuclide measurement of left ventricular function during rest and exercise. Circulation, 64, 586–601

Jones, R. H., Floyd, R. D., Austin, E. H., Sabiston, D. C. Jr. (1983). The role of radionuclide angiocardiography in the prolonged prediction of pain relief and prolonged survival following coronary artery bypass grafting. Ann. Surg., 197, 743–54

Kaliff, V., Rabinovitch, M. A., Chan, W., O'Neill, W., Stewart, J., Walton, J., Pitt, B. and Thrall, J. H. (1982). Baseline left-ventricular function during frequent ventricular or atrial ectopic beats: concise communication. J. Nucl. Med., 1076–9

Kamath, M. L., Hellman, C., Schmidt, D. H. and Johnson, W. D. (1979). Improvement of left ventricular function by coronary bypass surgery. Presented at The 59th Annual Meeting of the American Association of Thoracic Surgery, Boston, 1979

Kapelanski, D. P., Al-Sadir, J., Lamberti, J. J. and Anagnostopoulos, C. E. (1978). Ventriculographic features predictive of surgical outcome for left ventricular aneurysm. Circulation, 58 (6), 1167–1174

Kennedy, J. W., Yarnall, S. R., Murray, J. A. and Figley, M. M. (1970). Quantitative angiocardiography IV. Relationships of left atrial and ventricular pressure and volume in mitral valve disease. Circulation, 41, 817–24

Kent, K. M., Borer, J. S., Green, M. V., Bacharach, S. L., McIntosh, C. L., Conkle, D. M. and Epstein, S. E. (1978). Effects of coronary artery bypass on global and regional left ventricular function during exercise. N. Engl. J. Med., 298, 1434

Kent, K. M., Beutinoglio, L., Block, P. C. et al (1982). Percutaneous transluminal coronary angioplasty: report from the Registry of the National Heart, Lung, and Blood Institute. Am. J. Cardiol., 49, 2011–20

Kirlin, P. C., Das, S., Zinjnen, P. et al. (1984). The exercise response in idiopathic dilated cardiomyopathy. Clin. Cardiol., 7, 205–10

Kleinmann, L. H., Hill, R. C., Chitwood, W. R., Hammon, J. W., Jones, K. W. and Wechsler, A. S. (1979). Regional myocardial dimensions following coronary artery bypass grafting in patients. J. Thorac. Cardiovasc. Surg., 77, 13

Kloster, F. E., Herr, R. H., Starr, A. and Griswold, H. E. (1969). Hemodynamic evaluation of cloth-covered Starr–Edwards valve prosthesis. Circulation, 39–40 (Suppl. I), 119

Konstam, M. A., Idoine, J., Wynne, J., Grossman, W., Cohn, L., Beck, J. R., Kozlowski, J. and Holman, B. L. (1983). Right ventricular function in adults with pulmonary hypertension with and without atrial septal defect. Am. J. Cardiol., 51, 1144–8

Korr, K. S., Gandsman, E. J., Winkler, M. L., Shulman, R. S. and Bough, E. W. (1982) Hemodynamic correlates of right ventricular ejection fraction measured with gated radionuclide angiography. Am. J. Cardiol., 49, 71–7

Kremers, S., Kight, J. and Heck, L. (1978). Value of nitroglycerine radionuclide angiocardiography in preoperative evaluation of patients with coronary artery disease. 2nd international congress of nuclear medicine and biology, September 1978, p. 23

Kreuzer, E. (1984). Globale und regionale Dimensions- und Funktionsänderungen des Myokards während und nach Mitralklappeninsuffizienz. Experimentelle Untersuchungen mit dem Ultraschall-Laufzeitverfahren. (Stuttgart, New York: Thième. Copythek)

Kreuzer, E., Schad, B., Peters, D. and Reichart, B. (1984). Plastic and reconstructive surgery on the mitral valve – long term follow-up pilot study with the first pass technic. Fortschr. Med., 102/4, 57

Kuhajda, F. P., Moore, G. W. and Hutchins, G. M. (1981). Myocardial injury in patients with aortic stenosis. Abstracts of the 54th Scientific Sessions, Circulation, 64 (Suppl. IV)

Kutsche, L. M., Oyer, P. E., Shumway, N. E. and Baum, D. (1979). An important complication of Hancock mitral valve replacement in children. Circulation, 60 (Suppl. I), 98–103

Lanzer, P., Botvinick, E. H., Schiller, N. B., Crooks, L. E., Arakawa, M., Kaufmann, L., Davis, P. L., Herfkens, R., Lipton, M. J. and Higgins, Ch. B. (1984). Cardiac imaging using gated magnetic resonance. Radiology, 150, 121–7

Leighton, R. F., Pollack, M. E. and Welch, T. G. (1975).

Abnormal left ventricular wall motion at mid-ejection in patients with coronary heart disease. *Circulation, 52*, 238

Levine, H. J. (1980). Difficult problems in the diagnosis of chest pain. *Am. Heart. J., 100*, 108–18

Levine, H. J., Isner, J. M. and Salem, D. N. (1982). Primary versus secondary mitral valve prolapse: clinical features and implications. *Clin. Cardiol., 5*, 371–5

Levinson G. E., Frank, M. J. and Schwartz, C. J. (1970). The affect of rest and physical effort on the left ventricular burden in mitral and aortic regurgitation. *Am. Heart J., 80*, 791–801

Liberthson, R. R., Boucher, C. A., Strauss, H. W., Dinsmore, R. E., McKusick, K. A. and Pohost, G. M. (1981). Right ventricular function in adult atrial septal defect. Preoperative and postoperative assessment and clinical implications. *Am. J. Cardiol., 47*, 56–60

Liedtke, A. J., Gault, J. H., Leaman, D. M. and Blumenthal, M. S. (1973). Geometry of left ventricular contraction in the systolic click syndrome. Characterization of a segmental myocardial abnormality. *Circulation, 47*, 27–35

Lillehei, C. W., Gott, V. L., DeWall, R. A. and Varco, P. L. (1958). The surgical treatment of stenotic or regurgitant lesions of the mitral and aortic valves by direct vision utilizing a pump oxygenator. *J. Thorac. Surg., 35*, 154

Lindsay, J. Jr., Nolan, N. G., Goldstein, S. A. and Bacos, J. M. (1980). The usefulness of radionuclide ventriculography for the identification and assessment of patients with coronary heart disease. *Am. Heart. J., 99*, 310–18

McGoon, D. C. (1960). Repair of mitral insufficiency due to ruptured chordae tendineae. *J. Thorac. Cardiovasc. Surg., 39*, 357

McManus, Q., Grunkemeier, G. L., Lambert, L. E., Teply, J. F., Harlan, B. J. and Starr, A. (1980). Year of operation as a risk factor in the late results of valve replacement. *J. Thorac. Cardiovasc. Surg., 80*, 834

Maddahi, J., Berman, D. S. and Diamond, G. A. (1979). Evaluation of left ventricular ejection fraction and segmental wall motion by multiple gated equilibrium cardiac blood pool scintigraphy. *Comput. Tec. Cardiol., 4*, 389

Magilligan, D. J., Lewis, J. W., Jara, R. M., Lee, M. W., Alam, M., Riddle, J. M. and Stein, P. D. (1980). Spontaneous degeneration of porcine bioprosthetic valves. *Ann. Thorac. Surg., 30*, 259–66

Malcom, A. D., Cankovie-Darracott, S., Chayen, J., Jenkins, B. S. and Webb-Peploe, M. M. (1979). Biopsy evidence of left ventricular myocardial abnormality in patients with mitral-leaflet prolapse and chest pain. *Lancet, 1*, 1052–5

Manyari, D. E. and Kostuk, W. J. (1983). Left and right ventricular function at rest and during bicycle exercise in the supine and sitting positions in normal subjects and patients with coronary artery disease. *Am. J. Cardiol., 51*, 36–42

Marcus, M. L. (1983). *The Coronary Circulation in Health and Disease*, pp. 242–66. (New York: McGraw-Hill)

Marcus, M. L., Doty, D. B., Hiratzka, L. F., Wright, C. B. and Eastham, C. L. (1982). Decreased coronary reserve. A mechanism for angina pectoris in patients with aortic stenosis and normal coronary arteries. *N. Engl. J. Med., 307*, 1362–7

Markiewicz, W., Stoner, J., London, E., Hunt, S. A. and Popp, R. L. (1976). Mitral valve prolapse in 100 presumably healthy young females. *Circulation, 53*, 464–73

Mason, J. W., Koch, F. H., Billingham, M. E. and Winkle, R. A. (1978). Cardiac biopsy evidence for a cardiomyopathy associated with symptomatic mitral valve prolapse. *Am. J. Cardiol., 42*, 557–62

Massie, B., Botvinick, E. H., Shames, D., Taradash, M., Werner, J. and Schiller, N. (1978). Myocardial perfusion scintigraphy in patients with mitral valve prolapse. Its advantage over stress electrocardiography in diagnosing associated coronary artery disease and its implications for the etiology of chest pain. *Circulation, 57*, 19–26

Mathey, D. G., Decoodt, P. R., Allen, H. N. and Swan, H. J. C. (1977). Abnormal left ventricular contraction pattern in the systolic click-late systolic murmur syndrome. *Circulation, 56*, 311–15

Mehta, J. (1984). Role of platelet antagonists in coronary artery disease: implications in coronary artery bypass surgery and balloon-catheter dilatation. *Am. Heart J., 107*, 859–69

Meltzer, R. S., Vered, Z., Benjamin, P., Hegesh, J., Visser, C. A. and Neufeld, H. N. (1983). Diagnosing tricuspid regurgitation by direct imaging of the regurgitant flow in the right atrium using contrast echocardiography. *Am. J. Cardiol., 52*, 1050–3

Mena, I., Narahara, K. A. and de Jong, R. B. J. (1982). Clinical application of short lived Gold-195m in sequential first pass radionuclide studies. *J. Nucl. Med., 23*, 48

Mena, I., Narahara, K. A., de Jong, R. B. J. and Maublant, J. (1983). Gold 195m, an ultra-short-lived generator-produced radionuclide: Clinical application in sequential first pass ventriculography. *J. Nucl. Med., 24*, 139

Merendino, K. A. and Bruce, R. A. (1957). One hundred seventeen surgically treated cases of valvular stenotic heart disease. *J. Am. Med. Assoc., 164*, 179

Miller, G. A. H., Kirklin, J. W. and Swan, H. J. C. (1965). Myocardial function and left ventricular volumes in acquired valvular insufficiency. *Circulation, 23*, 374–84

Moore, G. W., Hutchins, G. M., Bulkley, B. H., Tseng, J. S. and Ping, F. Ki (1980). Constituents of the human ventricular myocardium: Connective tissue hyperplasia accompanying muscular hypertrophy. *Am. Heart J., 100*, 610–16

Moran, S. V., Tarazi, R. C., Urzua, J. U., Favoloro, R. G. and Effler, D. B. (1973). Effects of aorto coronary bypass on myocardial contractility. *J. Thorac. Cardiovasc. Surg., 65*, 335

Morganroth, J., Jones, R. H., Chen, C. C. and Naito, M. (1980). Two dimensional echocardiography in mitral, aortic and tricuspid valve prolapse. The clinical problem, cardiac nuclear imaging considerations and a proposed standard for diagnosis. *Am. J. Cardiol., 46*, 1164–77

Naggar, C. Z. and Arctz, H. T. (1984). Pathogenesis of mitral valve prolapse. *Med. Times, 112*, 27–35

Nakamaru, Y. and Schwartz, A. (1970). Possible control of intracellular calcium metabolism by H^+: sarcoplasmic reticulum of skeletal and cardiac muscle. *Biochem. Biophys. Res. Commun., 41*, 830

Neuhaus, K. L., Bornikoel, K., Kreuzer, H. and Niessen, H. W. (1976). Left ventricular myocardial function before and after coronary surgery. *Proc. 14th Congr. Eur. Soc. Cardiol.*, Amsterdam 1976, p. 249

Newman, G. E., Gibbons, R. J. and Jones, R. H. (1981). Cardiac function during rest and exercise in patients with mitral valve prolapse. Role of radionuclear angiocardiography. *Am. J. Cardiol., 47*, 14–19

Nickel, O. and Schad, N. (1978). Image analysis of the heart action recorded with a high speed multicrystal gamma camera. *Med. Progr. Technol., 5*, 1–7

Nickel, O., Schad, N., Andrews, E. J., Fleming, J. W. and Mello, M. (1982). Scintigraphic measurement of left ventricular volumes from the count-density distribution. *J. Nucl. Med., 23*, 404–10

Nicod, P., Corvett, J. R., Firth, B. G., Dehmer, C. I., Izquierdo, C., Markham, R. V., Hillis, L. D., Willerson, J. T. and Lewis, S. E. (1983). Radionuclide techniques for valvular regurgitant index: comparison in patients with normal and depressed ventricular function. *J. Nucl. Med., 23*, 763–9

Noelpp, U. M., Schad, N. and Roesler, H. (1977). Trendszintigraphie. *Nucl. Med.*, **5**, 232

Nutter, D. O., Wickliffe, C., Gilbert, C. A., Moody, C. and King, S. B. III (1975). The pathophysiology of idiopathic mitral valve prolapse. *Circulation*, **52**, 297–305

Okada, R. D., Kirshenbaum, H. D., Kushner, F. G., Strauss, H. W., Dinsmore, R. E., Newell, J. B., Boucher, C. A., Block, P. C. and Pohost, G. M. (1980). Observer variance in the quantitative evaluation of left ventricular wall motion and the quantitation of left ventricular ejection fraction using rest and exercise multi-gated blood pool imaging. *Circulation*, **61**, 128

O'Neill, W., Walton, J., Bates, E. *et al.* (1984). Successful coronary angioplasty as assessed by alterations in coronary vasodilatory reserve. *J. Am. Coll. Cardiol.*, **3**, 1382–90

O'Rourke, R. A. and Crawford, M. H. (1980). Timing of valve replacement in patients with chronic aortic regurgitation. *Circulation*, **61**, 493–5

Osbakken, M. D., Bove, A. A. and Spann, J. F. (1981). Left ventricular regional wall motion and velocity of shortening in chronic mitral and aortic regurgitation. *Am. J. Cardiol.*, **47**, 1005–9

Osbakken, M. D., Boucher, C. A., Okada, R. D., Bingham, J. B., Strauss, H. W. and Pohost, G. M. (1983). Spectrum of global left ventricular responses to supine exercise. Limitation in the use of ejection fraction in identifying patients with coronary artery disease. *Am. J. Cardiol.*, **51**, 28–35

Oyer, P. E., Miller, D. C., Stinson, E. B., Reitz, B. A., Moreno-Cabrol, R. J. and Shumway, N. E. (1980). Clinical durability of the Hancock porcine bioprosthetic valve. *J. Thorac. Cardiovasc. Surg.*, **80**, 824–33

Panek, K. J., Lindeyer, J., v.d. Vlught, H. C. (1982). A new generator system of production of short-living Au-195m radioisotope. *J. Nucl. Med.*, **23**, 108

Papapietro, S. E., Coghlan, H. C., Zissermann, D., Russel, R. O., Rackley, C. E. and Rogers, W. J. (1979). Impaired maximal rate of left ventricular relaxation in patients with coronary artery disease and left ventricular dysfunction. *Circulation*, **59**, 984

Parker, J. A. and Treves, S. (1977). Radionuclide detections, localization and quantization of intracardiac shunts and shunts between the great arteries. *Prog. Cardiovasc. Dis.*, **20**, 121–150

Pavel, D. G., Byrom, E., Lam, W., Meyer-Pavel, C., Swiryn, St. and Pietras, R. (1983). Detection and quantification of regional wall motion abnormalities using phase analysis of equilibrium gated cardiac studies. *Clin. Nucl. Med.*, **8**, 315–22

Peter, C. A., Austin, E. H. and Jones, R. H. (1981). Effect of valve replacement for chronic mitral insufficiency on left ventricular function during rest and exercise. *J. Thorac. Cardiovasc. Surg.*, **82**, 127

Phillips, H. R., Levine, F. H., Carter, J. E., Boucher, C. A., Osbakken, M. D., Okada, E. D., Akins, C. W., Daggett, W. M., Buckley, M. J. and Pohost, G. M. (1981). Mitral valve replacement for isolated mitral regurgitation: analysis of clinical course and late postoperative left ventricular ejection fraction. *Am. J. Cardiol.*, **48**, 647–54

Pichard, A. D., Gorlin, R., Smith, H., Ambrose, J. and Meller, J. (1981). Coronary flow studies in patients with left ventricular hypertrophy of the hypertensive type. Evidence for an impaired coronary vascular reserve. *Am. J. Cardiol.*, **47**, 547–54

Pikal, W. (1980). Die linksventrikuläre Wandbewegung vor und nach Nitroglyceringabe nach Myokardinfarkt. *Thesis*, Technical University, München

Pomerance, A. (1967). Ageing changes in human heart valves. *Br. Heart J.*, **29**, 222–31

Popp, R. L., Brown, O. R., Silverman, J. F. and Harrison, D. C. (1974). Echocardiographic abnormalities in the mitral valve prolapse syndrome. *Circulation*, **49**, 428–33

Port, S. T., McEwan, P., Cobb, F. R. and Jones, R. H. (1981). Influence of resting left ventricular function on the left ventricular response to exercise in patients with coronary artery disease. *Circulation*, **63**, 856–63

Prinzmetal, M., Corday, E., Bergman, H. C., Schwar, L. and Spritzler, R. J. (1948). Radiocardiography: A new method for studying blood flow through chambers of heart in human beings. *Science*, **108**, 340

Rabinowitz, M. and Zak, R. (1975). Mitochondria and cardiac hypertrophy. *Circ. Res.*, **36**, 367–76

Rahimtoola, S. H. (1977). Early valve replacement for preservation of ventricular function? *Am. J. Cardiol.*, **40**, 472–5

Raizada, V., Benchimol, A., Desser, K. B., Reich, F. D., Sheasky, C. and Graves, C. (1977). Mitral valve prolapse in patient with coronary artery disease. Echocardiographic–angiocardiographic correlation. *Br. Heart J.*, **39**, 53–60

Ranganathan, N., Silver, M. D., Robinson, T. I. *et al.* (1973). Angiographic–morphologic correlation in patients with severe mitral regurgitation due to prolapse of the posterior mitral valve leaflet. *Circulation*, **48**, 514–18

Ranganathan, N., Silver, M. D., Robinson, T. I. and Wilson, J. K. (1976). Idiopathic prolapsed mitral leaflet syndrome. Angiographic–clinical correlations. *Circulation*, **54**, 707–16

Rankin, J. S., Nichelas, L. M., Kouchoukos, N. T. (1975). Experimental mitral regurgitation: Effects of left ventricular function before and after elimination of chronic regurgitation in the dog. *J. Thorac. Cardiovasc. Surg.*, **70**, 478

Reale, A. and Romeo, F. (1983). Il destino dell'infartuato. *Atti del 44° Congresso della Società Italiana di Cardiologia*, Turin, June 1983

Reduto, L. A., Marshall, R. C., Berger, H. S., Gottschalk, A. and Zaret, B. L. (1978). Variability sequential measures of left ventricular performance assessed with radionuclide angiography. *Am. J. Cardiol.*, **41**, (3), 531–6

Reduto, L. A., Wickemeyer, W. J., Young, J. B., del Ventura, L. A., Reid, J. W., Glaeser, D. H., Quinones, M. A. and Miller, R. R. (1981). Left ventricular diastolic performance at rest and during exercise in patients with coronary artery disease. *Circulation*, **63**, 1228

Reichart, B., Schad, N., Nickel, O., Kemkes, B. M., Kreuzer, E. and Harrington, O. B. (1982). Regional left ventricular function in the three main coronary artery territories at rest and during exercise; non-invasive assessment after aortocoronary bypass surgery. *Klin. Wschr.*, **60**, 181–91

Reichart, B., Schad, N., Hartmann, A., Nickel, O. and Luther, M. (1983). Globale und regionale linksventrikuläre Myokardfunktion nach aortokoronarem Mehrfach-(5-,6-,7-) Bypass. Nichtinvasive Bestimmung mit der Technetium-99m-Pertechnetat-Szintigraphie. *Fortschr. Med.*, **44**, 101, 2003–60

Rembert, J. C., Kleinman, L. H., Fedor, J. M., Wechsler, A. S. and Greenfield, J. C. (1978). Myocardial blood flow distribution in concentric left ventricular hypertrophy. *J. Clin. Invest.*, **62**, 379–86

Rentrop, P., de Vivie, E. R., Karsch, K. R. and Kreuzer, H. (1978). Acute coronary occlusion with impending infarction as an angiographic complication relieved by guidewire recanalisation. *Clin. Cardiol.*, **1**, 1010

Rentrop, P., Blanke, H., Kostering, H. and Karsch, K. R. (1980). Intrakoronare Streptaseapplikation beim akuten Infarkt und Angina pectoris. *Dtsch. Med. Wschr.*, **105**, 221

Rerych, S. K., Scholz, P. M., Newman, G. E., Sabiston, D. C. and Jones, R. H. (1978a). Cardiac function at rest and during exercise in normals and in patients with coronary heart disease: Evaluation by radionuclide angiocardiography. *Ann. Surg.*, **187**, 449

Rerych, S., Anderson, P., Scholz, P., Newman, G. and Jones, R. (1978b). Accuracy of left ventricular end-diastolic volume determination using first-pass radionuclide technique. *J. Nucl. Med.*, **19**, 726

Rod, J. L., Foster, C. and Schmidt, D. H. (1984). Evaluation of percutaneous transluminal coronary angioplasty by symptom – limited graded exercise testing. *J. Cardiac. Rehabil.*, **4**, 70–3

Rodriguez, L. (1970). Hemodynamic and angiographic findings in patients with isolated aortic valvular disease before and after insertion of a Starr–Edwards aortic ball valve prosthesis. *Scand. J. Thorac. Cardiovasc. Surg.*, **4**, (Suppl. 5), 1

Rosing, D. R., Kent, K. M., Barow, R. *et al.* (1984). Three year anatomic and functional followup after successful percutaneous transluminal coronary angioplasty. *J. Am. Coll. Cardiol.*, **3**, 470

Ross, J., Sonnenblick, E. H., Taylor, R. R., Spotnitz, H. M. and Covell, J. W. (1971). Diastolic geometry and sarcomere lengths in the chronically dilated canine. *Circ. Res.*, **28**, 49

Ross, R. and Glomset, J. A. (1976). Prepathogenesis of atherosclerosis. *N. Engl. J. Med.*, **295**, 369–77

Rousseau, M. F., Poucer, H., Detry, J. R. and Brasseur, L. A. (1981). Relationship between changes in left ventricular inotropic state and relaxation in normal subjects and in patients with coronary artery disease. *Circulation*, **64**, 736

Rozanski, A., Diamond, G. A., Berman, D., Forrester, J. S., Morris, D. and Swan, H. C. J. (1983). The declining specificity of exercise radionuclide ventricular ventriculography. *N. Engl. J. Med.*, **309**, 518–22

Saltiel, J., Lesperance, J., Bourassa, M. G., Castonqua, Y., Campeau, L. and Grondin, P. (1970). Reversibility of left ventricular dysfunction following aorto coronary bypass grafts. *Am. J. Roentgenol.*, **110**, 739

Sandler, H. and Dodge, H. T. (1968). The use of single plane angiography for the calculation of left ventricular volume in man. *Am. Heart J.*, **75**, 325

Santos, A. D., Mathew, P. K., Hilal, A. *et al.* (1981). Orthostatic hypotension: a commonly unrecognized cause of symptoms in mitral valve prolapse. *Am. J. Med.*, **71**, 746

Savage, D. D., Garrison, R. J., Devereux, R. B. *et al.* (1983). Mitral valve prolapse in the general population. 1. Epidemiologic features: The Framingham Study. *Am. Heart J.*, **106**, 571–6

Savage, D. D., Devereux, R. B., Garrison, R. J. *et al.* (1983). Mitral valve prolapse in the general population. 2. Clinical features: The Framingham Study. *Am. Heart J.*, **106**, 577–81

Scampardonis, G., Yang, S. S., Maranhão, V., Goldberg, H. and Gooch, A. S. (1973). Left ventricular abnormalities in prolapsed mitral leaflet syndrome. Review of eighty-seven cases. *Circulation*, **48**, 287–97

Schad, N. (1968). *Die intermittierende Kontrastmittelinjektion in das Herz.* (Stuttgart: Georg Thieme Verlag)

Schad, N. (1976a). Dynamische Untersuchungen des Herzens nach Myokardinfarkt. *Radioaktive Isotope in Klinik und Forschung, Bad Gasteiner Intern Symposium,* **12**, 407

Schad, N. (1976b). Nichtinvasive Darstellung der Wandbewegung und Schlagvolumenverteilung des linken Ventrikels nach Myokardinfarkt. *ROFO*, **124**, 201

Schad, N. (1977). Non-traumatic assessment of left ventricular wall motion and regional stroke volume after myocardial infarction. *J. Nucl. Med.*, **18**, 333

Schad, N. (1982). L'imaging non invasivo della funzione ventricolare sinistra. *G. Ital. Cardiol.*, **12** (Sept. 1982)

Schad, N. (1984). First-pass radiocardiography with the multicrystal gamma camera. (Berlin: Springer) (In press)

Schad, N. and Nickel, O. (1978a). Radionuclide angiography in coronary heart disease: Where do we stand? *Cardiovasc. Radiol.*, **1**, 27–35

Schad, N. and Nickel, O. (1978b). Noninvasive radionuclide angiography in coronary heart disease. In *Coronary Heart Disease.* p. 98. (Stuttgart: Thième)

Schad, N. and Nickel, O. (1979a). Assessment of ventricular function with first pass angiocardiography. *Cardiovasc. Radiol.*, **2**, 149

Schad, N. and Nickel, O. (1979b). Detection of regional flow disturbances with the gamma-camera: Nuclear imaging of the heart – Practical considerations. In Schaper, W. (ed.) *The Pathophysiology of Myocardial Perfusion*, p. 43. (Amsterdam, New York: Elsevier North-Holland, Biomedical Press)

Schad, N. and Nickel, O. (1980a). Nichtinvasive Beurteilung der regionalen Funktion des linken Ventrikels. Erste Tracer-Passage. *Radiologe*, **20**, 56

Schad, N. and Nickel, O. (1980b). Nuklearmedizinische Herzdiagnostik im Kindesalter. In Hahn, K. (ed.) *Paediatrische Nuklearmedizin Bd 2.* (Mainz: Krichheim Verlag)

Schad, N. and Nickel, O. (1981). Noninvasive assessment of left ventricular function. In Donner, M. W. and Heuck, F. H. W. (eds.) *Radiology Today*, pp. 13–25. (Berlin, Heidelberg: Springer)

Schad, N., Reichart, B., Bougioukas, G., Kemkes, B. M., Bortolotti, U., Milano, A. and Gallucci, V. (1982). Noninvasive assessment of left and right ventricular function in patients with bioprosthetic mitral valves at long-term risk. Presented at the *International Symposium on Cardiac Bioprosthesis*, Rome, 17–19 May

Schad, N. and Nickel, O. (1983). Assessment of left ventricular performance by functional images. In Hipona, F. A. (ed.) *Heart*, p. 143. (New York: Grune & Stratton)

Schad, N., Nickel, O., Schön, H., Le Thi, O. and Bruzzone, F. (1983a). First pass card-angiography with the new radionuclide Au 195m. *Proceedings of the International Symposium on Ultrashort-lived Radionuclide*, Washington DC (In press)

Schad, N., Schepke, H., Nickel, O. and Bruzzone, F. (1983b). Intracoronary injections of the new radionuclide Au-195m. *Proceedings of the International Symposium on Ultrashort-lived Radionuclides*, Washington DC (In press)

Schad, N., Nickel, O., Schön, H., Bruzzone, F., Le Thi, O., Baumgartl, W. and Hartman, A. (1984a). Nichtinvasive First-pass Untersuchung des Herzens mit dem kurzlebigen Radionuklid Aurum 195m. *Radiologe*, **24**, 257

Schad, N., Bruzzone, F., Nickel, O. and Le Thi, O. (1984b). Studio radioisotopico (First pass) della funzione ventricolare sinistra in due proiezioni oblique con l'uso die Aurum 195m nello infarto miocardico pregresso. *Radiol. Med.* (In press)

Schad, N., Bruzzone, F., Fesl, H., Nickel, O. and Le Thi, O. (1984c). Noninvasive assessment of regional left ventricular function with first pass radionuclide functional imaging. *Cardiovasc. Intervent. Radiol.* (submitted)

Schad, N., Romeo, F., Fesl, H. and Nickel, O. (1984d). Noninvasive assessment of regional diastolic left ventricular function with first pass radionuclide functional imaging. *Eur. J. Cardiol.* (submitted)

Schelbert, H. R., Verba, J. W., Johnson, A. D. *et al.* (1975). Nontraumatic determination of left ventricular ejection fraction by radionuclide angiocardiography. *Circulation*, **51**, 902–9

Schlant, R. C., Felner, J. M., Miklozek, C. L., Lutz, J. F. and Hurst, J. W. (1980). Mitral valve prolapse. *DM*, **26**, 1–51

Schneider, J., Berger, H. J., Sands, M. J., Lachman, A. B.

and Zaret, B. L. (1983). Beat-to-beat left ventricular performance in atrial fibrillation; radionuclide assessment with the computerized nuclear probe. *Am. J. Cardiol.*, **51**, 1189–95

Scholz, P. M., Rerych, S. K., Moran, J. F., Newmann, G. E., Douglas, J. M., Sabiston, D. C. and Jones, R. H. (1980). Quantitative radionuclide angiography. *Cath. Cardiovasc. Diagn.*, **6**, 265–83

Schröder, R. (1983). Successful rate and time until recanalisation with systemic infusion. Presented at *Recanalization in acute myocardial infarction: A cooperative symposium of the German and Dutch working groups for fibrinolytic therapy in acute myocardial infarction*, Aachen 1983

Schuberl, F. (1978). Lokalisation und Ausdehnung des Myokardinfarktes: Radionuklidangiographie und Elektrokardiogramm. *Thesis*, Ludwig–Maximilian University München

Schuler, G., Peterson, K. L., Johnson, A., Francis, G., Dennish, G., Utley, J., Daily, P. O., Ashburn, W. and Ross, J. (1979). Temporal response of left ventricular performance to mitral valve surgery. *Circulation*, **59**, 1218

Selzer, A. (1976). Cardiac valve replacement: an unanswered question. *Am. J. Cardiol.*, **37**, 322–4

Sesto, M. and Schwar, F. (1979). Regional myocardial functions at rest and after rapid ventricular pacing in patients of myocardial revascularizations by coronary bypass graft or by collateral vessels. *Am. J. Cardiol.*, **43**, 920

Shah, D. K., Pichler, M., Berman, D. S., Singh, B. N. and Swan, H. J. (1980). Left ventricular ejection fraction determined by radionuclide ventriculography in early stage of first transmural myocardial infarction. Relation to short term prognosis. *Am. J. Cardiol.*, **45** (3), 542–6

Sigwart, U., Girbic, M., Rivief, J. L. *et al.* (1982). Improvement of left ventricular function after percutaneous transluminal coronary angioplasty. *Am. J. Cardiol.*, **49**, 651–7

Slutsky, R., Battler, A., Karliner, J. S., Foelicher, V. and Ashburn, W. (1980). First-third ejection fraction at rest compared with exercise radionuclide angiography in assessing patients with coronary artery disease. *Radiology*, **136**, 197–201

Staniloff, H. M., Huckell, V. F., Morch, J. E. *et al.* (1978). Abnormal myocardial perfusion defects in patients with mitral valve prolapse and normal coronary arteries. *Am. J. Cardiol.*, **41**, 433

Starr, A., Edwards, M. L., McGard, C. W. and Griswald, H. E. (1963). Aortic replacement: clinical experience with a semi-rigid ball valve prosthesis. *Circulation*, **27**, 779

Steingart, R. M., Yee, C., Weinstein, L. and Scheuer, J. (1983). Radionuclide ventriculographic study of adaptations to exercise in aortic regurgitation. *Am. J. Cardiol.*, **51**, 483–8

Strauer, B. E., Kramer, H., Bolte, H. and Riecker, C. (1975). Die Beziehungen zwischen Volumengrößen und der Auswurffraktion des linken Ventrikels bei Mitral- und Aortenklappenregurgitation. *Klin. Wschr.*, **53**, 975

Strauss, H. W. and Pitt, B. (1978). Gated cardiac blood-pool scan: Use in patients with coronary heart disease. In Holman, B. L., Sonnenblick, E. H. and Lesch, M. (eds.). *Principles of Cardiovascular Nuclear Medicine*, pp. 161–70. (New York: Grune & Stratton)

Sutton, M. G., Frye, R. L., Smith, H. C., Chesebro, J. H. and Ritman, E. L. (1978). Relation between left coronary artery stenosis and regional left ventricular function. *Circulation*, **58**, 491

Swiryn, S., Pavel, D., Byrom, E., Witham, D., Meyer-Paval, C., Wyndham, C. R. C., Handler, B. and Rosen, K. M. (1981). Sequential regional phase mapping of radionuclide gated biventriculograms in patients with left bundle branch block. *Am. Heart J.*, **102**, 1000–10

Tenant, R. and Wiggers, C. J. (1935). Effect of coronary occlusion on myocardial contraction. *Am. J. Physiol.*, **112**, 351

Towne, W. (1978). Mitral valve prolapse: part I. *J. Contin. Educ. Cardiol.*, **13**, 23–45

Towne, W. (1978). Mitral valve prolapse: part II. *J. Contin. Educ. Cardiol.*, **13**, 11–29

Tu'meh, S. S., Tracy, D. A., Wynne, J., Konstam, M. A., Kozlowski, J. F., Neumann, A. L. and Holman, R. L. (1982). Scintigraphic diagnosis of tricuspid regurgitation. *Radiology*, **145**, 463–6

Upton, M. T., Rerych, S. K., Newmann, G. E., Bounous, E. P. and Jones, R. H. (1980). The reproducibility of radionuclide angiographic measurement of left ventricular function in normal subjects at rest and during exercise. *Circulation*, **62**, 126–32

Uschel, C. W., Cowell, J. W., Sonnenblick, E. H., Ross, J. and Braunwald, E. (1968). Myocardial mechanics in aortic and mitral valvular regurgitation. The concept of instantaneous impedance as a determinant of the performance of the intact heart. *J. Clin. Invest.*, **47**, 867

Verani, M. S., Carroll, R. J. and Falsetti, H. L. (1976). Mitral valve prolapse in coronary artery disease. *Am. J. Cardiol.*, **37**, 1–6

Vos, P. H., Vossepoel, A. M. and Pauwels, E. K. (1983). Quantitative assessment of wall motion in multiple gated studies using temporal Fourier analysis. *J. Nucl. Med.*, **24**, 388

Wackers, F., Giles, R. and Hoffer, P. (1982). Gold 195m, a new generator produced short-lived radionuclide for sequential assessment of ventricular performance by first pass radionuclide angiography in man using Gold 195m (T½ 30.5 sec). *J. Nucl. Med.*, **23**, 48

Wackers, F., Stein, R., Pytlik, L., Plankey, M., Lange, R., Hoffer, P. B., Sands, M., Zaret, B. L. and Berger, H. J. (1983). Gold-195m for serial first pass radionuclide angiocardiography during upright exercise in patients with coronary artery disease. *J. Am. Coll. Cardiol.*, **2**, 497

Waller, B. F., McManus, B. M., Garfinkel, J. *et al.* (1983). Status of the major epicardial coronary arteries 80 to 150 days after percutaneous coronary angioplasty: analysis of three necropsy patients. *Am. J. Cardiol.*, **51**, 81–4

Wangler, R. D., Peters, K. G., Marcus, M. L. and Tomanek, R. J. (1982). Effects of duration and severity of arterial hypertension and cardiac hypertrophy on coronary vasodilator reserve. *Circ. Res.*, **51**, 10–18

Watson, L. E., Dickhaus, D. W. and Martin, R. H. (1975). Left ventricular aneurysm. Preoperative hemodynamics, chamber volume, and results of aneurysmectomy. *Circulation*, **52**, 868–73

Weisfeldt, M. L. (1984). A total occlusion, two 70 percent lesions and normal ventricular function. *J. Engl. J. Med.*, **310**, 850–51

Weisfeldt, M. L., Armstrong, P., Sully, H. E., Sanders, C. A. and Daggett, W. M. (1974). Incomplete relaxation between beats after myocardial hypoxia and ischemia. *J. Clin. Invest.*, **53**, 1626

Wexler, J., Steingart, R. M. and Blaufox, D. (1981). Assessment of ventricular function: physiological interventions. *Semin. Nucl. Med.*, **11**, 8–79

Williams, D. O., Riley, R., Sing, A. *et al.* (1980). Restoration of normal coronary hemodynamics and myocardial metabolism after percutaneous transluminal coronary angioplasty. *Circulation*, **62**, 653–6

Winkle, R. A., Lopes, M. G., Popp, R. L. *et al.* (1976). Life-threatening arrhythmias in the mitral valve prolapse syndrome. *Am. J. Med.*, **60**, 961

Winzelberg, G. G., Boucher, C. A., Pohost, G. M.,

McKusick, K. A., Bingham, J. B., Ikada, R. D. and Strauss, H. W. (1981). Right ventricular function in aortic and mitral valve disease. Relation of gated first-pass radionuclide angiography to clinical and hemodynamic findings. *Chest*, **79**, 520–8

Wolf, N. M., Kreuten, T. H., Bove, A. A., McDonough, M. T., Kessler, K. H., Strong, M., LeMole, G. and Spann, J. F. (1978). Left ventricular function following coronary bypass surgery. *Circulation*, **58**, 63

Wong, C. Y. H and Spotnitz, H. M. (1979). Diastolic compliance and systolic mechanisms of mitral regurgitation. *Surg. Forum*, **30**, 233

Wooler, G. H., Nixon, P. C. G., Grinshaw, V. A. and Watson, D. A. (1962). Experiences with the repair of the mitral valve in mitral incompetence. *Thorax*, **17**, 49

Wright, C., White, C., Furda, J., Doty, D., Eastham, C., Laughlin, D. and Marcus, M. (1980). Can the coronary arteriogram predict the functional significance of a coronary stenosis? *Circulation*, **62**, 214

Zaret, B. L., Strauss, H. W., Hurley, P. J., Natarajan, T. K. and Pitt, B. (1971). A noninvasive scintiphotographic method for detecting regional ventricular function in man. *N. Engl. J. Med.*, **284**, 1165

INDEX